Lecture Notes in Computer Science　　7359

Commenced Publication in 1973
Founding and Former Series Editors:
Gerhard Goos, Juris Hartmanis, and Jan van Leeuwen

Editorial Board

David Hutchison
  Lancaster University, UK
Takeo Kanade
  Carnegie Mellon University, Pittsburgh, PA, USA
Josef Kittler
  University of Surrey, Guildford, UK
Jon M. Kleinberg
  Cornell University, Ithaca, NY, USA
Alfred Kobsa
  University of California, Irvine, CA, USA
Friedemann Mattern
  ETH Zurich, Switzerland
John C. Mitchell
  Stanford University, CA, USA
Moni Naor
  Weizmann Institute of Science, Rehovot, Israel
Oscar Nierstrasz
  University of Bern, Switzerland
C. Pandu Rangan
  Indian Institute of Technology, Madras, India
Bernhard Steffen
  TU Dortmund University, Germany
Madhu Sudan
  Microsoft Research, Cambridge, MA, USA
Demetri Terzopoulos
  University of California, Los Angeles, CA, USA
Doug Tygar
  University of California, Berkeley, CA, USA
Gerhard Weikum
  Max Planck Institute for Informatics, Saarbruecken, Germany

W0227503

Benoît M. Dawant
Gary E. Christensen
J. Michael Fitzpatrick
Daniel Rueckert (Eds.)

Biomedical Image Registration

5th International Workshop, WBIR 2012
Nashville, TN, USA, July 7-8, 2012
Proceedings

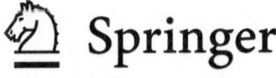 Springer

Volume Editors

Benoît M. Dawant
J. Michael Fitzpatrick
Vanderbilt University
Department of Electrical Engineering and Computer Science
2301 Vanderbilt Place, Nashville, TN 37235, USA
E-mail: {benoit.dawant, j.michael.fitzpatrick}@vanderbilt.edu

Gary E. Christensen
University of Iowa
Department of Electrical and Computer Engineering
4324 Seamans Center for the Engineering Arts and Sciences
Iowa City, IA 52242, USA
E-mail: gary-christensen@uiowa.edu

Daniel Rueckert
Imperial College London
Department of Computing
London, SW7 2AZ, UK
E-mail: d.rueckert@imperial.ac.uk

ISSN 0302-9743   ISSN 1611-3349
ISBN 978-3-642-31339-4   ISBN 978-3-642-31340-0 (eBook)
DOI 10.1007/978-3-642-31340-0
Springer Heidelberg Dordrecht London New York

Library of Congress Control Number: 2012940274

CR Subject Classification (1998): I.4.3, I.4, I.5, J.3, G.3, G.1

LNCS Sublibrary: SL 6 – Image Processing, Computer Vision, Pattern Recognition,
and Graphics

Typesetting: Camera-ready by author, data conversion by Scientific Publishing Services, Chennai, India

Printed on acid-free paper

Springer is part of Springer Science+Business Media (www.springer.com)

Preface

The 5th Workshop on Biomedical Image Registration (WBIR) was held on the Vanderbilt University campus in Nashville, Tennessee, USA. It followed a series of workshops that were held in Bled, Slovenia (1999), in Philadelphia, USA (2003), in Utrecht, The Netherlands (2006), and in Lübeck, Germany (2010).

This workshop series brings together researchers involved in developing new registration methods and users of these methods. Papers submitted to the workshop were reviewed blindly by three members of the workshop's international Program Committee. This year, 44 papers were submitted, 20 papers were accepted for oral presentation and 11 papers were accepted for poster presentation. All papers presented at the workshop are published in this volume. The program clearly shows that medical image registration is a vibrant research area. Papers were submitted by researchers from many parts of the world and address fundamental algorithmic issues as well as issues related to the translation of these algorithms to the medical imaging community at large. The keynote speakers also discussed a spectrum of topics. Dr. J. Michael Fitzpatrick presented a historical overview covering more than 20 years of theoretical developments aiming at elucidating the relation between target registration error (TRE), fiducial registration error (FRE), and fiducial localization error (FLE). Dr. John Gore, Director of the Vanderbilt Institute of Imaging Science, discussed registration needs and challenges in large imaging institutes involved in small animal and human imaging research. Dr. Nassir Navab discussed registration needs and challenges to support research in the area of computer-assisted procedures.

We are grateful to those who contributed to the success of WBIR 2012. In particular, we would like to thank the organization staff and members of the Program Committee for their work. We also thank Medtronic Surgical Technologies, the Vanderbilt Initiative for Surgery and Engineering, and NDI (Northern Digital Inc.) for their generous support. Last but not least, we thank all the participants of this workshop for their contributions to the many discussions. We hope they found the workshop stimulating and enjoyed Nashville and the Vanderbilt Campus. For those who could not attend the workshop, we hope that this volume will provide you with valuable information and that you will be able to participate to the next WBIR workshop.

July 2012

Benoît M. Dawant
Gary E. Christensen
J. Michael Fitzpatrick
Daniel Rueckert

Organization

Chairs

Benoît M. Dawant	Vanderbilt University, USA
Gary E. Christensen	University of Iowa, USA
J. Michael Fitzpatrick	Vanderbilt University, USA
Daniel Rueckert	Imperial College London, UK

Program Committee

Paul Aljabar	Imperial College, London, UK
Christian Barillot	INRIA Rennes, France
Mirsa Faisal Beg	Simon Fraser University, Canada
Nathan Cahill	Rochester Institute of Technology, USA
Bernd Fischer	University of Lübeck, Germany
Jim Gee	University of Pennsylvania, USA
Christoph Guetter	Siemens Corporate Research, Princeton, USA
David Haynor	University of Washington, USA
Tobias Heimann	German Cancer Research Center, Germany
Joachim Hornegger	Pattern Recognition Lab, Erlangen, Germany
Ali Kamen	Siemens Corporate Research, Princeton, USA
Stefan Klein	Erasmus MC, Rotterdam, The Netherlands
Sebastian Kurtek	Florida State University, USA
Jan Kybic	Czech Technical University, Prague, Czech Republic
Rasmus Larsen	Technical University of Denmark (DTU), Denmark
Xia Li	Vanderbilt University, USA
Bostjan Likar	University of Ljubljana, Slovenia
Tommaso Mansi	Siemens Corporate Research, Princeton, USA
Marc Modat	University College London, UK
Jan Modersitzki	University of Lübeck, Germany
Kensaku Mori	Nagoya University, Japan
Nassir Navab	Technische Universität München, Germany
Jack Noble	Vanderbilt University, USA
Yangming Ou	University of Pennsylvania, USA
Sebastien Ourselin	University College London, UK
Xavier Pennec	INRIA Sophia, France
Graeme Penney	King's College London, UK
Franjo Pernus	University of Ljubljana, Slovenia
Josien Pluim	University Medical Center, Utrecht, The Netherlands

Kilian Pohl	University of Pennsylvania, USA
Joseph Reinhardt	University of Iowa, USA
Torsten Rohlfing	SRI International, USA
Karl Rohr	University of Heidelberg, Germany
Julia Schnabel	University of Oxford, UK
Dinggang Shen	University of North Carolina, Chapel Hill, USA
Anuj Srivastava	Florida State University, USA
Colin Studholme	University of Washington, USA
Philippe Thévenaz	Ecole Polytechnique Fédérale de Lausanne (EPFL), Switzerland
Simon Warfield	Children's Hospital, Boston, USA
Wolfang Wein	Technische Universität München, Germany
Sandy Wells	Harvard Medical School and Brigham and Women's Hospital, USA
Jay West	Accuray, Inc., USA
Andrew Wiles	NDI, Inc., USA

Sponsors

Medtronic Surgical Technologies, Louisville, Colorado, USA (Gold Sponsor)
Vanderbilt Initiative in Surgery and Engineering, Vanderbilt University,
    Nashville, Tennessee, USA (Gold Sponsor)
NDI (Northern Digital Inc), Waterloo, Ontario, Canada (Silver Sponsor)

Table of Contents

Multiple Image Sets

Poster Session

Brain

Non-rigid Anatomy I

Non-rigid Anatomy II

Frameworks and Similarity Measures

Robust Global Registration through Geodesic Paths on an Empirical Manifold with Knee MRI from the Osteoarthritis Initiative (OAI)

Claire R. Donoghue[1], Anil Rao[1], Anthony M.J. Bull[2], and Daniel Rueckert[1]

[1] Department of Computing, Imperial College London, London, UK
[2] Department of Bioengineering, Imperial College London, London, UK

Abstract. Accurate affine registrations are crucial for many applications in medical image analysis. Within the Osteoarthritis Initiative (OAI) dataset we have observed a failure rate of approximately 4% for direct affine registrations of knee MRI without manual initialisation. Despite this, the problem of robust affine registration has not received much attention in recent years. With the increase in large medical image datasets, manual intervention is not a suitable solution to achieve successful affine registrations. We introduce a framework to improve the robustness of affine registrations without prior manual initialisations. We use 10,307 MR images from the large dataset available from the OAI to model the low dimensional manifold of the population of unregistered knee MRIs as a sparse k-nearest-neighbour graph. Affine registrations are computed in advance for nearest neighbours only. When a pairwise image registration is required the shortest path across the graph is extracted to find a geodesic path on the empirical manifold. The precomputed affine transformations on this path are composed to find an estimated transformation. Finally a refinement step is used to further improve registration accuracy. Failure rates of geodesic affine registrations reduce to 0.86% with the registration framework proposed.

1   Introduction

Many applications of medical image analysis rely on a sufficiently accurate affine registration, including multi-atlas segmentation [1], statistical shape models [2], atlas building [3], non-rigid registration [4] and many more applications for computer aided diagnosis which need spatial information [5]. Within many experiments we have found that affine registration algorithms frequently fail if not given an adequate initialisation where patient position and anatomical structures can vary significantly. Such initialisation is typically provided as an initial manual guess by a user for every pair of images to be registered. More robust automated initialisation methods could dramatically reduce this burden.

With the dawn of large datasets of medical images, any form of manual intervention is quickly becoming infeasible and full automation is important. The dataset used within this work is from a large, longitudinal imaging study of the knee provided by the Osteoarthritis Initiative (OAI). In total 10,307 MRI

B.M. Dawant et al. (Eds.): WBIR 2012, LNCS 7359, pp. 1–10, 2012.
© Springer-Verlag Berlin Heidelberg 2012

scans of the knee are used here, at such scales it is indisputable that automatic accurate initialisation of registrations is crucial.

We present a data driven framework to reduce the affine registration failure rate. It takes advantage of the large number of knee MRI which are acquired in a variety of orientations, scales and positions (in addition to many non-rigid variations). The population of these images can be modelled as a low dimensional manifold in high dimensional space, where each image is a sample on or near the low dimensional manifold and samples close together are more "similar" to each other. We assume that similar images which are closer together on the manifold should have an increased likelihood of a successful registration. Since this space is well sampled, we can travel between a pair of images embedded in the manifold on a shortest geodesic path, passing similar images at each sampled point. An affine registration can be defined by composing transformations between each image on the path. The proposed method suggests a way for a small number of registrations between similar images to be precomputed, which means the run time computational cost is low.

2   Related Work

Accurate affine registration is required for many previous works for medical image analysis of knee MRI [1,3,2,4,5]. However, most recent works assume affine registrations are a solved problem and few focus on improving success rates.

Registration across geodesic paths of a manifold has been previously performed for non-rigid registration for large deformations by [9], where, like in this method, the population is modelled as a graph. A similar approach is taken for atlas-based segmentation [11], registrations are computed via the near neighbours in a learnt low dimensional Laplacian eigenmap embedding. Learning an embedding has the drawback of restricting the dimensionality to a fixed value across the entire space. For both [9,11] registrations are not precomputed which means run time costs are higher than the method presented here. Manifold learning has been applied to medical image analysis in a variety of applications. For example, Isomap has been used to learn the manifold structure of brain images to reconstruct images at new locations on the manifold [10]. Additionally, ABSORB has also been proposed to create unbiased atlases through learning a manifold of images [12].

Previously, affine registration initialisation has been proposed by extracting features to locate key landmark points followed by an iterative closest point algorithm (ICP) [6]. Due to severe disease in some subjects potentially dominating image appearance, selecting landmark points might not be sufficiently resilient. A thorough review of image registration techniques can be found in [7]. The affine registration algorithm employed in this article is based on [8].

3 Method

3.1 Overview

Upon registering images in a large dataset it has been noted that the failure rate of affine registration between pairs of images without prior manual initialisation is high at 4.08%, where failure is defined in section 3.2. Many registrations fail because a large component of registration is an optimisation, which only finds the local minima and will not reliably locate the global minimum. We hypothesise that pairs of images with greater similarities are closer to their global optimum. Therefore, we assume that images with high similarity will generally achieve a good affine registration. We propose a registration framework where affine registration is only considered reliable when the similarity between two images is high. An empirical manifold of the space of unregistered knee MRI is estimated. From this low dimensional representation registrations between similar images are precomputed. When a registration between a pair of image is required a series of transformations are composed to achieve a strong global geodesic affine registration. Figure 1 depicts an overview of this framework.

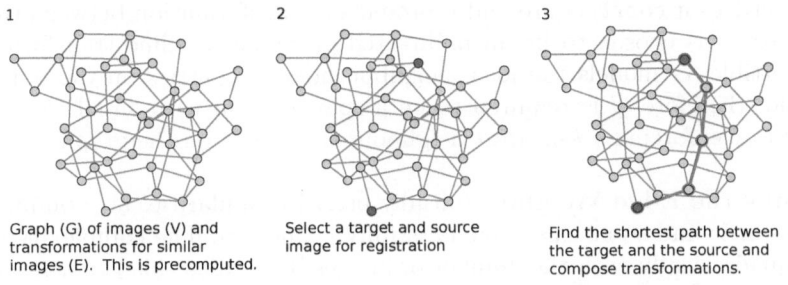

1   2   3

Graph (G) of images (V) and transformations for similar images (E). This is precomputed.

Select a target and source image for registration

Find the shortest path between the target and the source and compose transformations.

Fig. 1. Diagram of the proposed registration framework

3.2 Dataset

Image Data. The experiments presented use 10,307 MRI scans of left and right knees, which are obtained from the Osteoarthritis Initiative (OAI) database, available for public access at http://www.oai.ucsf.edu/. Specific datasets used are 1.C.0 and 1.E.0 at baseline and 1.C.1 and 1.E.1 at 12 months after the baseline date. The fat-suppressed, sagittal 3D dual-echo in steady state (DESS) sequence with selective water excitation (WE) has been selected since it has both high in plane resolution (0.36 by 0.36mm) and a small slice thickness (0.7mm). Further information regarding the imaging protocol can be found in [13].

Validation Data. For validation of registration accuracy, 97 MRIs were randomly selected and annotated with landmark points. Each image is landmarked with four distinct points, at the ACL and PCL ligament insertions on the femur and the tibia. The middle voxel of each ligament is selected just before it meets the bone. These landmarks are selected as they visible in most subjects and due to high landmark placement reproducibility by reader.

Since the ligaments are thin and cylindrical, the landmarks were found to be reproducible. The error for validation is computed as mean euclidean distance between the set of landmark points. A reproducibility study was performed to test how reproducible landmark placement was, 13 subjects were annotated twice, the mean error computed between landmarks was 1.1mm. An intra-subject pose study was performed for 13 subjects by measuring the error between a subject registered affinely at two time points, the mean error is 2.1mm. In the latter case it is probable that the errors cannot be entirely attributed to reader error but also to non-rigid pose variations or anatomical changes. Based on these experiments, registrations with error greater than 10mm are defined as failures.

3.3   Geodesic Registration Framework

Representation of the Population. A graph $G = (V, E)$ is constructed to model the low dimensional manifold space of all MRI scans in native space for an anatomical site of interest (in this case the knee) using a prespecified acquisition protocol. Each vertex in V is a sample on the manifold and represents an image in the dataset. Each edge in E is weighted based on how similar the two images at the vertices it connects are and represents a transformation between the pair of images. G is chosen to be an undirected graph since affine transformations are invertible. G models the local neighbourhood properties on the non-linear manifold, therefore G is required to be a sparse graph with small $|E|$. This is achieved by enforcing a k-nearest neighbour constraint on the graph.

Choosing the Edge Weights. Initially pairwise similarities are computed for all pairs in V and so at this stage G is fully connected. The complexity clearly grows quadratically with the number of images $|V|$ and so this is not feasible at full image resolution. Therefore the images are blurred and downsampled. Since the goal of the method is to achieve a strong global transformation, pairwise similarities of images at this lower resolution are sufficient.

We choose the smallest k such that there is only one connected component and thus all vertices can be reached from any selected vertex. When k is very large, G is fully connected and thus as k grows the shortest path across the graph is more likely to be equivalent to a direct registration. Improvements upon computing k-nearest neighbours are discussed in section 5.1.

Local Registrations. For each edge in E, affine registrations are computed between the images at the vertices it connects. The direction of the affine registration is stored such that an inversion can be computed should the registration be required in the opposite direction. These registrations are all precomputed and so any local registration can be retrieved instantaneously.

Global Pairwise Registrations. An affine registration between any target image and source image is derived by finding the shortest path in G between the two corresponding vertices. The shortest path is computed using Dijkstra's algorithm [14]. The geodesic path across the empirical manifold is comprised of n

edges, each edge is composed to create the global geodesic affine transformation T_G. As local registrations are computed in advance the composition is simply a short series of matrix multiplications, which means that any pairwise registration can be retrieved rapidly.

$$T_G = T_1 \circ T_2 \ldots \circ T_n \qquad (1)$$

When affine transformations are composed, small errors at each edge in the path will be propagated and accumulate. Therefore the geodesic transformation T_G is suboptimal and might not reflect the true transformation. A further refinement step can be employed, T_G is considered to be an initialisation for a further affine registration and serves as a good estimate for the desired registration. The refined geodesic transformation is referred to as $T_{G'}$, illustrated in figure 2.

$$T_{G'} = T_G \circ T_{refine} \qquad (2)$$

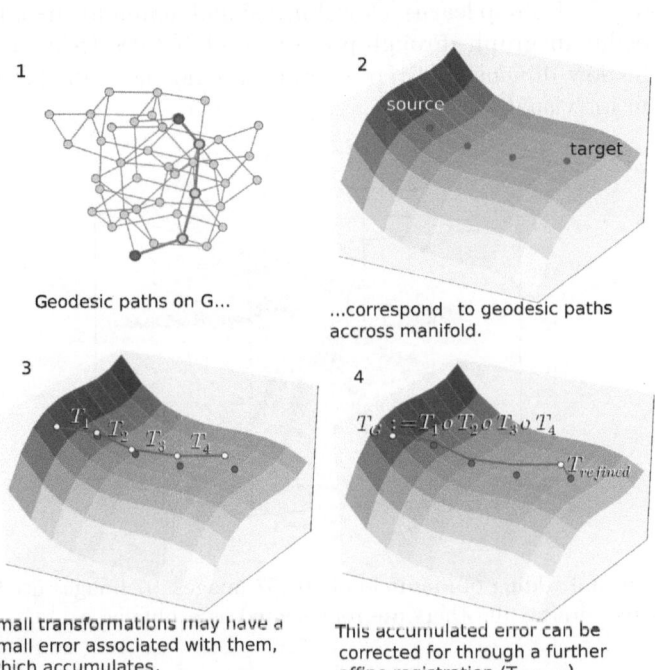

Fig. 2. Illustration of accumulation of affine registration error and refinement step to eradicate error

4   Results

4.1   Parameter Selection

For the graph construction any similarity metric that reflects registration quality could be applied, in this work both normalised cross correlation and normalised mutual information were tried. For the dataset in question, normalised cross correlation outperformed normalised mutual information. For consistency normalised cross correlation was also used as a similarity metric for affine registrations.

All similarity computations and registrations assume that the central voxel of the two images are aligned as an initialisation. Experiments regarding the number of degrees of freedom appropriate for affine registration with this dataset was performed and nine degrees of freedom were deemed sufficient.

4.2   Visualisation

In this work an empirical manifold is constructed to represent a population of unregistered knee MRI. Figure 3 is a visualisation of the manifold in a low dimensional space which can be used to help understand the structure of the data. Since geodesic paths are the basis of this work the visualisation is created using Isomap [15]. Isomap learns a low dimensional manifold embedding from the k-nearest neighbour graph through preserving global geodesic distances. Please note that this low dimensional representation is not used in the method but is simply useful for visualisation.

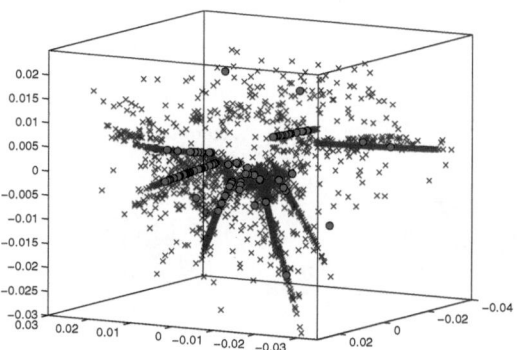

Fig. 3. Isomap Embedding of Manifold of 10,307 images. 97 images used for validation indicated by red circles, all others are represented as a blue cross.

4.3   Validation

In this section the validation of the method is discussed. Validation is carried out using the pairwise registration accuracy between a set of 97 randomly selected and annotated images. Since the graph is symmetric 4656 registrations are tested. The registrations are validated by computing the error as the mean euclidean distance between sets of landmarked points in two registered images, specifically

$$ err = \frac{1}{N} \sum_{i}^{N} ||T_{G'}(\boldsymbol{p}_i) - \boldsymbol{q}_i|| \tag{3} $$

where $\boldsymbol{p}_i$ and $\boldsymbol{q}_i$ are the ith landmark vectors of a set of N landmarks for the source and target image respectively. $||.||$ indicates an L_2^{norm}.

Figure 4 shows the distribution of errors for all the pairwise registration.

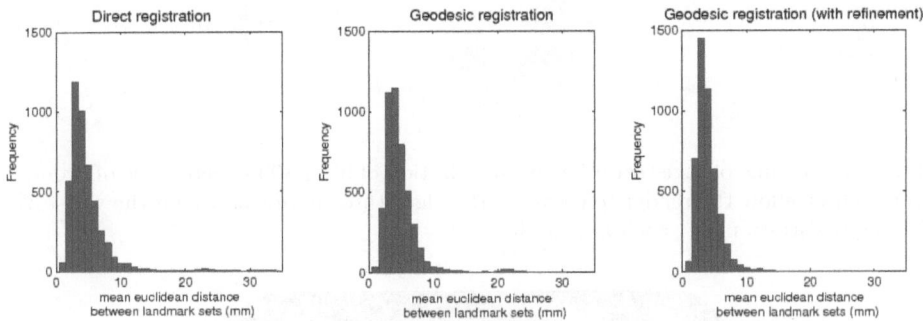

Fig. 4. Histograms of registration error (mean euclidean distance between a set of landmarked points) distribution for all pairwise registrations

Table 1 shows the mean and variance of the registration errors and the proportion of failed registrations. As can be seen from the results the geodesic registration improves upon direct registration. However it does accumulate errors as the composed transformations are added at each vertex in the geodesic path, therefore the resultant transformation does not achieve an excellent registration. When the geodesic registration is considered to be an approximation or initialisation of affine registration, the results are improved through this refinement. This is evident in the statistics and histograms presented.

Table 1. Mean and variance of registration error and the percentage of failed registrations. A failed registration is considered to have an error of greater than 10mm.

Affine registration algorithm	mean euclidean distance [mean(var)] (mm)	failed registrations (%)
direct registration [8]	4.71 (9.05)	4.08%
geodesic registration	4.72 (7.19)	2.94%
geodesic registration (refined)	3.92 (2.73)	0.86%

The focus of this work is to reduce the failure rate of affine registration, figure 5 shows the error distribution across the worst 5% of affine registration (the 95th - 100th percentile). It can be observed that the geodesic registration method proposed here improves upon the direct registration, reducing the number of failed registrations, this is also evident in the statistics reported in table 1.

Figure 6 gives a qualitative example of failed direct affine registration which was improved by the geodesic registrations framework.

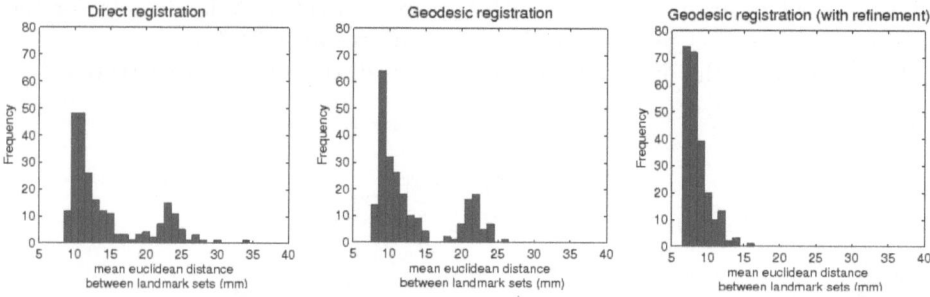

Fig. 5. Histograms of registration error distribution of 95th-100th percentile of ordered errors. These allow the reader to compare the algorithms performance on the worst 5% of affine registrations for each approach.

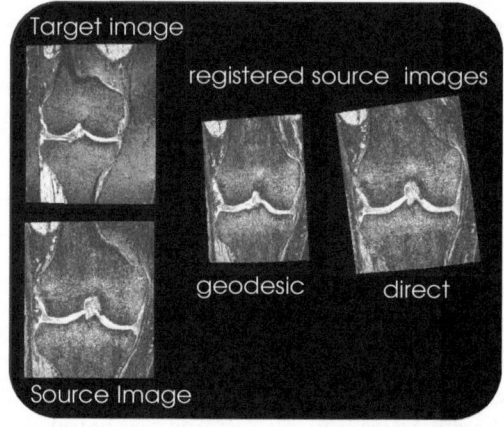

Fig. 6. Qualitative example of bad registrations improved by geodesic framework

5   Conclusions

We propose modelling the population of unregistered knee MRI as an empirical manifold using a graph, where the local properties of the manifold are modelled at each vertex. This enables registrations to be precomputed at each edge of the graph. Since the graph is a sparse k-nearest neighbour graph, where k is small, the maximum number of registration required would be $k * |V|$. However it is frequently observed that nearest neighbours might be common between vertices and so this upper bound is unlikely to be reached. Since all of these registrations can be precomputed as part of the learning process and Dijkstra's shortest path algorithm is highly efficient, the run time computational cost is low. A request for an initialisation between any pair of images can be retrieved quickly. A refinement step is also proposed, leading to to dramatically increased registration accuracy relative to direct affine registrations.

In this work the manifold space of unregistered knee images is represented as a graph, in contrast, a manifold learning method could have been used to find shortest paths in the learnt manifold space [11]. However, with the geodesic approach proposed here all registrations required are precomputed and so any pairwise registration can be requested on the fly. This speed could not be achieved across a learnt manifold since the number of potential paths increases vastly, registrations in the shortest path in the learnt manifold would need to be computed when requested. Additionally, a manifold learning approach requires the user to choose the intrinsic dimensionality of the manifold embedding in advance. In contrast to this work where the dimensionality of the graph is implicitly defined by the number of connections or degree at each vertex. This means the dimensionality effectively varies across the embedding space.

5.1   Future Work and Improvements

The search for k-nearest neighbours for the graph construction is exhaustive and the number of comparisons grows quadratically with the number of images. There are many contributions in the literature which discuss improvements, including hashing [16] or tree based searches [17]. However since the graph only needs to be constructed once, this was considered out of the scope of this work.

An out-of-sample extension could be added to this framework, where an unseen image could be accurately registered to any image in the population. Initially the nearest neighbour of the unseen image would need to be determined, then the method proposed here can be applied to find the registration. This scenario would benefit from an efficient nearest neighbour algorithm to find the nearest image in the empirical manifold, a sub-linear search would be preferable to an exhaustive linear search.

Similarity metrics computed at low resolutions appear to be sufficient in these experiments. However the effect of similarities at higher resolutions could be explored using a multiscale approach. The l-nearest neighbours of G determined by pairwise similarity of low resolution images can be found, where $|V| \gg l > k$. From the set of l selected neighbours, the k-nearest neighbours can be determined using similarity metrics of higher resolution images.

Upon manually investigating poor registrations using the geodesic framework, it appears the failure is typically due to a singular erroneous edge on the graph. Future work could explore approaches to omit such erroneous edges or improve paths through more sophisticated machine learning algorithms.

References

1. Tamez-Pena, J., Gonzalez, P., Farber, J., Baum, K., Schreyer, E., Totterman, S.: Atlas based method for the automated segmentation and quantification of knee features: Data from the osteoarthritis initiative. In: 2011 IEEE International Symposium on Biomedical Imaging: From Nano to Macro, pp. 1484–1487 (2011)
2. Fripp, J., Crozier, S., Warfield, S.K., Ourselin, S.: Automatic segmentation and quantitative analysis of the articular cartilages from magnetic resonance images of the knee. IEEE Transactions on Medical Imaging 29(1), 55–64 (2010)

3. Carballido-Gamio, J., Majumdar, S.: Atlas-based knee cartilage assessment. Magnetic Resonance in Medicine 66(2), 575–581 (2011)
4. Rueckert, D., Sonoda, L., Hayes, C., Hill, D., Leach, M., Hawkes, D.: Nonrigid registration using free-form deformations: application to breast mr images. IEEE Transactions on Medical Imaging 18(8), 712–721 (1999)
5. Donoghue, C., Rao, A., Bull, A.M.J., Rueckert, D.: Manifold learning for automatically predicting articular cartilage morphology in the knee with data from the osteoarthritis initiative (oai). In: SPIE Medical Imaging 2011: Image Processing, Proc., vol. 7962, p. 12 (2011)
6. Yang, G., Stewart, C.V., Sofka, M., Tsai, C.L.: Registration of challenging image pairs: Initialization, estimation, and decision. IEEE Transactions on Pattern Analysis and Machine Intelligence 29, 1973–1989 (2007)
7. Hill, D.L.G., Batchelor, P.G., Holden, M., Hawkes, D.J.: Medical image registration. Physics in Medicine and Biology 46(3), R1–R45 (2001)
8. Studholme, C.: An overlap invariant entropy measure of 3d medical image alignment. Pattern Recognition 32(1), 71–86 (1999)
9. Hamm, J., Ye, D.H., Verma, R., Davatzikos, C.: Gram: A framework for geodesic registration on anatomical manifolds. Medical Image Analysis 14(5), 633–642 (2010)
10. Gerber, S., Tasdizen, T., Thomas Fletcher, P., Joshi, S., Whitaker, R.: Manifold modeling for brain population analysis. Medical Image Analysis 14(5), 643–653 (2010)
11. Wolz, R., Aljabar, P., Hajnal, J.V., Hammers, A., Rueckert, D.: Leap: learning embeddings for atlas propagation. NeuroImage 49(2), 1316–1325 (2010)
12. Jia, H., Wu, G., Wang, Q., Shen, D.: Absorb: Atlas building by self-organized registration and bundling. NeuroImage 51(3), 1057–1070 (2010)
13. Peterfy, C., Schneider, E., Nevitt, M.: The osteoarthritis initiative: report on the design rationale for the magnetic resonance imaging protocol for the knee. Osteoarthritis and Cartilage 16(12), 1433–1441 (2008)
14. Dijkstra, E.W.: A note on two problems in connexion with graphs. Numerische Mathematik 1(1), 269–271 (1959)
15. Tenenbaum, J.B.: A global geometric framework for nonlinear dimensionality reduction. Science 290(5500), 2319–2323 (2000)
16. Indyk, P., Motwani, R.: Approximate nearest neighbors: Towards removing the curse of dimensionality. In: STOC 1998 Proceedings of the Thirtieth Annual ACM Symposium on Theory of Computing, pp. 604–613 (1998)
17. Bentley, J.L.: Multidimensional binary search trees used for associative searching. Communications of the ACM 18(9), 509–517 (1975)

Simple Geodesic Regression
for Image Time-Series

Yi Hong[1], Yundi Shi[1], Martin Styner[1], Mar Sanchez[2], and Marc Niethammer[1]

[1] University of North Carolina (UNC), Chapel Hill NC 27599-3175, USA
yundiuu@gmail.com, {yihong,styner,mn}@cs.unc.edu
[2] Emory University, Atlanta GA 30322, USA
mmsanch@emory.edu

Abstract. Geodesic regression generalizes linear regression to general Riemannian manifolds. Applied to images, it allows for a compact approximation of an image time-series through an initial image and an initial momentum. Geodesic regression requires the definition of a squared residual (squared distance) between the regression geodesic and the measurement images. In principle, this squared distance should also be defined through a geodesic connecting an image on the regression geodesic to its respective measurement. However, in practice only standard registration distances (such as sum of squared distances) are used, to reduce computation time. This paper describes a simplified geodesic regression method which approximates the registration-based distances with respect to a fixed initial image. This results in dramatically simplified computations. In particular, the method becomes straightforward to implement using readily available large displacement diffeomorphic metric mapping (LDDMM) shooting algorithms and decouples the problem into pairwise image registrations allowing parallel computations. We evaluate the approach using 2D synthetic images and real 3D brain images.

Keywords: Geodesic regression, time-series, image registration.

1 Introduction

The increasing availability of longitudinal image time-series to study aging processes, brain development, or disease progression requires image analysis methods, and in particular image registration methods, customized for longitudinal data. A standard approach is to directly extend methods devised for pair-wise image registration to image time-series. In the case of LDDMM registration [1] a spatio-temporal velocity field is estimated over the full time-duration of the available measurements, with image similarity terms at the measurement time-points. This results in a piece-wise geodesic interpolation path [2,3] with jumps of the velocity field caused by the measurements.

To avoid these jumps, two directions have been pursued: (i) spline(-like) interpolations or general temporal smoothness terms (primarily for shapes) [4,5] or methods based on kernel regression [6] and (ii) approximations of time-series

B.M. Dawant et al. (Eds.): WBIR 2012, LNCS 7359, pp. 11–20, 2012.

12	Y. Hong et al.

through geodesic regression [7, 8]. While the former models are more flexible, geodesic regression directly yields a simple generative model which compactly parameterizes a full spatio-temporal trajectory using only an initial image and an initial momentum.

Geodesic regression seeks to minimize the sum of squared distances of the measurements to the regression geodesic. Closed-form solutions are generally not available. However, for some spaces analytical expressions for the "forces" exerted by the measurements on the regression geodesic (the equivalent to the model residuals for linear regression) can be computed [8]. Unfortunately, this is not the case when working with diffeomorphisms for image-valued geodesic regression [7]. Here, the squared distances can either be defined by registrations themselves, which is computationally expensive, or by using standard similarity measures for image registration (such as sum of squared intensity differences) assuming that all measurements are close to the regression geodesic.

This paper proposes an approximation to image-valued geodesic regression [7] *with registration-based distances* using a distance approximation for image-to-image registration proposed in [9]. This approximation allows for the computation of the regression geodesic (for a fixed initial image) by a weighted average of the initial momenta obtained by registering the initial image with the measurement images pairwise. Hence, standard shooting-based LDDMM implementation methods can be used for the computation of the regression geodesic and its computation decouples into pairwise registrations (see Fig. 1 for an illustration) which can be solved in parallel.

We motivate the weighting of the initial momenta for the image-valued case by illustrating the concept for linear regression in Sec. 2. Sec. 3 describes the image-valued case. To demonstrate the effectiveness of our scheme, we apply it to both synthetic and real image time-series in Sec. 4. We conclude and discuss future work in Sec. 5.

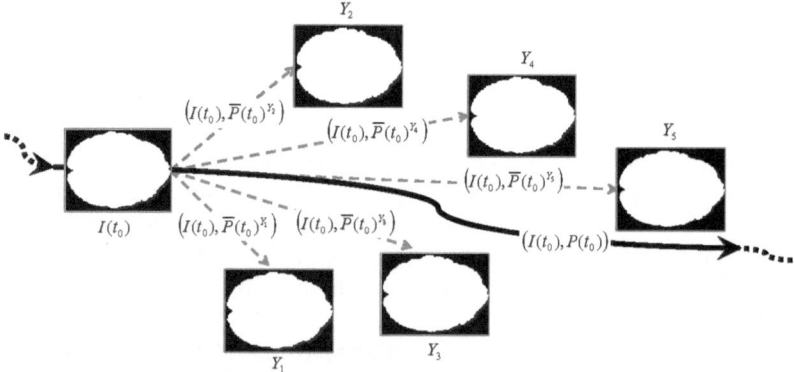

Fig. 1. Simple geodesic regression: the regression geodesic (bold) is determined by pairwise registrations between the base image, $I(t_0)$, and the measurement images, Y_i

2 Linear Regression (w/ fixed base-point) Reformulated

Given a set of N measurements $\{y_i\}$ at time instants $\{t_i\}$ we want to find the slope, a, and the y-intercept, b, of the best fitting line $y = at + b$ in a least squares sense. We assume that one point on this line is known[1]. Without loss of generality, we assume this point to be at the origin. Hence, we want to minimize

$$E(a) = \frac{1}{2} \sum_{i=1}^{N} (at_i - y_i)^2 \;\Rightarrow\; a = \frac{\sum_i y_i t_i}{\sum_i t_i^2}. \tag{1}$$

Assume that instead of fitting one line to all the measurements, we fit lines from the origin to all the measurement points individually. This amounts to independently minimizing

$$E_i(a_i) = \frac{1}{2}(a_i t_i - y_i)^2 \;\Rightarrow\; a_i = \frac{y_i}{t_i}. \tag{2}$$

Since $y_i = a_i t_i$, we obtain upon substitution in (1)

$$a = \frac{\sum_i t_i^2 a_i}{\sum_i t_i^2} = \sum_i w_i a_i, \quad \text{with } w_i = \frac{t_i^2}{\sum_i t_i^2}, \quad \sum_i w_i = 1. \tag{3}$$

Hence, the slope of the regression line can be computed as a weighted average of the slopes of the individual lines. What remains to be shown is that a similar averaging procedure can be used for the image-valued case.

3 Simple Geodesic Regression

Geodesic regression for image time-series generalizes linear regression to the space of images [7]. It uses a shooting formulation to LDDMM registration [11] and is based on the minimization of

$$E(I(t_0), p(t_0)) = \frac{1}{2} \langle p(t_0) \nabla I(t_0), K(p(t_0) \nabla I(t_0)) \rangle + \sum_i w_i d^2(I(t_i), Y_i), \quad (4)$$

$$\text{s.t.} \quad I_t + \nabla I^T v = 0, \; p_t + div(pv) = 0, \; v + K(p\nabla I) = 0, \quad (5)$$

where $I(t_0)$ and $p(t_0)$ are the unknown initial image and the unknown initial Hamiltonian momentum respectively, K is a chosen smoothing kernel, $w_i > 0$ scalar weights and Y_i is the measured image at time t_i; $d^2(A, B)$ denotes a squared distance(-like) image similarity measure between the two images A and B and can be one of the standard image similarity measures or can be based on image registration itself to allow for large deviations between the geodesic regression line and the Y_i [7]. A numerical scheme using registration-based distances can be derived, but is impractical, because it would require frequent

---

[1] This is a simplifying assumption akin to formulating a growth model with respect to an initial image.

costly recomputations of the distances in an iterative solution scheme. Hence, an approximation of the registration-based distance is desirable. We define the squared distance [1] as

$$d^2(A, B) = \frac{1}{2} \int_0^1 \|v^*\|_L^2 \, dt, \text{ where} \tag{6}$$

$$v^* = \underset{v}{argmin} \, \frac{1}{2} \int_0^1 \|v\|_L^2 \, dt + \frac{1}{\sigma^2} \|I(1) - B\|_2^2, \text{ s.t. } I_t + \nabla I^T v = 0, \ I(0) = A.$$

This is an inexact matching formulation since an exact matching is typically impossible by a spatial transformation alone due to noise and appearance changes[2].

To simplify the geodesic regression formulation (4) we use a first order approximation of pairwise distances [9]. In contrast to [9], the time-series aspect of the images has to be considered. For all pairwise distances, $I(t_0)$ becomes the base image. For two images A, B and given spatial transformations $\Phi_t^{v_0^A}$ and $\Phi_t^{v_0^B}$ which map $I(t_0)$ to A and B in time t, the composition $\Phi_t = \Phi_t^{v_0^B} \circ (\Phi_t^{v_0^A})^{-1}$ maps A to B. Since both transformations are parameterized by initial velocity fields v_0^A and v_0^B respectively, we approximate Φ_t to first order as

$$\Phi_t = \text{Exp}_{\text{Id}}(tv_0^B) \circ \text{Exp}_{\text{Id}}(-tv_0^A) \approx \text{Exp}_{\text{Id}}(t(v_0^B - v_0^A)). \tag{7}$$

Then the squared distance can be approximated as

$$d^2(A, B) \approx \frac{1}{2} t^2 \langle K^{-1}(v_0^B - v_0^A), v_0^B - v_0^A \rangle \tag{8}$$

or in momentum form

$$d^2(A, B) \approx \frac{1}{2} t^2 \langle (p(t_0)^B - p(t_0)^A)\nabla I(t_0), K((p(t_0)^B - p(t_0)^A)\nabla I(t_0)) \rangle. \tag{9}$$

Using this approximation to rewrite the geodesic regression formulation (4) yields

$$E(I(t_0), p(t_0)) = \frac{1}{2} \langle p(t_0)\nabla I(t_0), K(p(t_0)\nabla I(t_0)) \rangle$$

$$+ \sum w_i \frac{1}{2}(t_i - t_0)^2 \langle (p(t_0)^{Y_i} - p(t_0))\nabla I(t_0), K((p(t_0)^{Y_i} - p(t_0))\nabla I(t_0)) \rangle. \tag{10}$$

We assume that $I(t_0)$ is on the geodesic[3]. All $p(t_0)^{Y_i}$ are precomputed by pairwise registrations with $I(t_0)$. The approximated energy only depends on the initial momentum $p(t_0)$. Taking the variation of (10) with respect to $p(t_0)$ results in

$$\delta E(I(t_0), p(t_0); \delta p) = \langle \nabla I(t_0)^T K m(t_0), \delta p \rangle$$

$$+ \sum w_i (t_i - t_0)^2 \langle \nabla I(t_0)^T K(m_i(t_0) - m(t_0)), -\delta p \rangle, \tag{11}$$

---

[2] A metamorphosis approach [10] could be used instead.

[3] Otherwise registrations between $I(t_0)$ and all other images would be required when $I(t_0)$ changes, providing no benefit over the original geodesic regression method. This is a simplifying assumption, which transforms the model into a type of growth model described by a geodesic.

where K is assumed to be a symmetric kernel, $m(t_0) = p(t_0)\nabla I(t_0)$ and $m_i(t_0) = p(t_0)^{Y_i} \nabla I(t_0)$. Collecting terms yields

$$\delta E(I(t_0), p(t_0); \delta p) = \langle \nabla I(t_0)^T K[m(t_0) + \sum w_i(t_i - t_0)^2 (m(t_0) - m_i(t_0))], \delta p \rangle. \tag{12}$$

For a candidate minimizer δE needs to vanish for any admissible δp. Hence,

$$m(t_0) + \sum w_i(t_i - t_0)^2 (m(t_0) - m_i(t_0)) = 0 \tag{13}$$

or in momentum space

$$p(t_0) + \sum w_i(t_i - t_0)^2 (p(t_0) - p(t_0)^{Y_i}) = 0. \tag{14}$$

Solving for $p(t_0)$ results in

$$p(t_0) = \frac{\sum w_i(t_i - t_0)^2 p(t_0)^{Y_i}}{1 + \sum w_i(t_i - t_0)^2}. \tag{15}$$

In practice most frequently, $w_i = w = const$ and $w >> 1$ simplifying (15) to

$$p(t_0) \approx \frac{\sum (t_i - t_0)^2 p(t_0)^{Y_i}}{\sum (t_i - t_0)^2}, \tag{16}$$

which is a simple averaging of the initial momenta with weights $g_i = \frac{(t_i - t_0)^2}{\sum (t_i - t_0)^2}$. This formulation recovers the original image-to-image registration result for the special case of two images. To obtain the initial momenta $p(t_0)^{Y_i}$ which are needed to approximate the registration distance at time t_i one could modify the registration problem (6) by integrating between t_0 and t_i and solve it with the algorithm proposed in [1]. However, such an approach would suffer from two short-comings: (i) it would not guarantee geodesic solutions and (ii) the relative weighting of the image similarity measure would be influenced by the different time-periods used to perform the deformations (since $\|v\|_L^2$ is integrated over time, the same deformation becomes cheaper for a longer time interval). We therefore use (i) a shooting method [11] to compute the registrations and (ii) compute $\bar{p}(t_0)^{Y_i}$ by registering $I(t_0)$ to Y_i in unit time followed by a rescaling of the momentum to account for the original time duration: $p(t_0)^{Y_i} = \frac{1}{t_i - t_0} \bar{p}(t_0)^{Y_i}$. Using the momenta computed for a unit time, the initial momentum for the regression geodesic can be written as

$$p(t_0) \approx \frac{\sum (t_i - t_0) p(t_0)^{Y_i}}{\sum (t_i - t_0)^2}. \tag{17}$$

Given the base image $I(t_0)$ and $p(t_0)$, we can integrate Eq. (5) forward or backward in time to obtain the regression geodesic. Our approximate geodesic regression results in a dramatic simplification of the optimization method for geodesic regression. Pairwise registrations can be computed in parallel if desired.

4   Experiments

Implementation. In the following experiments, the smoothing kernel K is set as the weighted sum of N Gaussian kernels K_{σ_n} [12]: $K(x) = \sum_{n=1}^{N} c_n K_{\sigma_n}(x)$, $c_n = c'_n / g(K_{\sigma_n}, I_S, I_T)$. Usually we set $c'_n = 1$. We first compute c_n for image pairs (following [12]) and then take the average of all the c_n as the weights for the kernels. All images are slightly blurred before registration.

Synthetic Images. In the first experiment, we synthesized the movement of a bull's eye using a series of 2D binary images (32×32 pixels, spacing 0.04) as shown in Fig. (2). The white circle inside of the eye grows at a constant speed while the outside white loop shrinks. We used four images at time instants 0, 10, 20, 30s, $I(0)$ as the base image, and 7 Gaussian kernels for K, $\{K_{0.5}, K_{0.4}, K_{0.3}, K_{0.2}, K_{0.15}, K_{0.1}, K_{0.05}\}$; $\sigma^2 = 0.01$. The simple geodesic regression result (2nd row of Fig. (2)) shows that changes are captured well.

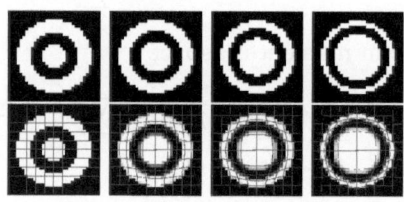

Fig. 2. Synthetic bull's eye experiment (top row) and results for simple geodesic regression (bottom row). The movement is well captured.

To quantify the regression accuracy we compute the overlay error between measurement images and the images on the geodesic:

$$E_{overlay}(I(t_i), Y_i) = \frac{1}{|\Omega|} \|\epsilon(I(t_i), Y_i)\|_{L^1}, \quad \epsilon(I, J)(x) = |I(x) - J(x)|. \quad (18)$$

Table 1. Comparison of overlay errors among image pairs, the original geodesic regression, and our simple geodesic regression

Measurement Images	$E_{overlay}(I(t_i), Y_i)$			
	Y_0	Y_1	Y_2	Y_3
Image pairs($I(t_i) = Y_0, Y_i$)	0	0.0820	0.1914	0.3242
OGR(fixed initial image: Y_0)	0	0.0247	0.0306	0.0311
SGR(base image: Y_0)	0	0.0274	0.0329	0.0261

Tab. 1 shows the overlay errors between the initial image and all other measurements, the results of the original geodesic regression (OGR) and of the simple geodesic regression (SGR) regression respectively. The regression models are comparable in accuracy indicating that SGR works correctly in this experiment.

To illustrate the necessity of using a registration-based distance rather than the squared L^2 distance of two images, two test cases in Fig. 3 are employed for comparing the results of the original geodesic regression and our method. In the cases, five binary images (64×64 pixels, spacing 0.02) are generated to describe a square moving from left to right at uniform speed without oscillation (subfigure (a)) and with strong vertical oscillation by a constant amplitude (subfigure (b)). Here, K is $\{K_1, K_{0.75}, K_{0.5}, K_{0.4}, K_{0.3}, K_{0.2}, K_{0.15}, K_{0.1}\}$.

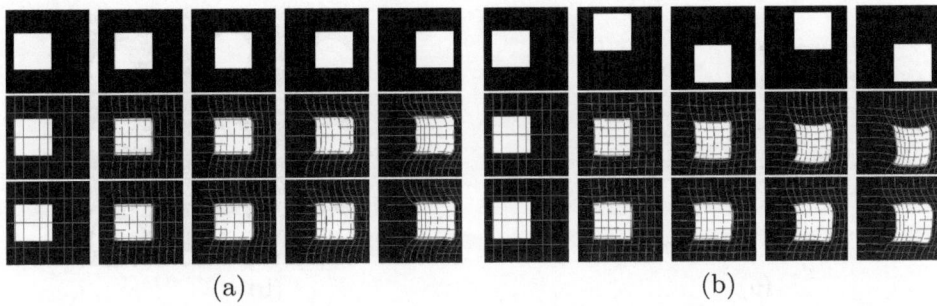

Fig. 3. Square moving from left to right without oscillation (a) and with vertical oscillation (b). Top: original images. Middle: the results of the original geodesic regression. Bottom: the results of our method.

When there is no oscillation in the movement (Fig. 3(a)), the original geodesic regression has comparable performance to our method. In case (b), similar to the regression lines for the scalar case (Fig. 4), the square is expected to move to the right while moving down slightly, which is consistent with the SGR result (bottom row of subfigure (b)). However, the square in the original geodesic regression (using the L^2 distance) leads to a stronger shape deformation and deviation from the horizontal line.

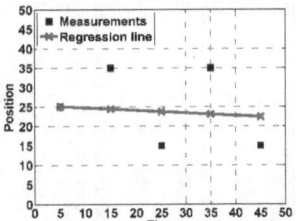

Fig. 4. Scalar experiment

Fig. 5 compares the proposed weighting of initial momenta for SGR (Eq. (16)) to a direct arithmetic average for a set of 3 images (64×64 pixels; spacing 0.02) at time points 0, 10, 40s respectively. The images at 10s and 40s are displaced by an equal distance vertically with respect to the image at 0s, but the horizontal displacements differ by a factor of 3. We chose the same multi-Gaussian kernel as in the first experiment. The SGR weighting is clearly more appropriate.

Real Images. We also evaluated SGR on two sets of longitudinal magnetic resonance images: 2D slices of a longitudinal dataset from the OASIS database and a 3D longitudinal dataset from a macaque monkey. One K, $\{K_{3.0}, K_{1.5}, K_{0.5}, K_{0.4}, K_{0.3}, K_{0.2}, K_{0.1}, K_{0.05}\}$, was applied to all the real images[4].
The four images in the first row of Fig. 6(a) are slices from an OASIS data set (161×128 pixels, spacing 0.5) for a subject scanned at age 67, 68, 71, and 73. We applied SGR with the youngest slice as the base image. The changes between the base image and other measurements are subtle, as illustrated by the difference images in the left column of Fig. 6(b) and the overlay errors in the first row of Tab. 2. However, our method successfully captures the variations in the brain images, especially the ventricle expansion, which is supported by the generated images (Fig. 6(a), 2nd row) and the difference images (right column Fig. 6(b)).

---

[4] Slightly better results may be achievable by data-set-dependent tuning of the kernel.

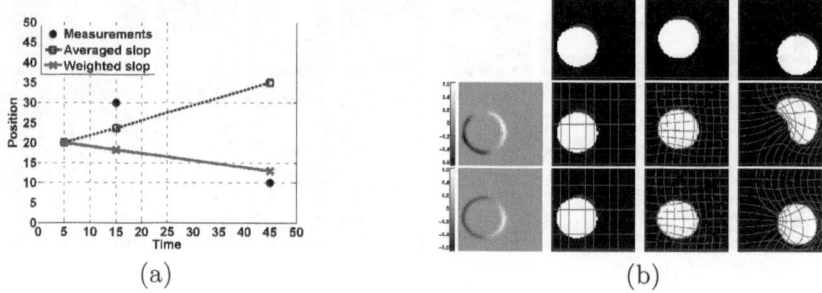

Fig. 5. Scalar and image-valued cases comparing arithmetic averaging and the proposed weighting approach for initial momenta. (a) Scalar case. (b) Image case: image time-series (0, 10, 40s) (top), the initial momentum and the images generated by simply averaging the initial momenta (middle) and by our weighting method (bottom).

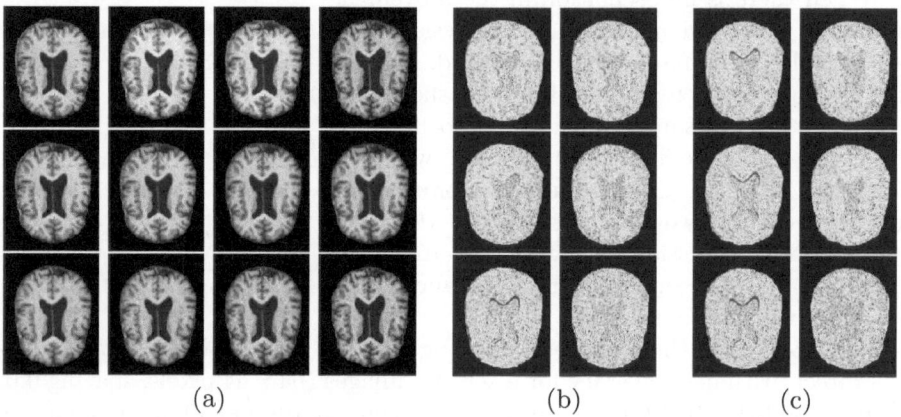

Fig. 6. OASIS data: (a): Original images (top, left to right: 67, 68, 71, 73 [years]), geodesic I with youngest slice as base image (middle), and geodesic II with oldest slice as base image (bottom). (b): Difference images of measurement images (up to down: 68, 71, 73 [years]) with youngest image (left) and images on geodesic I (right). (c): Difference images of measurement images (up to down: 71, 68, 67 [years]) with oldest image (left) and images on the geodesic II (right).

We also took the oldest slice as the base image to verify the efficiency of our model. As shown by the generated trajectory (Fig. 6(a), 3rd row), the difference images (Fig. 6(c)), and overlay errors in Tab. 2, our method works well.

The images ($150 \times 125 \times 100$ pixels with spacing 0.5468) in Fig. 7 are from a longitudinal data-set of a macaque monkey at the age of 3, 6, 12 and 18 months respectively[5]. We set the image at 3 months as the base image and applied our approach to capture the changes of the ventricle marked by the magenta

---

[5] Note that this is a time-range of active brain myelination for the macaque. Hence image intensities for the white matter are not constant over time and therefore a perfect image match is not expected.

Table 2. Overlay error among image pairs, the original geodesic regression (OGR), and our simple geodesic regression (SGR) for longitudinal subject data shown in Fig. 6

	$E_{overlay}(I(t_i), Y_i)$			
Measurement Images [Years]	$Y_0 = 67$	$Y_1 = 68$	$Y_2 = 71$	$Y_3 = 73$
Image pairs ($I(t_i) = Y_0, Y_i$)	0	0.0468	0.0342	0.0472
OGR (fixed initial image: Y_0)	0	0.0452	0.0298	0.0313
SGR (base image: Y_0)	0	0.0449	0.0304	0.0286
Measurement Images [Years]	$Y_0 = 73$	$Y_1 = 71$	$Y_2 = 68$	$Y_3 = 67$
Image pairs ($I(t_i) = Y_0, Y_i$)	0	0.0536	0.0631	0.0472
OGR (fixed initial image: Y_0)	0	0.0448	0.0457	0.0284
SGR (base image: Y_0)	0	0.0438	0.0432	0.0258

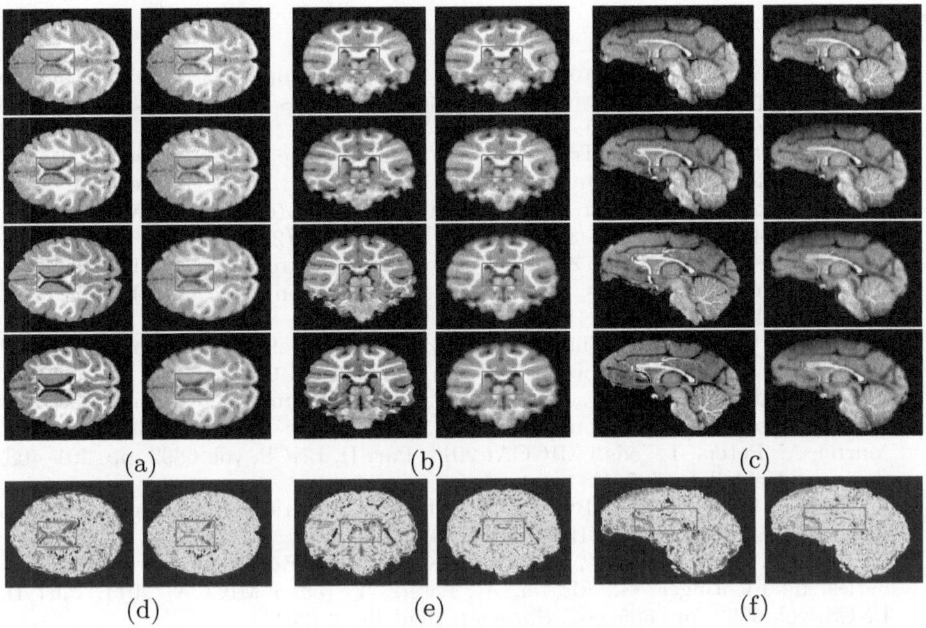

Fig. 7. Results for the macaque monkey data (up to down: 3, 6, 12, 18 [months], the youngest one as base image). (a-c): axial, coronal and sagittal slices of the original images (left) and images on the geodesic (right). (d-f): difference images of the oldest image with the youngest one (left) and with the images on the geodesic (right).

windows. As the monkey's age increases, the ventricle gradually approaches the edges of the windows, which is well captured by SGR.

5   Discussion and Conclusions

We developed a simplified geodesic regression model by approximating the squared distances between the regression geodesic and the measurement images.

In contrast to the original geodesic regression formulation for images, SGR can be efficiently computed. In fact, it only requires pair-wise registrations of the measurement images with respect to a chosen base-image (typically either the first or the last image of a time-series). The regression geodesic is then determined by the base image and the initial momentum obtained by appropriate averaging of the initial momenta of the pairwise registrations. Future work will focus on using this regression model for longitudinal image-based population-studies and on extending it to capture spatial and appearance changes simultaneously.

Acknowledgments. This work was sponsored by NSF EECS-1148870, NSF EECS-0925875, NIH NIHM 5R01MH091645-02, NIH NIBIB 5P41EB002025-28, NIH NHLBI 5R01HL105241-02 and U54 EB005149.

References

1. Beg, M.F., Miller, M.I., Trouvé, A., Younes, L.: Computing large deformation metric mappings via geodesic flows of diffeomorphisms. International Journal of Computer Vision 61(2), 139–157 (2005)
2. Durrleman, S., Pennec, X., Trouvé, A., Gerig, G., Ayache, N.: Spatiotemporal Atlas Estimation for Developmental Delay Detection in Longitudinal Datasets. In: Yang, G.-Z., Hawkes, D., Rueckert, D., Noble, A., Taylor, C. (eds.) MICCAI 2009, Part I. LNCS, vol. 5761, pp. 297–304. Springer, Heidelberg (2009)
3. Niethammer, M., Hart, G., Zach, C.: An optimal control approach for the registration of image time series. In: Conference on Decision and Control (CDC), pp. 2427–2434. IEEE (2009)
4. Trouvé, A., Vialard, F.X.: Shape splines and stochastic shape evolutions: A second order point of view. Arxiv preprint arXiv:1003.3895 (2010)
5. Fishbaugh, J., Durrleman, S., Gerig, G.: Estimation of Smooth Growth Trajectories with Controlled Acceleration from Time Series Shape Data. In: Fichtinger, G., Martel, A., Peters, T. (eds.) MICCAI 2011, Part II. LNCS, vol. 6892, pp. 401–408. Springer, Heidelberg (2011)
6. Davis, B.C., Fletcher, P.T., Bullitt, E., Joshi, S.: Population Shape Regression from Random Design Data. In: 11th IEEE ICCV (2007)
7. Niethammer, M., Huang, Y., Vialard, F.-X.: Geodesic Regression for Image Time-Series. In: Fichtinger, G., Martel, A., Peters, T. (eds.) MICCAI 2011, Part II. LNCS, vol. 6892, pp. 655–662. Springer, Heidelberg (2011)
8. Fletcher, P.T.: Geodesic regression on Riemannian manifolds. In: Proceedings of International Workshop on Mathematical Foundations of Computational Anatomy, MFCA (2011)
9. Yang, X., Goh, A., Qiu, A.: Approximations of the Diffeomorphic Metric and Their Applications in Shape Learning. In: Székely, G., Hahn, H.K. (eds.) IPMI 2011. LNCS, vol. 6801, pp. 257–270. Springer, Heidelberg (2011)
10. Trouvé, A., Younes, L.: Metamorphoses through Lie group action. Foundations of Computational Mathematics 5(2), 173–198 (2005)
11. Vialard, F.X., Risser, L., Rueckert, D., Cotter, C.J.: Diffeomorphic 3D image registration via geodesic shooting using an efficient adjoint calculation. International Journal of Computer Vision, 1–13 (2011)
12. Risser, L., Vialard, F.-X., Wolz, R., Murgasova, M., Holm, D.D., Rueckert, D.: Simultaneous Multi-Scale Registration Using Large Deformation Diffeomorphic Metric Mapping. IEEE Transcations on Medical Imaging 30(10), 1746–1759 (2011)

Automatic Detection of the Magnitude and Spatial Location of Error in Non-rigid Registration

Ryan D. Datteri and Benoît M. Dawant

Department of Electrical Engineering and Computer Science,
Vanderbilt University, Nashvile, TN 37235, USA
{ryan.d.datteri,benoit.dawant}@vanderbilt.edu

Abstract. Non-rigid image registration is used pervasively in medical image analysis for applications ranging from anatomical and functional studies to surgical assistance. Error in specific instances of a non-rigid registration process, however, is often not determined. In this paper, we propose a method to determine the magnitude and spatial location of error in non-rigid registration. The method is independent of the registration method and similarity measure used. We show that our algorithm is capable of detecting the distribution and magnitude of registration error in a simulated case. Using real data, our algorithm also is able to identify registration error that is consistent with error that can be seen visually.

Keywords: Image registration, registration circuits, non-rigid registration, error detection.

1   Introduction

Detection of error in non-rigid registration has been detailed in various studies as a difficult and important problem [1,2,3]. Intensity-based image registration algorithms, which are the most commonly used methods for non-rigid registration tasks, depend on similarity measures to estimate how well two images match. However, registration algorithms are unable to determine the quality of their results based on image intensity alone. The problem of correspondence error and its potential negative effect on studies that use voxel-based morphometry is described in [1]. The paper was published in 2003 and, to the best of our knowledge no method has yet to be developed in response to the problem they pose, that is "most widely used methods are essentially dumb in that, for a particular registration task, they report only a measure of image similarity which does not allow a judgment of 'success' or 'failure' to be made. Worse the magnitude and spatial distribution of errors in NRR are unknown". The aim of this paper is to begin to address this problem.

Analytical solutions to calculate error have been developed for the rigid-body registration case when fiducial markers are available [4]. It has been shown, however, that it does not allow for the estimation of error in individual cases [5]. Other attempts at quantifying error in cases without fiducial markers simplify the registration problem and are therefore un-applicable to most medical image registration problems.

B.M. Dawant et al. (Eds.): WBIR 2012, LNCS 7359, pp. 21–30, 2012.

Möller et al. [6] developed a method in computer vision that quantifies the quality of a registration, yet the method is restricted to translations. Simonson et al. [7] developed a statistical method that gives a measure of confidence for a given registration, yet, this method is restricted to affine, rigid body and translational transformations and can only be applied to binary images. Simpson et al. [8] recently proposed a method that estimates the uncertainty at each voxel, and then utilizes this uncertainty value to regularize the deformation field that results from the registration algorithm. While novel, this technique requires the usage of a specific registration framework the group has developed and requires voxel-level similarity metrics.

The following section details our algorithm which we call AQUIRC for Assessing Quality Using Image Registration Circuits. AQUIRC was recently proposed in [9] where it was utilized to estimate error in rigid registrations and [10] where it was used for atlas selection. AQUIRC utilizes the deformation fields that result from a registration algorithm, and thus can be applied to any registration algorithm. In this paper, we describe AQUIRC applied at the voxel-level, which differs from previous work that has utilized a global metric. We apply our algorithm to identify error in a simulated problem as well as to identify error in a registration between two images. We will show that AQUIRC is able to identify the magnitude and spatial location of registration error, discuss regions in which AQUIRC is not able to identify registration error, and propose future applications and avenues of research.

2   AQUIRC

AQUIRC builds on the idea of registration circuits which was proposed as a consistency measure by Woods et al. [11] and Holden et al. [12]. A registration circuit involves three images A, B, and C and three transformations T_{AB}, T_{BC}, and T_{CA}. As discussed by Fitzpatrick [13], using only one registration circuit can lead to an underestimation of registration error because the error made along one edge in the circuit may correct error introduced from a separate edge in the circuit.

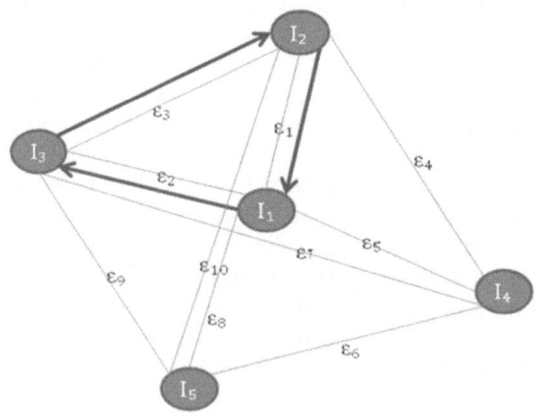

Fig. 1. Example complete graph with one circuit shown in red arrows

In this work, we expand upon the idea of registration circuits to multiple circuits. We start with a set of images and compute pair-wise registrations between all elements in the set, creating a complete graph as shown in Figure 1. The complete graph of registrations is similar to what is done by Christensen [14]. In [14], however, they used the complete graph of registrations as an overall measure of the quality of a registration algorithm, rather than as a method to determine the quality of individual registrations as we have done here. If our initial set contains N images, the graph contains $\binom{N}{2}$ edges. There are $\binom{N}{3}$ unique registration circuits that can be formed from a complete graph (we have used registration circuits of size 3; the circuit size can be increased to form more registration circuits but this was not explored here). With each edge in this graph, we associate an initially unknown measure of registration quality called ε that we wish to solve for. In this work, we solve for a registration quality at each voxel, $\bar{\varepsilon} = [\varepsilon^1, \varepsilon^2, . . ., \varepsilon^Q]$, with Q equal to the number of voxels in the common image space. Thus, $\bar{\varepsilon}$ represents a rasterised vector of registration quality for each voxel in an image.

Next, we define a measure of registration error that can be computed across a circuit. We compute this error for every voxel in the image. This requires a common coordinate system for each of the images in the network, thus if all the images in the network do not have the same dimension or voxel size, they are re-sampled. To compute the error we take the set of coordinates in an image, call it $\mathbf{X}$. We then compute the transformed coordinates $\mathbf{X}'$ as $\mathbf{X}' = T_{AB}(T_{BC}(T_{CA}(\mathbf{X})))$. The error across circuit A, B, C, is then defined for each voxel i, as $E_C^i = distance(\mathbf{X}_i, \mathbf{X}'_i)$. $\bar{E}_C = \left[E_C^1, E_C^2, . . ., E_C^Q\right]$ is then defined as a vector of errors across a circuit. The values in $\bar{E}_C$ are affected by the error of three registrations, i.e., the registration error between A and B, the registration error between B and C, and the registration error between C and A. With only one circuit the contribution of each component cannot be computed. It can, however, be estimated with more than one circuit. To achieve this we make the assumption that each registration affects the quality measure multiplicatively, i.e., $\log(\varepsilon_{ABC}) = \log(\varepsilon_A) + \log(\varepsilon_B) + \log(\varepsilon_C)$. An additive model may also be applicable, but this was not explored here. Computing this expression for all unique circuits and rearranging them in matrix form, we obtain

$$
\begin{bmatrix} 1\,1\,1\,0\,..\,0 \\ 1\,0\,1\,1\,..\,0 \\ 1\,1\,0\,1\,..\,0 \\ 0\,1\,1\,1\,..\,0 \\ \cdot \\ \cdot \\ \cdot \\ \end{bmatrix} \begin{bmatrix} \log\left([\varepsilon_1^1, \varepsilon_1^2, ..., \varepsilon_1^Q]\right) \\ \log\left([\varepsilon_2^1, \varepsilon_2^2, ..., \varepsilon_2^Q]\right) \\ \log\left([\varepsilon_3^1, \varepsilon_3^2, ..., \varepsilon_3^Q]\right) \\ \cdot \\ \cdot \\ \cdot \\ \log\left(\left[\varepsilon_{\binom{N}{2}}^1, \varepsilon_{\binom{N}{2}}^2, ..., \varepsilon_{\binom{N}{2}}^Q\right]\right) \end{bmatrix} = \begin{bmatrix} \log\left([E_{C_1}^1, E_{C_1}^2, ..., E_{C_1}^Q]\right) \\ \log\left([E_{C_2}^1, E_{C_2}^3, ..., E_{C_2}^Q]\right) \\ \log\left([E_{C_3}^1, E_{C_3}^2, ..., E_{C_3}^Q]\right) \\ \cdot \\ \cdot \\ \cdot \\ \log\left(\left[E_{C_{\binom{N}{3}}}^1, E_{C_{\binom{N}{3}}}^2, ..., E_{C_{\binom{N}{3}}}^Q\right]\right) \end{bmatrix} \quad (1)
$$

in which E_{Cp}^i is defined as the $distance(\mathbf{X}, \mathbf{X}')$ value around circuit p at voxel i and ε_l^i is defined as the quality of the registration l at voxel l. This expression can be rewritten as $\bar{\bar{P}} \log(\bar{\varepsilon}) = \log(\bar{E}_c)$. Where $\bar{\bar{P}}$ is a matrix that represents the links utilized for each circuit, with the value of $\bar{\bar{P}}$ set to 1 if the link is utilized in the circuit and 0 otherwise. As a result of the multiplicative assumption, $\log(\bar{\varepsilon})$ can be solved for using a linear least squares solution

$$
\log(\bar{\varepsilon}) = \left(\bar{\bar{P}}^T \bar{\bar{P}}\right)^{-1} \bar{\bar{P}}^T \log(\bar{\bar{E}}_c) \quad (2)
$$

and solving for $\bar{\bar{\varepsilon}}$

$$\bar{\bar{\varepsilon}} = e^{\log (\bar{\bar{\varepsilon}})} \qquad (3)$$

In this implementation, we calculate $\bar{\bar{\varepsilon}}$ separately for the x, y, and z directions. Thus we calculate equation (3) using three different distance metrics, i.e. $\bar{\bar{\varepsilon}}_x$ is calculated using $distance(\mathbf{X}, \mathbf{X}') = \mathbf{X}_x - \mathbf{X}'_x$, $\bar{\bar{\varepsilon}}_y$ is calculated using $distance(\mathbf{X}, \mathbf{X}') = \mathbf{X}_y - \mathbf{X}'_y$, and $\bar{\bar{\varepsilon}}_z$ is calculated using $distance(\mathbf{X}, \mathbf{X}') = \mathbf{X}_z - \mathbf{X}'_z$. This results in an estimation of error for the x, y, and z directions at each and every voxel. We then calculate the magnitude error for each registration as $\bar{\bar{\varepsilon}}_{mag} = \sqrt{\left(\bar{\bar{\varepsilon}}_x{}^2 + \bar{\bar{\varepsilon}}_y{}^2 + \bar{\bar{\varepsilon}}_z{}^2\right)}$. We are currently working on a proof of conditions on the registration circuits for when $\bar{\bar{P}}$ is full rank and therefore $\left(\bar{\bar{P}}^T\bar{\bar{P}}\right)$ is invertible. Experimentally $\bar{\bar{P}}$ has been observed to be full rank when N $\geq$ 5. We define $\bar{\bar{P}}$ to be all unique circuits in the graph of size 3, although it may be possible to utilize fewer circuits to eliminate redundancy. There are two known instances where AQUIRC is not able to identify the error in a registration between two images.

- First, if each of the registrations in a complete graph resulted in identical transformations then the metric E_c would be the same for each registration circuit and AQUIRC would be unable to identify a relevant error value for each registration.
- Secondly, if there is an error that is the same across all registrations into one image, AQUIRC is unable to account for this error. This is because for every possible circuit, the error is first added to, and then subtracted from the resulting combination of transformations. No circuit is thus able to account for that error since it is always removed from the final error value of a circuit.

We do not believe these two instances are likely to appear often in practice, but their impact is under continuing evaluation.

2.1   Image Information and Registration Method

In the experiments discussed in this article, we used 5 MR images that are T1-weighted sagittal volumes with 256x256x170 voxels 1mm in each direction acquired with the parameters TE = 2.4 ms, TR = 12.2 ms. The images were acquired with the SENSE parallel imaging technique (T1 W/3D/TFE) from Phillips on a 3 Tesla scanner. The images were registered utilizing the Adaptive Bases Algorithm (ABA) [15], which uses Normalized Mutual Information (NMI) [16] as its similarity measure. Briefly, ABA computes a deformation field that is modeled as a linear combination of radial basis functions with finite support. This results in a transformation with thousands of degrees of freedom. Two transformations (one from the atlas to the subject and the other from the subject to the atlas) are computed simultaneously and constrained to be inverses of each other. When calculating a circuit, $T_{AB}(T_{BC}(T_{CA}(\mathbf{X})))$, the deformation fields are interpolated using tri-linear interpolation.

3   Experiments

In this work we perform three experiments. In the first experiment we simulate error and apply AQUIRC to estimate this error. We compare the estimated error and the known simulated error visually and statistically. In the second experiment, we add simulated error to a non-rigid registration between two randomly chosen images. We then apply AQUIRC to estimate the error. Finally we estimate the error in a non-rigid registration between two images without adding any simulated error. For all experiments, 5 separate images are pair-wise non-rigidly registered to each other. We visually show AQUIRC 's overall magnitude estimation of error for each experiment. We do not show the estimation of directional error due to space considerations. In general, the quality of the results for the magnitude error estimation are representative of the results for the directional error.

3.1   Experiment 1

In the first experiment, we create a simulated image which is a deformed copy of an image from our data set. We call the original image I_1 and the deformed image I_{1d}. The simulated image is deformed using a radially symmetric growth model. There are three sizes of deformations that are utilized in the growth model in three different locations in the image. The largest deformation in the center of the image has a radius of 30mm with a maximum displacement of 8mm, the moderately sized deformation has a radius of 15mm with a maximum displacement of 5mm, and the smallest deformation has a radius of 10mm with a maximum displacement of 3mm. The simulated image and the growth model can be seen in Figure 2. The transformation between the simulated image and the image it was copied from is defined to be the identity transformation. This simulates a case in which the two images are mis-registered by the growth added to the deformed image. The other images in our data set are then non-rigidly registered to the simulated image, creating a network of 6 images as illustrated in Figure 3. AQUIRC is then applied, calculating a voxel-level error estimation of the simulated error. We calculate the correlation between the growth model and the error estimation and show a scatter plot of the values.

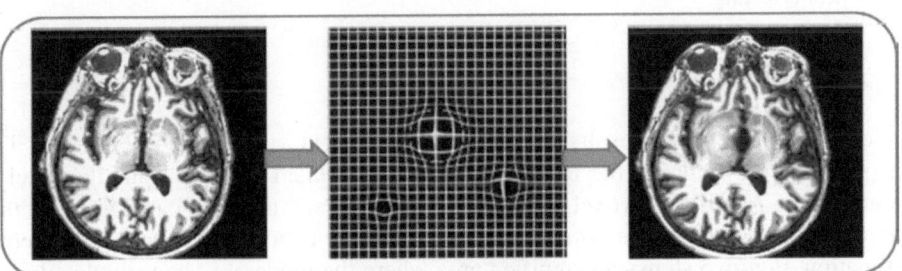

Fig. 2. Left: Original image. Middle: Grid deformed by the simulated growth model. Right: Simulated image

3.2   Experiment 2

In the second experiment, two images are chosen, which we call images I_1 and I_2. The images I_1 and I_2 are non-rigidly registered to each other. Then I_1 is deformed utilizing the same growth model that was used in Experiment 1, resulting in I_{1d}. The non-rigid registration between I_1 and I_2 is used for the transformation between I_{1d} and I_2, but the other images within the data set are re-registrered to I_{1d} as can be seen in Figure 3. This simulates a case in which the growth model adds a known mis-registration to an unknown base mis-registration. AQUIRC is run and we compare the voxel-wise error that the algorithm detects with the simulated error. Because we do no know the base mis-registration, we present qualitative and visual results for this experiment.

3.3   Experiment 3

In the third experiment, we run AQUIRC across the reference set images. We consider the images, I_1 and I_2, and the error in the registration between them is estimated. This is illustrated in the right panel of Figure 3. Through this experiment we investigate the ability of AQUIRC to localize mis-registration errors in practical situations.

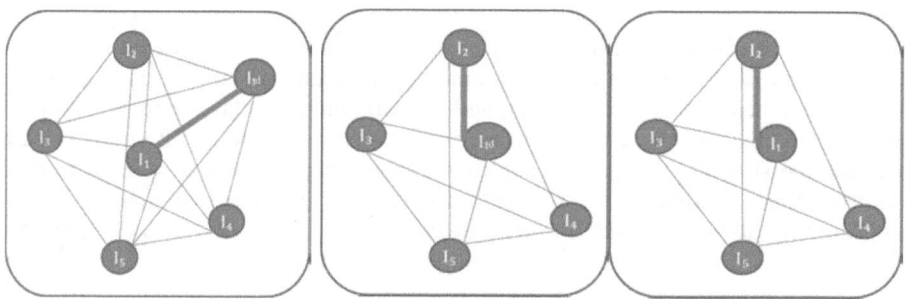

Fig. 3. Diagram illustrating the 3 experiments performed. Left: Experiment 1, Middle: Experiment 2, Right: Experiment 3. The larger link represents the registration that each experiment is testing.

4   Results

An example slice of the results obtained in Experiment 1 is shown in Figure 4. The left panel of the figure is the magnitude of the simulated error, the middle panel is magnitude of AQUIRC 's voxel-wise error estimation and the right panel is a grid that has been deformed by the simulated growth model overlayed on top of the error estimation. Figure 5 shows a magnified area where the moderate sized simulated error was added, alongside the original image and the deformed image. We also calculated the correlation between the magnitude of AQUIRC's error estimation and the magnitude of the simulated growth that was added to the image, and find a strong correlation with an $r = 0.7008$ that is statistically significant with a $p < 0.001$.

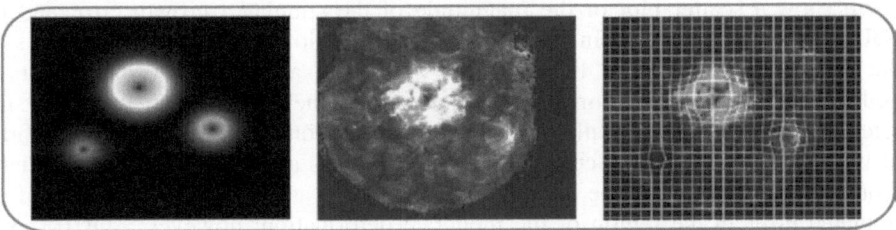

Fig. 4. Left: magnitude of the growth model. Middle: Error estimation. Right: overlay of the error estimation onto a grid that has been deformed by the growth model.

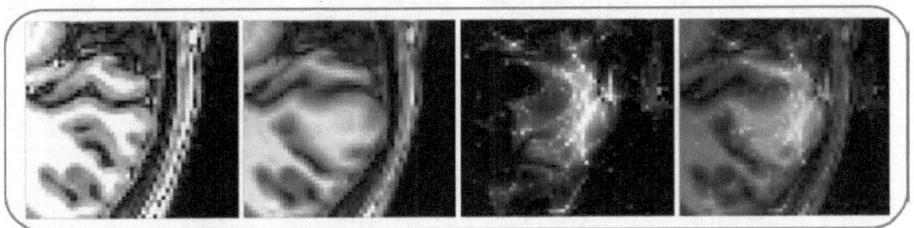

Fig. 5. Left: the original image. Middle Left: region of moderate deformation. Middle Right: Error estimation. Right: overlay of the error estimation onto the deformed image.

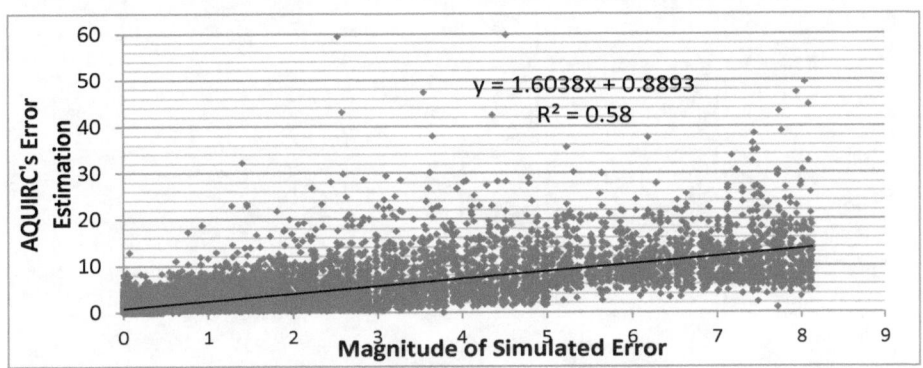

$$y = 1.6038x + 0.8893$$
$$R^2 = 0.58$$

Fig. 6. Scatter plot comparing the estimation of error to the magnitude of the simulated deformation field. Voxels within the head and in one transverse slice were included.

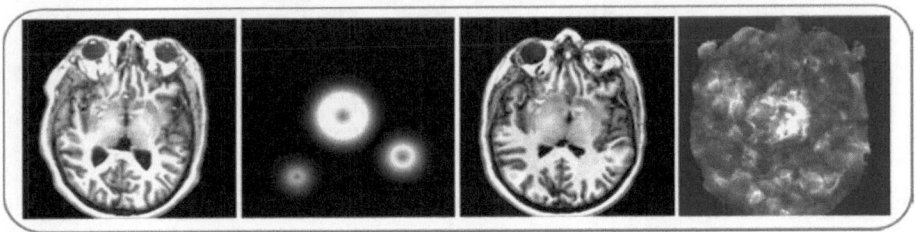

Fig. 7. Left: I_2 registered to I_1. Middle Left: magnitude of the growth model. Middle Right: I_{1d}. Right: Error estimation of the registration between I_{1d} and I_2.

We show a scatter plot of the magnitude of the simulated growth error and the AQUIRC's error estimation in Figure 6. The scatter plot utilizes data from one slice (the slice shown in Figure 4) since otherwise there are too many data points to produce a useful visualization of the results (note, the r-correlation from the slice differs slightly than the overall correlation). We only consider voxels within the brain for both the scatter plot and correlation. AQUIRC was able to identify the simulated error well in the region of the large deformation and was able to identify some of the simulated error in the region of the moderate deformation; however, AQUIRC was unable to identify the simulated error in the region of the small deformation.

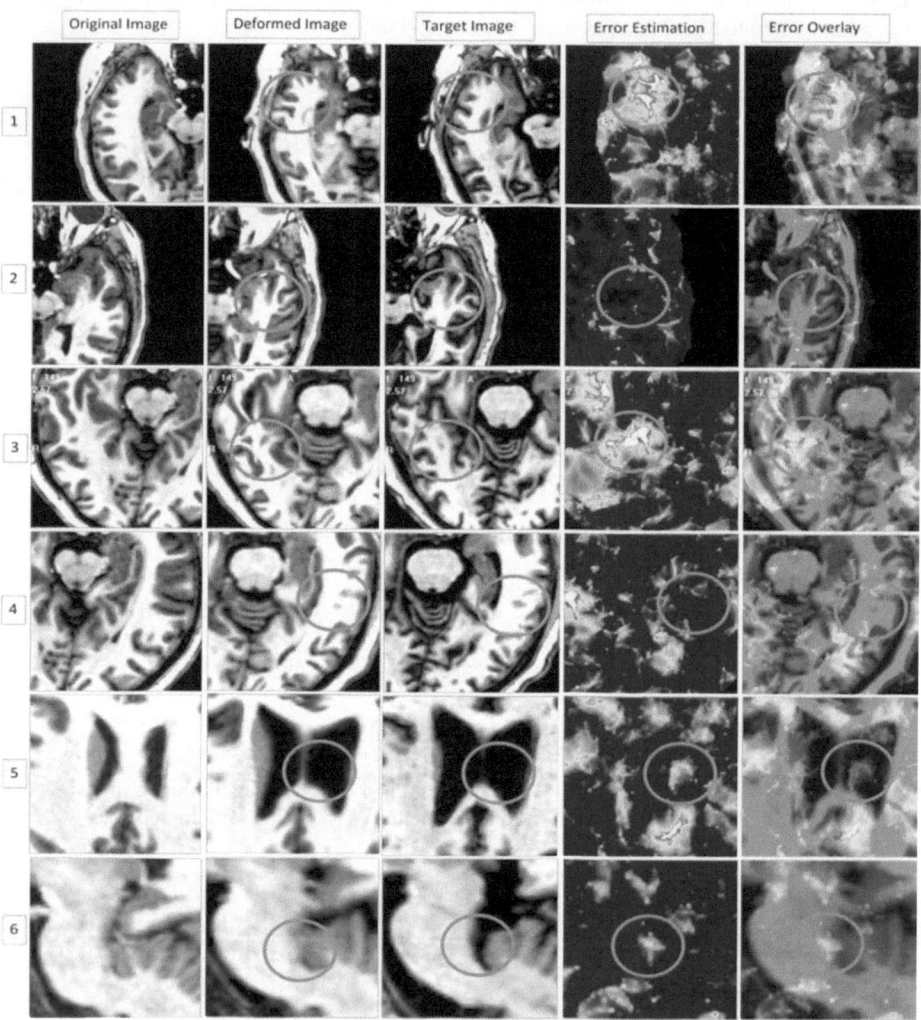

Fig. 8. Row 1-5 shows the transverse plane and row 6 shows the sagittal plane. From left to right the column rows are the original image, the original image registered to the target, the target image, estimation of the error, and error overlayed on top of the original image registered to the target image. Areas of interest are highlighed with an orange circle.

The results from Experiment 2 are show in Figure 7. The image on the left is I_2 registered to I_1, the left middle image is the magnitude of the growth model, the image in the middle right is the image I_{1d}, and on the right is the final error estimation of the registration between I_{1d} and I_2. As can be seen in Figure 7, the added simulation error is apparent in the center of AQUIRC's error estimation figure, although it is difficult to identify the medium and small growth deformations from the background registration error estimation.

The results from Experiment 3 are shown in Figure 8. In the very left column of Figure 8 we show the original image, followed by the original image registered to the target, followed by the target image, followed by AQUIRC's estimation of the error and finally the error overlayed on top of the original image registered to the target image. In rows 1-5 we show the results in the transverse plane and row 6 shows the results in the sagittal plane. We found that most of the highest registration error levels were found in the sulci of the brain, which is logical since there is a high level of inter-patient variability in sulci regions. In rows 1 and 2 we show the left and right side of the head in the same image slice. AQUIRC estimates a high amount of registration error for the left side of the head, and a small amount of error for the other. Rows 3 and 4 also show the left and right side of the same image slice, and we again find a high estimated error on the left side compared to a small amount of estimated error on the right side. Qualitatively, it appears that regions with low estimated error are better registered than the regions of high estimated error. In row 5 we show a region in the CSF where the registration appears correct, but that AQUIRC identifies as having some registration error. A potential cause for this is that in the CSF region there is no contrast to direct the registration, and without a consistent possible correspondence, AQUIRC may mis-identify error. In row 6 of Figure 8 we see an example in the brainstem where visually we can identify a clear registration error that AQUIRC is also able to identify as being a registration error.

5   Discussion and Future Work

We have presented an algorithm to estimate voxel-wise registration error. In Experiment 1 AQUIRC is able to identify simulated errors, with a high correlation ($r = 0.7008$) between the estimated and actual error. In Experiment 2, AQUIRC is able to identify the large registration error that has been added to the center of an inter-patient registration. However, it is not obvious whether or not AQUIRC is able to identify the moderate and small simulated deformations. In Experiment 3, AQUIRC has identified areas that are visually mis-registered, but the results in this instance are qualitative because the ground truth is unknown.

Our results suggest that AQUIRC is able to identify regions of simulated error better when the growth model affects regions with contrast. This can be seen in Figure 5 in the region of moderate growth where the simulated error affects a region with contrast as well as a homogeneous region. AQUIRC is not able to identify the simulated growth in the homogeneous region but is able to identify the simulated growth in the area with contrast. When the growth region is larger and contains homogeneous regions as well as regions with contrast, AQUIRC is able to identify error in both types of regions.

We are continuing to explore the sensitivity of our technique to a variety of parameters and situations. We are currently extending the method to voxel-level atlas selection and are testing AQUIRC using a larger number of images and with various error combination metrics.

Acknowledgments. This work was partially supported by NSF grant DMS-0334769 and by NIH Grant No. R01EB006193 from the National Institute of Biomedical Imaging and Bioengineering.

References

1. Crum, W.L., Hill, D.L.G., Hawkes, D.J.: Zen and the art of medical image registration: correspondence, homology, and quality. Neuroimage 20(3), 1425–1437 (2003)
2. West, J., et al.: Comparison and evaluation of retrospective intermodality brain image registration techniques. Journal of Computer Assisted Tomography 21, 554–566 (1997)
3. Rohlfing, T.: Image Similarity and Tissue Overlaps as Surrogates for Image Registration Accuracy: Widely Used but Unreliable. IEEE Transactions on Medical Imaging 99 (2011)
4. Fitzpatrick, J.M., West, J.B., Maurer Jr., C.R.: Predicting error in rigid-body point-based registration. IEEE Transactions on Medical Imaging 17, 694–702 (1998)
5. Fitzpatrick, J.M., West, J.B.: The distribution of target registration error in rigid-body point-based registration. IEEE Transactions on Medical Imaging 20, 917–927 (2001)
6. Möller, B., Garcia, R., Posch, S.: Towards Objective Quality Assessment of Image Registration Results. In: Proceedings of Int. Conf. on Computer Vision Theory and Applications (VISAPP), Barcelona, Spain, pp. 233–240 (2007)
7. Simonson, K.M., Drescher, S.M., Tanner, F.R.: A Statistics-Based Approach to Binary Image Registration with Uncertainty Analysis. IEEE Transactions on Pattern Analysis and Machine Intelligence 29, 112–125 (2007)
8. Simpson, I., Woolrich, M., Schnabel, J.: Probabilistic segmentation propagation. Medical Image Understanding and Analysis (2011)
9. Datteri, R.D., Dawant, B.M.: Estimation of Rigid-Body Registration Quality Using Registration Networks. In: Proc. SPIE, Medical Imaging 2011: Image Processing (2011)
10. Datteri, R.D., Asman, A.J., Landman, B.A., Dawant, B.M.: Estimation of Registration Quality Applied to Multi-Atlas Segmentation. In: MICCAI (2011)
11. Woods, R.P., Grafton, S.T., Holmes, C.J., Cherry, S.R., Mazziotta, J.C.: Automated image registration: I. General methods and intrasubject, intramodality validation. J. Comput. Assist. Tomogr. 22, 139–152 (1998)
12. Holden, M., Hill, D.L.G., Denton, E.R.E., Jarosz, J.M., Cox, T.C.S., Rohlfing, T., Goodey, J., Hawkes, D.J.: Voxel similarity measures for 3D serial MR brain image registration. IEEE Transactions on Medical Imaging 19, 94–102 (2000)
13. Fitzpatrick, J.M.: Detecting failure, assessing success. In: Hajnal, J.V., Hill, D.L.G., Hawkes, D.J. (eds.) Medical Image Registration, pp. 117–139. CRC Press, Baton Rouge (2001)
14. Christensen, G.E.: Transitivity ErrorNon-Rigid Image Registration Evaluation Project (NIREP) (2006), http://www.nirep.org/te
15. Rohde, G.K., Aldroubi, A., Dawant, B.M.: The adaptive bases algorithm for intensity-based nonrigid image registration. IEEE Trans. On Medical Imaging 22(11), 1470–1479 (2003)
16. Studholme, C., Hill, D.L.G., Hawkes, D.J.: An overlap invariant entropy measure of 3D medical image alignment. Pattern Recognition 32(1), 71–86 (1999)

Diffeomorphic Directly Manipulated Free-Form Deformation Image Registration via Vector Field Flows

Nicholas J. Tustison[1] and Brian B. Avants[2]

[1] University of Virginia, Charlottesville VA 22903, USA
ntustison@virginia.edu
[2] University of Pennsylvania, Philadelphia PA 18104,USA
avants@picsl.upenn.edu

Abstract. Motivated by previous work [16] and recent diffeomorphic image registration developments in which the characteristic velocity field is represented by spatiotemporal B-splines [3], we present a diffeomorphic B-spline-based image registration algorithm combining and extending these techniques. The advancements of the proposed framework over previous work include a preconditioned gradient descent algorithm and potential weighting of the metric gradient permitting, among other things, enforcement of stationary boundary conditions. In addition to theoretical and practical discussions of our contribution, we also describe its parallelized implementation as open source in the Insight Toolkit and perform an evaluation on publicly available brain data.

Keywords: B-splines, DMFFD, diffeomorphisms, image registration, ITK.

1 Introduction

Significant algorithmic developments characterizing modern intensity-based image registration research include the B-spline parameterized approach (so called *free-form deformation*) with early contributions including [10,11,7]. Amongst the variant extensions, the *directly manipulated free-form deformation* approach [16] addressed the hemstitching issue associated with steepest descent traversal of problematic energy topographies during the course of optimization.

Other important image registration research reflected increased emphasis on topological transformation considerations in modeling biological/physical systems where topology is consistent throughout the course of deformation or a homeomorphic relationship is assumed between image domains. Methods such as LDDMM [2] optimize time-varying velocity field flows to yield diffeomorphic transformations. Alternatively, the FFD variant reported in [8] enforced diffeomorphic transforms by concatenating multiple FFD transforms, each of which is constrained to describe a one-to-one mapping. Another FFD registration incorporated the recent log-Euclidean framework for enforcing diffeomorphic

B.M. Dawant et al. (Eds.): WBIR 2012, LNCS 7359, pp. 31–39, 2012.
© Springer-Verlag Berlin Heidelberg 2012

transformations [5]. Recently, the work of [3] combined these registration concepts into a single framework called *temporal free-form deformation* in which the time-varying velocity field characteristic of LDDMM-style algorithms is modeled using a 4-D B-spline object (3-D + time). Integration of the velocity field yields the mapping between parameterized time points.

In this work, we describe our extension to these methods. Similar to [3], we also use an N-D + time B-spline object to represent the characteristic velocity field. However, we use the directly manipulated free-form deformation optimization formulation to improve convergence during the course of optimization. This also facilitates modeling temporal periodicity and the enforcement of stationary boundaries consistent with diffeomorphic transforms. We also incorporate B-spline mesh multi-resolution capabilities for increased control during registration progression. Most importantly, we also describe the parallelized algorithmic implementation as open source available through the Insight Toolkit.[1]

We first describe the methodology by laying out a mathematical description of the various algorithmic elements coupled with implementation details where appropriate. This is followed by an evaluation on publicly available brain data.

2   Methods: Formulae and Implementation

In this section, we explain the underlying theory focusing on differences with previous work. We first explain how B-spline velocity fields can be used to produce diffeomorphisms through numerical integration involving the B-spline basis functions. We then show how our previous work involving optimization in B-spline vector spaces [16] can be used for optimization of diffeomorphisms. Additional insight is then gleaned by illustrating correspondence between theory and implementation.

2.1   B-Spline Velocity Field Transform

Briefly, as with other diffeomorphic formulations based on vector flows, we assume the diffeomorphism, ϕ, is defined on the image domain, Ω, with stationary boundaries such that $\phi(\partial\Omega) = \mathbf{Id}$. ϕ is generated as the solution of the ordinary differential equation

$$\frac{d\phi(\mathbf{x}, t)}{dt} = v(\phi(\mathbf{x}, t), t), \ \ \phi(\mathbf{x}, 0) = \mathbf{x} \tag{1}$$

where v is a (potentially) time-dependent smooth field, $v : \Omega \times t \to \mathrm{R}^d$ parameterized by $t \in [0, 1]$. Diffeomorphic mappings between parameterized time points $\{t_a, t_b\} \in [0, 1]$ are obtained from Eq. (1) through integration of the transport equation, viz.

$$\phi(\mathbf{x}, t_b) = \phi(\mathbf{x}, t_a) + \int_{t_a}^{t_b} v(\phi(\mathbf{x}), t)dt. \tag{2}$$

---

[1] http://www.itk.org/

In the case of d-dimensional registration, we can represent the time-dependent velocity field as a $(d+1)$-dimensional B-spline object

$$v(\mathbf{x}, t) = \sum_{i_1=1}^{X_1} \cdots \sum_{i_d=1}^{X_d} \sum_{i_t=1}^{T} v_{i_1,\ldots,i_d,i_t} B_{i_t}(t) \prod_{j=1}^{d} B_{i_j}(x_j) \tag{3}$$

where $v_{i_1,\ldots,i_d,i_t}$ is a $(d+1)$-dimensional control point lattice characterizing the velocity field and $B(\cdot)$ are the univariate B-spline basis functions separately modulating the solution in each parametric dimension.

Although various methods exist for solving Eqns. (1) and (2), we use 4th-order Runge-Kutta, i.e.

$$\phi_{n+1} = \phi_n + \frac{1}{6}\left(k_1 + 2k_2 + 2k_3 + k_4\right) \tag{4}$$

$$t_{n+1} = t_n + \Delta t \tag{5}$$

$$\phi_0 = \phi(t_0) \tag{6}$$

where

$$k_1 = v\left(\phi_n, t_n\right) \Delta t \tag{7}$$

$$k_2 = v\left(\phi_n + \frac{k_1}{2}, t_n + \frac{\Delta t}{2}\right) \Delta t \tag{8}$$

$$k_3 = v\left(\phi_n + \frac{k_2}{2}, t_n + \frac{\Delta t}{2}\right) \Delta t \tag{9}$$

$$k_4 = v\left(\phi_n + k_3, t_n + \Delta t\right) \Delta t \tag{10}$$

which provides a more stable and reliable alternative than other numerical methods [6].

2.2 Directly Manipulated Free-Form Deformation Optimization of the B-Spline Velocity Field

In [16] it was observed that optimization of FFD registration with gradient descent is intrinsically susceptible to problematic energy topographies. However, a well-understood preconditioned gradient was proposed based on the work described in [14] which we denote as directly manipulated free-form deformation (DMFFD) image registration. This alternative demonstrates improved performance over the steepest descent equivalent [16].

Similarly, for the time-varying velocity field case we propose the following preconditioned gradient, $\delta v_{i_1,\ldots,i_d,i_t}$, given the similarity metric, Π,[2]

---

[2] Current options include neighborhood cross correlation (CC), mutual information (MI), and sum of squared differences (SSD).

$$\delta v_{i_1,\dots,i_d,i_t} = \left(\sum_{c=1}^{N_\Omega \times N_t} \left(\frac{\partial \Pi}{\partial \mathbf{x}} \right)_c B_{i_t}(t^c) \prod_{j=1}^{d} B_{i_j}(x_j^c) \right.$$

$$\cdot \left. \frac{B_{i_t}^2(t^c) \prod_{j=1}^{d} B_{i_j}^2(x_j^c)}{\sum_{k_1=1}^{r+1} \cdots \sum_{k_d=1}^{r+1} \sum_{k_t=1}^{r+1} B_{k_t}^2(t^c) \prod_{j=1}^{d} B_{k_j}^2(x_j^c)} \right)$$

$$\cdot \left(\sum_{c=1}^{N_\Omega \times N_t} B_{i_t}^2(t^c) \prod_{j=1}^{d} B_{i_j}^2(x_j^c) \right)^{-1} \tag{11}$$

which is a slight modification of Eqn. (21) in [16] which takes into account the temporal locations of the dense gradient field sampled in $t \in [0,1]$. N_t and N_Ω are the number of time point samples and the number of voxels in the reference image domain, respectively. r is the spline order in all dimensions[3] and c indexes the spatio-temporal dense metric gradient sample.

Additionally, in [14] it was shown that one could associate each metric gradient sample, $\left(\frac{\partial \Pi}{\partial \mathbf{x}} \right)_c$ with a confidence weighting. Thus, in order to enforce stationary boundaries, we assign image boundary metric gradients a value of zero with a corresponding large confidence value.

2.3 Implementation

As mentioned previously, the registration algorithm has been implemented and introduced into the Insight Toolkit and consists of the following major classes:

- `itk::TimeVaryingVelocityFieldIntegrationImageFilter` — Implementation of the Runge-Kutta integration. Given a sampled velocity field derived from the control point lattice as input and the lower and upper integration limits, integration is performed in a multi-threaded fashion (since each point in the domain can be integrated separately).
- `itk::TimeVaryingBSplineVelocityFieldTransform`: Handles the mapping of geometric primitives using the transform described in this work. It is defined by the velocity field control point lattice which is sampled prior to being integrated to yield the resulting displacement field.
- `itk::TimeVaryingBSplineVelocityFieldImageRegistrationMethod`: Coordinates the optimization using gradient descent given an user-specified number of resolution levels, shrink factors, and smoothing choices.
- `itk::TimeVaryingBSplineVelocityFieldTransformParametersAdaptor`: Handles the decomposition of the B-spline mesh resolution during the multi-resolution optimization given a user-specified scheduling.
- `itk::BSplineScatteredDataPointSetToImageFilter`: Calculates the similarity metric gradient (cf. Eqn. 11) which takes as input the dense similarity metric gradient and an optional weighting for each gradient sample. As described earlier, this permits enforcement of stationary physical boundaries.

---

[3] In terms of implementation spline orders can be specified separately for each dimension but, for simplicity, we only specify a single spline order.

Access to the new ITK registration framework (including the B-spline velocity field transform) is facilitated via the command line module antsRegistration available both in ANTs[4] and accompanied by a technical report offered through the Insight Journal [12].[5]

3   LPBA40 Evaluation

As a preliminary evaluation for our algorithm we used a portion of the approach of Klein et al. [4] in which various open brain data sets were used to evaluate different segmentation algorithms. Specifically, we used the first 20 subjects of the LPBA40 data set [9][6] publicly available from the Laboratory of Neuro Imaging at the University of California, Los Angeles. Preprocessing included brain extraction using the provided masks and N4 bias correction [15].

A portion of the batch script used to produce the registrations is found in Listing 1.1. Each image was histogram- matched prior to application of an initial affine transform using the Demons metric. The resulting transform was composed with the proposed work using a neighborhood cross correlation similarity metric [1] of radius = 4. A multi-resolution strategy was employed where the initial B-spline velocity field mesh size was $24 \times 24 \times 12 \times 1$ which was doubled at each level. Other registration parameters can be gleaned from the Listing 1.1. Batch

```
# Register the n4 corrected moving LPBA subject to the
# n4 corrected fixed LPBA subject.

antsRegistration --dimensionality 3 \
                 --output ${prefix} \
                 --use-histogram-matching 1 \
                 --transform Affine[0.5] \                    # affine stage
                 --metric Demons[${fixed_n4},${moving_n4},1,0,Regular,0.01] \
                 --iterations 100x100x100 \
                 --smoothing-sigmas 4.0x3.0x2.0 \
                 --shrink-factors 4x3x2 \
                 --transform tvdmffd[0.75,24x24x12x1,4] \ # tv dmffd stage
                 --metric CC[${fixed_n4},${moving_n4},1,4] \
                 --iterations 40x50x2 \
                 --smoothing-sigmas 1.0x0.5x0.0 \
                 --shrink-factors 3x2x1

# Apply the resulting transforms (affine + tvdmffd) to the
# moving labels.

antsApplyTransforms --dimensionality 3 \
                    --input ${moving_labels} \
                    --reference-image ${fixed_n4} \
                    --output ${moving_warped_labels} \
                    --n NearestNeighbor \
                    --transform ${prefix}1Warp.nii.gz \
                    --transform ${prefix}0Affine.mat \
                    --default-value 0
```

Listing 1.1. Representative script used for the LPBA40 evaluation

---

[4] http://www.picsl.upenn.edu/ANTs
[5] http://hdl.handle.net/10380/3334
[6] http://www.loni.ucla.edu/Atlases/LPBA40

processing was performed on the linux cluster at the University of Virginia with allocation of 4 nodes for each job multi-threading purposes. Each registration took approximately 3 hours.

Registration assessment used the average target overlap [13] for each of the 56 LPBA40 labeled regions. The numerical values of this assessment are given in Table 1. These values were projected onto LBPA40 Subject 1 for display in Fig. 1 which can be compared to a similar display given in [4] with the caveat that the colormap is slightly different.

Table 1. Average target overlap values for cross-registration of the first 20 subjects of the LPBA40 data set. A visual depiction of these values is given in Figure 1.

Region	Overlap	Region	Overlap
L superior frontal gyrus	0.802	L inferior occipital gyrus	0.621
R superior frontal gyrus	0.810	R inferior occipital gyrus	0.637
L middle frontal gyrus	0.790	L cuneus	0.622
R middle frontal gyrus	0.778	R cuneus	0.624
L inferior frontal gyrus	0.753	L superior temporal gyrus	0.750
R inferior frontal gyrus	0.728	R superior temporal gyrus	0.737
L precentral gyrus	0.687	L middle temporal gyrus	0.660
R precentral gyrus	0.674	R middle temporal gyrus	0.644
L middle orbitofrontal gyrus	0.687	L inferior temporal gyrus	0.662
R middle orbitofrontal gyrus	0.671	R inferior temporal gyrus	0.674
L lateral orbitofrontal gyrus	0.669	L parahippocampal gyrus	0.711
R lateral orbitofrontal gyrus	0.607	R parahippocampal gyrus	0.707
L gyrus rectus	0.654	L lingual gyrus	0.694
R gyrus rectus	0.652	R lingual gyrus	0.681
L postcentral gyrus	0.604	L fusiform gyrus	0.703
R postcentral gyrus	0.620	R fusiform gyrus	0.719
L superior parietal gyrus	0.709	L insular cortex	0.812
R superior parietal gyrus	0.701	R insular cortex	0.768
L supramarginal gyrus	0.619	L cingulate gyrus	0.691
R supramarginal gyrus	0.623	R cingulate gyrus	0.676
L angular gyrus	0.594	L caudate	0.704
R angular gyrus	0.620	R caudate	0.717
L precuneus	0.668	L putamen	0.773
R precuneus	0.659	R putamen	0.761
L superior occipital gyrus	0.548	L hippocampus	0.753
R superior occipital gyrus	0.561	R hippocampus	0.742
L middle occipital gyrus	0.671	cerebellum	0.935
R middle occipital gyrus	0.696	brainstem	0.899

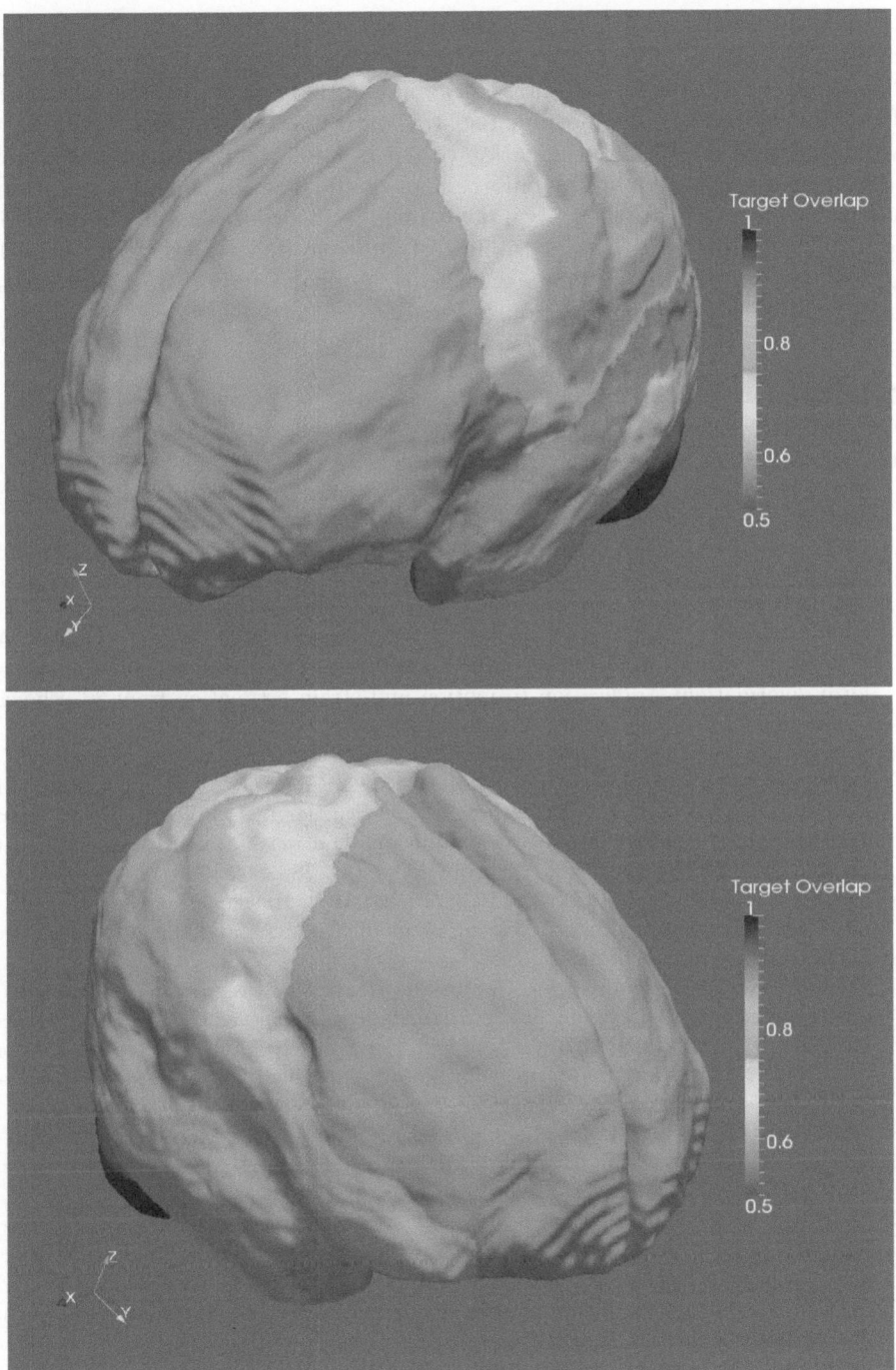

Fig. 1. Average regional total overlap measures mapped onto Subject 1 of the LPBA40 data set

4   Discussion and Conclusions

This work constitutes an advantageous combination of the continuous aspects of B-splines with the diffeomorphic registration framework via vector field flows. We incorporate DMFFD optimization of the B-spline velocity field which facilitates convergence and permits enforcement of stationary boundary conditions. While not discussed, further advantages include incorporation of temporal periodicity in dealing with the possibility of multiple images describing periodic motion (e.g. cardiac or pulmonary motion). A future publication will explore these possibilities in greater detail.

References

1. Avants, B.B., Epstein, C.L., Grossman, M., Gee, J.C.: Symmetric diffeomorphic image registration with cross-correlation: evaluating automated labeling of elderly and neurodegenerative brain. Med. Image Anal. 12(1), 26–41 (2008)
2. Beg, M.F., Miller, M.I., Trouvé, A., Younes, L.: Computing large deformation metric mappings via geodesic flows of diffeomorphisms. Int. J. Comput. Vision 61, 139–157 (2005), http://dl.acm.org/citation.cfm?id=1026574.1026580
3. De Craene, M., Piella, G., Camara, O., Duchateau, N., Silva, E., Doltra, A., D'hooge, J., Brugada, J., Sitges, M., Frangi, A.F.: Temporal diffeomorphic free-form deformation: Application to motion and strain estimation from 3d echocardiography. Med. Image Anal. (November 2011)
4. Klein, A., Andersson, J., Ardekani, B.A., Ashburner, J., Avants, B., Chiang, M.C., Christensen, G.E., Collins, D.L., Gee, J., Hellier, P., Song, J.H., Jenkinson, M., Lepage, C., Rueckert, D., Thompson, P., Vercauteren, T., Woods, R.P., Mann, J.J., Parsey, R.V.: Evaluation of 14 nonlinear deformation algorithms applied to human brain MRI registration. Neuroimage 46(3), 786–802 (2009)
5. Modat, M., Ridgway, G.R., Daga, P., Cardoso, M.J., Hawkes, D.J.: Log-Euclidean free-form deformation. In: Progress in Biomedical Optics and Imaging - Proceedings of SPIE, vol. 7962 (2011)
6. Press, W.H.: Numerical recipes. Cambridge University Press, code cd-rom v 2.06 edn. (1996), http://www.loc.gov/catdir/description/cam0210/99382414.html
7. Rueckert, D., Sonoda, L.I., Hayes, C., Hill, D.L., Leach, M.O., Hawkes, D.J.: Non-rigid registration using free-form deformations: application to breast MR images. IEEE Trans. Med. Imaging 18(8), 712–721 (1999)
8. Rueckert, D., Aljabar, P., Heckemann, R.A., Hajnal, J.V., Hammers, A.: Diffeomorphic registration using B-splines. Med. Image Comput Comput. Assist. Interv. 9(pt. 2), 702–709 (2006)
9. Shattuck, D.W., Mirza, M., Adisetiyo, V., Hojatkashani, C., Salamon, G., Narr, K.L., Poldrack, R.A., Bilder, R.M., Toga, A.W.: Construction of a 3D probabilistic atlas of human cortical structures. Neuroimage 39(3), 1064–1080 (2008)
10. Szeliski, R., Coughlan, J.: Spline-based image registration. International Journal of Computer Vision 22, 199–218 (1997), http://dx.doi.org/10.1023/A:1007996332012, doi:10.1023/A:1007996332012
11. Thévenaz, P., Ruttimann, U.E., Unser, M.: A pyramid approach to subpixel registration based on intensity. IEEE Trans.Image Process 7(1), 27–41 (1998)
12. Tustison, N.J., Avants, B.B.: The TVDMFFDVR algorithm. Insight Journal (2012)

13. Tustison, N.J., Gee, J.C.: Introducing Dice, Jaccard, and other label overlap measures to ITK. Insight Journal (2009)
14. Tustison, N.J., Gee, J.C.: Generalized n-D C^k B-Spline Scattered Data Approximation with Confidence Values. In: Yang, G.-Z., Jiang, T., Shen, D., Gu, L., Yang, J. (eds.) MIAR 2006. LNCS, vol. 4091, pp. 76–83. Springer, Heidelberg (2006)
15. Tustison, N.J., Avants, B.B., Cook, P.A., Zheng, Y., Egan, A., Yushkevich, P.A., Gee, J.C.: N4ITK: improved N3 bias correction. IEEE Trans. Med. Imaging 29(6), 1310–1320 (2010)
16. Tustison, N.J., Avants, B.B., Gee, J.C.: Directly manipulated free-form deformation image registration. IEEE Trans. Image Process 18(3), 624–635 (2009)

Multi-modal Image Registration Using Polynomial Expansion and Mutual Information

Daniel Forsberg[1,2,3], Gunnar Farnebäck[1],
Hans Knutsson[1,2], and Carl-Fredrik Westin[4]

[1] Department of Biomedical Engineering, Linköping University, Sweden
[2] Center for Medical Image Science and Visualization, Linköping University, Sweden
[3] Sectra Imtec, Linköping, Sweden
[4] Laboratory of Mathematics in Imaging, Brigham and Women's Hospital,
Harvard Medical School, Boston, MA, USA

Abstract. The use of polynomial expansion in image registration has previously been shown to be beneficial due to fast convergence and high accuracy. However, earlier work has only been for mono-modal image registration. In this work, it is shown how polynomial expansion and mutual information can be linked to achieve multi-modal image registration. The proposed method is evaluated using MRI data and shown to have a satisfactory accuracy while not increasing the computation time significantly.

1 Introduction

The use of image registration within the medical image domain is vast and includes various tasks, such as; surgical planning, radiotherapy planning, image-guided surgery, disease progression monitoring and image fusion. Especially image fusion is becoming more and more important in several clinical work-flows, since patients tend to have multiple examinations from different imaging modalities that need to be registered before image fusion is possible. Intensity-based similarity metrics, such as; sum-of-squared-difference or normalized cross-correlation, are often inadequate for handling multi-modal image registration. A frequently applied measure that can handle multi-modal registration is mutual information. Since the introduction of mutual information in image registration by Collignon et al. [1] and by Viola and Wells [10], it has become a well-established similarity metric for multi-modal image registration [8].

Polynomial expansion was introduced by Farnebäck [3] as a method to locally approximate a signal with a polynomial. It was later shown by Farnebäck and Westin [4] how polynomial expansion could be used to perform both linear (e.g. translation and affine) and non-rigid image registration. The idea of image registration using polynomial expansion was further developed by Wang et al. [11]. Both Farnebäck and Westin [4] and Wang et al. [11] showed that image registration using polynomial expansions has some valuable qualities. Firstly, since it is

B.M. Dawant et al. (Eds.): WBIR 2012, LNCS 7359, pp. 40–49, 2012.

based on an analytical solution, the convergence rate is fast, typically only needing a few iterations per scale. Secondly, also the accuracy of the registration has been demonstrated to be on a similar or even better level than some of the algorithms included in ITK. However, thus far, image registration using polynomial expansion has only been applicable for mono-modal image registration.

The contribution of this paper, is to present how mutual information can be integrated into polynomial expansion in order to achieve multi-modal image registration, thus, making image registration based on polynomial expansion feasible for not only mono-modal registration but also for multi-modal image registration.

2   Background

2.1   Polynomial Expansion

The basic idea of polynomial expansion is to locally approximate each signal value with a polynomial. In case of a linear polynomial, this approximation can be expressed as $f(\mathbf{x}) \sim \mathbf{b}^T\mathbf{x} + c$, where the coefficients are determined by a weighted least squares fit to the local signal. The weighting depends on two factors, certainty and applicability. These terms are the same as in normalized convolution [3,6], which forms the basis for polynomial expansion.

2.2   Image Registration Using Polynomial Expansion

Global Translation. Let both the fixed and the moving images be locally approximated with a linear polynomial expansion and assume that the moving image is a globally translated version of the fixed image, thus,

$$I_{\mathrm{f}}(\mathbf{x}) = \mathbf{b}_f^T\mathbf{x} + c_f, \tag{1}$$

$$I_{\mathrm{m}}(\mathbf{x}) = \mathbf{b}_m^T\mathbf{x} + c_m = I_{\mathrm{f}}(\mathbf{x} - \mathbf{d}) = \mathbf{b}_f^T(\mathbf{x} - \mathbf{d}) + c_f, \tag{2}$$

which gives $c_m = c_f - \mathbf{b}_f^T\mathbf{d}$ and hence, the translation $\mathbf{d}$ can be is estimated as

$$\mathbf{d} = (\mathbf{b}_f\mathbf{b}_f^T)^{-1}\mathbf{b}_f(c_f - c_m). \tag{3}$$

In practice, a point-wise polynomial expansion is estimated, i.e. $\mathbf{b}_f(\mathbf{x})$, $c_f(\mathbf{x})$, $\mathbf{b}_m(\mathbf{x})$, and $c_m(\mathbf{x})$. Since it cannot be expected that $\mathbf{b}_f(\mathbf{x}) = \mathbf{b}_m(\mathbf{x})$ holds, they are replaced with the average

$$\mathbf{b}(\mathbf{x}) = \frac{\mathbf{b}_f(\mathbf{x}) + \mathbf{b}_m(\mathbf{x})}{2}. \tag{4}$$

Also, set

$$\Delta c(\mathbf{x}) = c_f(\mathbf{x}) - c_m(\mathbf{x}) \tag{5}$$

and thus, the primary constraint is given by:

$$\mathbf{b}(\mathbf{x})^T\mathbf{d} = \Delta c(\mathbf{x}) \tag{6}$$

To solve (6), compute $\mathbf{d}$ by minimizing the squared error in the constraint over the whole image,

$$\epsilon^2 = \sum_{\mathbf{x}} \|\mathbf{b}(\mathbf{x})\mathbf{d} - \boldsymbol{\Delta}c(\mathbf{x})\|^2. \tag{7}$$

Affine Registration. If a space-variant displacement is assumed, then the previous solution can be extended to handle affine registration. Let $\mathbf{d}(\mathbf{x}) = \mathbf{S}(\mathbf{x})\mathbf{p}$, where

$$\mathbf{S}(\mathbf{x}) = \begin{pmatrix} x\ y\ 0\ 0\ 1\ 0 \\ 0\ 0\ x\ y\ 0\ 1 \end{pmatrix}, \tag{8}$$

$$\mathbf{p} = \begin{pmatrix} a_1\ a_2\ a_3\ a_4\ a_5\ a_6 \end{pmatrix}^T. \tag{9}$$

To estimate the parameters of the affine displacement field, replace $\mathbf{d}$ with $\mathbf{d}(\mathbf{x}) = \mathbf{S}(\mathbf{x})\mathbf{p}$ in (7),

$$\epsilon^2 = \sum_{\mathbf{x}} \|\mathbf{b}(\mathbf{x})^T \mathbf{S}(\mathbf{x})\mathbf{p} - \boldsymbol{\Delta}c(\mathbf{x})\|^2 \tag{10}$$

and the parameters $\mathbf{p}$ are given by the least squares solution of (10).

Non-rigid Registration. A non-rigid registration algorithm can be achieved if the assumption about a global translation is relaxed and we instead sum over a neighborhood around each pixel in (7), thereby obtaining an estimate for each pixel. In this case, a local translation is assumed but it could easily be changed to a local affine transformation as is done by Wang *et al.* [11]. More precisely (7) is changed to

$$\epsilon^2(\mathbf{x}) = \sum_{\mathbf{y}} w(\mathbf{y}) \left(\|\mathbf{b}(\mathbf{x} - \mathbf{y})^T \mathbf{d}(\mathbf{x}) - \boldsymbol{\Delta}c(\mathbf{x} - \mathbf{y})\|^2 \right), \tag{11}$$

where w weights the points in the neighborhood around each pixel. This weight can be any low-pass function, but here it is assumed to be Gaussian. This equation can be interpreted as a convolution of the point-wise contributions to the squared error in (7) with the low-pass filter w. The solution is given as

$$\mathbf{G}(\mathbf{x}) = \mathbf{b}(\mathbf{x})\mathbf{b}(\mathbf{x})^T, \tag{12}$$

$$\mathbf{h}(\mathbf{x}) = \mathbf{b}(\mathbf{x})\boldsymbol{\Delta}c(\mathbf{x}), \tag{13}$$

$$\mathbf{G}_{\text{avg}}(\mathbf{x}) = (\mathbf{G} * w)(\mathbf{x}), \tag{14}$$

$$\mathbf{h}_{\text{avg}}(\mathbf{x}) = (\mathbf{h} * w)(\mathbf{x}), \tag{15}$$

$$\mathbf{d}(\mathbf{x}) = \mathbf{G}_{\text{avg}}(\mathbf{x})^{-1}\mathbf{h}_{\text{avg}}(\mathbf{x}). \tag{16}$$

Note that in this work only a linear polynomial expansion have been used, but as shown in [4,11] a quadratic polynomial expansion along with similar derivations can also be used for image registration. In fact, it is possible to combine both in order to obtain a more robust solution. Further, the described method for non-rigid registration can be extended to handle diffeomorphic deformations by using diffeomorphic field accumulation as described by Forsberg *et al.* [5].

2.3 Mutual Information

Mutual information is typically based on the *Shannon Entropy* and defined as

$$H = \sum_i p_i \log \frac{1}{p_i} = -\sum_i p_i \log p_i, \tag{17}$$

where p_i is the probability that event e_i occurs. Based on the Shannon entropy we can define the mutual information of the random variables A and B as

$$MI(A, B) = H(A) + H(B) - H(A, B), \tag{18}$$

where $H(A, B)$ is the joint entropy of A and B. The Shannon entropy for the joint distribution is given by

$$-\sum_{i,j} p_{i,j} \log p_{i,j}. \tag{19}$$

3 Polynomial Expansion and Mutual Information

3.1 Algorithm Overview

The basic idea of combining polynomial expansion and mutual information lies in replacing $\boldsymbol{\Delta}c(\mathbf{x})$ in (5). The term $\boldsymbol{\Delta}c(\mathbf{x})$ can be interpreted as how much $I_f(\mathbf{x})$ should change in order to match $I_m(\mathbf{x})$ based on intensity-difference. Instead, estimate $\boldsymbol{\Delta}c(\mathbf{x})$ as how much $I_f(\mathbf{x})$ should change in order to match $I_m(\mathbf{x})$ but based on a pixel-wise minimization of the conditional entropy, i.e. a pixel-wise maximization of the mutual information. This is estimated according to the following scheme:

- Estimate the joint distribution $p(I_f, I_m)$ given I_f and I_m.
- For each $\mathbf{x}$:
  - Retrieve the corresponding pixel values $i_f = I_f(\mathbf{x})$ and $i_m = I_m(\mathbf{x} + \mathbf{d})$.
  - Estimate the conditional distribution $p(I_f | I_m = i_m)$.
  - Estimate how the conditional entropy $H(I_f | I_m = i_m)$ is affected by i_f.
  - Find $i^\star$ for which the conditional entropy has a local minimum and estimate $\boldsymbol{\Delta}c(\mathbf{x})$ as $i_f - i^\star$.

Knowing that mutual information can also be defined as

$$MI(A, B) = H(A) - H(A|B), \tag{20}$$

ensures that the last step is reasonable for finding a $\boldsymbol{\Delta}c(\mathbf{x})$ that matches I_f and I_m based on mutual information, since minimizing $H(I_f | I_m)$ will maximize $MI(I_f, I_m)$ in a point-wise manner.

3.2   Channel Coding and Probability Distribution Estimation

A well-known issue with mutual information is how to estimate the needed probability distributions, since the straightforward solution of using a standard histogram is insufficient. A common approach is to use some sort of *soft histograms* where the intensity of each pixel is distributed fractionally over multiple bins. This will give a more stable and often close to continuous result. In this work, channel coding and B-splines have been used to achieve this, which in practice is similar to *kernel density estimation* introduced by Rosenblatt and Parzen to estimate probability density functions [7,9].

The basic concept of channel coding consists of representing a value x by passing it through a set of localized basis functions $\{B\,(x-k)\}_1^K$. The output signal from each basis function is called a channel, thus, the channel representation of x is given by a vector of a set of channel values

$$\varphi(x) = [B\,(x-1)\ B\,(x-2)\ \ldots\ B\,(x-K)]^T. \tag{21}$$

A suitable basis function is the quadratic B-spline function, defined as the unit rectangle convolved with itself two times. A B-spline of degree two, $B_2(x)$, is chosen because it is continuously differentiable and has compact support.

The probability distribution of an image, using K channels, is, thus, estimated as:

1. Map each intensity value $I(\mathbf{x})$ to $[1, K-1]$, $\tilde{I}(\mathbf{x})$.
2. Compute the channel representation of each mapped value $\varphi(\tilde{I}\,(\mathbf{x}))$.
3. Compute the bins h_k of the soft histogram as the element-wise sum of the channel representations.
4. Estimate a probability distribution p_k by normalizing the soft histogram.

The fractional bins of the joint histogram can then be estimated as the sum of the element-wise products of the channel representations over the respective images

$$h_{k,l} = \sum_{\mathbf{x}} \varphi_k\left(\tilde{I}_f\,(\mathbf{x})\right) \varphi_l\left(\tilde{I}_m\,(\mathbf{x+d})\right), \tag{22}$$

which is then normalized to obtain the joint probability distribution, $p_{k,l}$.

3.3   Conditional Entropy

To estimate $\boldsymbol{\Delta}c(\mathbf{x})$ for the corresponding pixel values $i_f = I_f\,(\mathbf{x})$ and $i_m = I_m\,(\mathbf{x+d(x)})$, we start by estimating the conditional probability distribution $p_k\,(I_f|I_m = i_m)$ as

$$p_k\,(I_f|I_m = i_m) = \frac{h_k\,(I_f|I_m = i_m)}{\sum_{k=1}^K h_k\,(I_f|I_m = i_m)} \tag{23}$$

where

$$h_k\,(I_f|I_m = i_m) = \sum_{l=1}^L \varphi_l\left(\tilde{i}_m\right) p_{k,l}\,(I_f, I_m) \quad \text{for} \quad k = 1\ldots K, \tag{24}$$

and where $\tilde{i}_m$ is the mapped i_m value. Here $\varphi_l\left(\tilde{i}_m\right) p_{k,l}\left(I_f, I_m\right)$ acts as a sub-channel interpolation term.

Given the conditional probability distribution $p_k\left(I_f | I_m = i_m\right)$, the conditional entropy is estimated as

$$H\left(I_f | I_m = i_m\right) = -\sum_k p_k\left(I_f | I_m = i_m\right) \log p_k\left(I_f | I_m = i_m\right). \qquad (25)$$

However, in our case we are interested in understanding how i_f affects the conditional entropy. This can be investigated by an infinite small addition of the intensity value i_f to create a new distribution

$$p_k\left(i_f\right) = \frac{p_k\left(I_f | I_m = i_m\right) + \epsilon \times \varphi_k\left(\tilde{i}_f\right)}{1 + \epsilon}, \qquad (26)$$

where ϵ is small. Thus, the modified entropy is given by

$$H\left(i_f\right) = -\sum_k p_k\left(i_f\right) \log p_k\left(i_f\right) = \frac{1}{1+\epsilon}\bigg(H\left(I_f | I_m = i_m\right) -$$

$$\epsilon \sum_k \varphi_k\left(\tilde{i}_f\right)\left(1 + \log p_k\left(I_f | I_m = i_m\right)\right)\bigg) + O\left(\epsilon^2\right). \qquad (27)$$

Differentiating (27) with respect to i_f and omitting $O\left(\epsilon^2\right)$ gives

$$\frac{\partial H\left(i_f\right)}{\partial i_f} = \frac{\epsilon}{1+\epsilon}\bigg(\sum_k \varphi_k\left(\tilde{i}_f\right)\left(1 + \log p_k\left(I_f | I_m = i_m\right)\right)\bigg). \qquad (28)$$

Using the expressions in (27) and in (28), it is straightforward to find a $i^\star$, which minimizes $H\left(i^\star\right)$. This in turn, can be viewed as a pixel-wise minimization of the conditional entropy. The found $i^\star$ is used to estimate $\Delta c(\mathbf{x})$ as

$$\Delta c(\mathbf{x}) = i_f - i^\star. \qquad (29)$$

The term $\Delta c(\mathbf{x})$ can, as previously explained, be interpreted as how much i_f should change in order to match i_m in a mutual information sense, instead of in a intensity-difference sense. The estimated $\Delta c(\mathbf{x})$ can now be used for image registration as previously described in Sect. 2.2, but with the difference that $\mathbf{b}(\mathbf{x}) = \mathbf{b}_f(\mathbf{x})$ instead of as defined in (4).

4   Results

The proposed method was evaluated using both affine and non-rigid image registration as described in Sect. 2.2 and 2.2. For the non-rigid registration, diffeomorphic field accumulation was used for achieving diffeomorphic deformations. For some of the performed experiments, the proposed method was compared with its mono-modal counterpart on mono-modal data. The image data used in the experiments were obtained from BrainWeb [2].

In the first experiment, the proposed multi-modal method was compared with the previously presented mono-modal method using a linear polynomial expansion [4]. A single T1-weighted brain image was used as moving image. From the moving image, 20 fixed images were created using known affine transforms. The affine transforms were obtained according the following schema: the scaling factors within $[0.80, 1.30]$, the rotation factor within $[-\pi/4, \pi/4]$, and the translation factors within $[-15, 15]$. The moving image was then registered to each of the 20 fixed images using affine registration. The obtained affine transforms where then compared with the known transforms, yielding the results in Table 1, comparing the average error for each parameter type. The experiment was run twice, one time where noise was added (Gaussian noise with $\sigma = 200$) and one time without any added noise. Timing the experiment showed that the computation time increased with a mere 40% for adding the computational steps for multi-modal image registration, i.e. from approximately 1.0 seconds to 1.4 seconds.

Table 1. Results (average error and its standard deviation) for comparing accuracy per parameter type (scale, rotation and translation) of affine mono-modal registration with the proposed multi-modal registration on mono-modal data

Transformation factor	Scale	Rotation	Translation
Mono-modal (noise added)	1.0e-5 ± 1.1e-3	-5.8e-4 ± 2.4e-3	2.0e-4 ± 3.2e-2
Mono-modal	-4.1e-6 ± 4.9e-5	1.8e-5 ± 1.4e-4	6.9e-4 ± 3.2e-3
Multi-modal (noise added)	7.4e-4 ± 1.7e-3	-1.0e-3 ± 4.1e-3	1.6e-4 ± 5.3e-2
Multi-modal	-2.9e-5 ± 1.3e-4	-2.1e-6 ± 5.7e-5	6.3e-4 ± 3.3e-3

In the second experiment, the proposed multi-modal method was evaluated in the same manner as in the first experiment but on multi-modal data, i.e. on a T1-weighted image and a T2-weighted image, where the T2-weighted image was transformed according to a set of known affine transforms (in this experiment the rotation factor was limited to $[-\pi/6, \pi/6]$), and without running the mono-modal registration algorithm. The experiment was also executed twice, one time where noise was added and one time without any added noise (Gaussian noise with $\sigma = 200$). The results for this experiment are given in Table 2. Example images from the second experiment are depicted in Fig. 1. In both the experiments for affine registration, the number of scales and iterations per scale were kept constant, five scales and ten iterations per scale.

To evaluate the accuracy for non-rigid registration, a similar setup was used as for affine registration. A single image was deformed using 20 known displacement fields (randomly created and with an average displacement of 5 pixels and maximum displacement of 15 pixels). The original image was then registered to the deformed images and the obtained displacements fields were compared with the known displacement fields using the target registration error (TRE). As before, the experiment was first run on mono-modal data to compare the accuracy of multi-modal registration with mono-modal registration (with and without added

Table 2. Results (average error and its standard deviation) for comparing accuracy per parameter type (scale, rotation and translation) of affine multi-modal registration on multi-modal 2D data

Transformation factor	Scale	Rotation	Translation
With added noise	-4.1e-3 ± 6.8e-3	-5.5e-4 ± 4.3e-3	1.3e-2 ± 4.9e-2
Without added noise	-9.82e-4 ± 2.0e-4	-2.8e-4 ± 4.9e-4	-8.7e-3 ± 9.0e-3

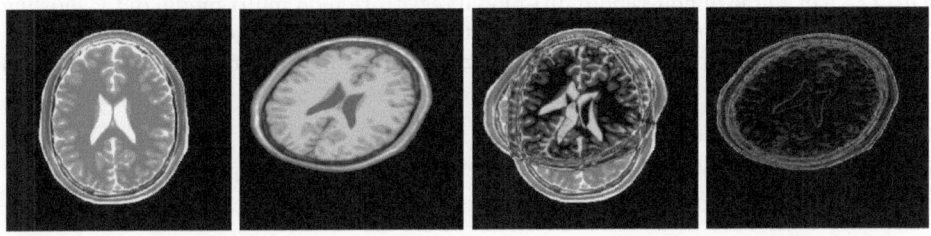

Fig. 1. An example of affine multi-modal registration, showing from left the moving image (T2-weighted), the fixed image (T1-weighted), the absolute difference between fixed and moving, and fixed and deformed for T2-weighted images

noise) and then it was run on multi-modal data (also with and without added noise). Also here Gaussian noise with $\sigma = 200$ was used. The results for this experiment are given in Table 3 and some example images are shown in Fig. 2. Also in this experiment, the number of scales and iterations per scale were kept constant, four scales and ten iterations per scale. Timing the experiment further showed that for non-rigid registration the computation time increased with only 30% for adding the computational steps for multi-modal image registration, i.e. from approximately 3.0 seconds to 3.8 seconds per registration.

Table 3. Average target registration error (TRE) of 20 non-rigid 2D registrations, comparing accuracy of multi-modal registration on mono-modal and multi-modal data with mono-modal registration on mono-modal data, with and without added noise. TRE is given in pixels.

Registration	Mono	Multi	Multi
Data	Mono	Mono	Multi
With added noise	0.59	0.68	1.16
Without added noise	0.35	0.42	0.91

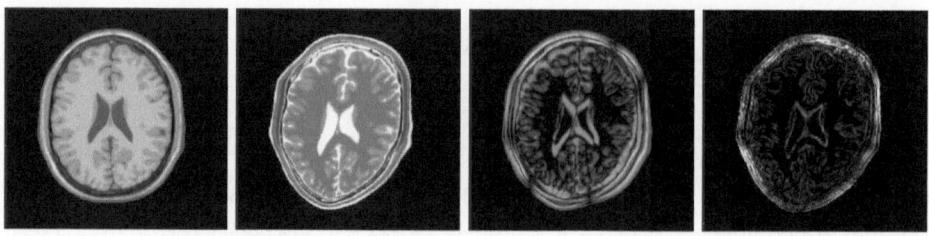

Fig. 2. An example of non-rigid multi-modal registration on multi-modal data, showing from left the moving image (T1-weighted), the fixed image (T2-weighted), the absolute difference image between fixed and moving, and fixed and deformed for T1-weighted images

5   Discussion

In this work, we have presented how polynomial expansion can be utilized for multi-modal image registration (both linear and non-rigid). This is achieved by incorporating a pixel-wise minimization of the conditional entropy, in order to estimate a pixel-wise intensity change that maximizes the mutual information.

The results in Tables 1 and 2 demonstrate the accuracy of the proposed method for multi-modal image registration but also when compared to its mono-modal counterpart in mono-modal image registration. In the case of affine registration of mono-modal image data, both algorithms achieves a descent registration accuracy. The accuracy of the registration decreases with a factor of approximately ten when adding Gaussian noise to the images but is still sufficient. For affine registration of multi-modal data, the accuracy is on a similar level as for registration of mono-modal data, hence sufficient for achieving a good registration. One thing that differed between the multi-modal registration of mono-modal data and multi-modal data was that the capture range for rotations decreased from $[-\pi/4, \pi/4]$ to $[-\pi/6, \pi/6]$ when running the registration on multi-modal data.

In the case of non-rigid registration, see Table 3, the accuracy of mono-modal registration and multi-modal registration of mono-modal data is also on similar levels and achieving sub-pixel accuracy. For non-rigid registration of multi-modal data the accuracy decreased by a factor of two and reached an average TRE of approximately one pixel.

A difference that could be noted between the mono-modal registration and the multi-modal registration was that the multi-modal was more iterative in its nature, i.e. the mono-modal algorithm converged within a few iterations, whereas the multi-modal often required at least twice as many iterations. Hence, the large number of iterations per scale used in the experiments.

Future work includes a more thorough investigation of how the number of channels affect the end result of the registration. In our experiments we only empirically decided how to set the number of channels, typically eight channels for coarse scales and step-wise increasing up to 24 or 32 for the finest scales. For instance, a better use of the number of channels might decrease the TRE further for non-rigid registration and making sub-pixel accuracy also possible for multi-modal registration. Further evaluation and implementation in 3D will also be of interest to better compare with other existing algorithms for multi-modal image registration and on various types of multi-modal data.

Acknowledgment. This work was funded by the Swedish Research Council (grant 2007-4786) and the National Institute of Health (grants R01MH074794, P41RR013218, and R01MH092862).

References

1. Collignon, A., Maes, F., Delaere, D., Vandermeulen, D., Suetens, P., Marchal, G.: Automated multimodality image registration based on information theory. In: XIVth International Conference on Information Processing in Medical Imaging, IPMI 1995, vol. 3, pp. 263–274. Kluwer Academic Publishers (1995)
2. Collins, D., Zijdenbos, A., Kollokian, V., Sled, J., Kabani, N., Holmes, C., Evans, A.: Design and construction of a realistic digital brain phantom. IEEE Transactions on Medical Imaging 17(3), 463–468 (1998)
3. Farnebäck, G.: Polynomial expansion for orientation and motion estimation. Ph.D. thesis, Linköping University, Sweden (2002)
4. Farnebäck, G., Westin, C.-F.: Affine and Deformable Registration Based on Polynomial Expansion. In: Larsen, R., Nielsen, M., Sporring, J. (eds.) MICCAI 2006, Part I. LNCS, vol. 4190, pp. 857–864. Springer, Heidelberg (2006)
5. Forsberg, D., Andersson, M., Knutsson, H.: Non-rigid diffeomorphic image registration of medical images using polynomial expansion (2012), Accepted at the International Conference on Image Analysis and Recognition
6. Knutsson, H., Westin, C.F.: Normalized and differential convolution: Methods for interpolation and filtering of incomplete and uncertain data. In: Proceedings of Computer Vision and Pattern Recognition 1993, New York City, USA, pp. 515–523 (1993)
7. Parzen, E.: On Estimation of a Probability Density Function and Mode. The Annals of Mathematical Statistics 33(3), 1065–1076 (1962)
8. Pluim, J., Maintz, J., Viergever, M.: Mutual-information-based registration of medical images: A survey. IEEE Transactions on Medical Imaging 22(8), 986–1004 (2003)
9. Rosenblatt, M.: Remarks on some nonparametric estimates of a density function. The Annals of Mathematical Statistics 27, 832–837 (1956)
10. Viola, P., Wells III., W.M.: Alignment by maximization of mutual information. In: Proceedings of Fifth International Conference on Computer Vision, pp. 16–23 (1995)
11. Wang, Y.J., Farnebck, G., Westin, C.F.: Multi-affine registration using local polynomial expansion. Journal of Zhejiang University - Science C 11, 495–503 (2010)

Bayesian Characterization of Uncertainty in Multi-modal Image Registration

Firdaus Janoos, Petter Risholm, and William Wells (III)

Harvard Medical School, Boston, USA
{fjanoos,pettri,sw}@bwh.harvard.edu

Abstract. Understanding and quantifying the uncertainty involved when registering images is an important problem in medical imaging, where clinical decisions are made based on the registered solution. This is especially important in non-rigid registration where the higher degrees of freedom may provide unwarranted confidence in the results, through over-fitting. The Bayesian approach, which defines uncertainty as the posterior distribution on deformations, requires a generative model of the image formation process where the fixed image is modeled as a deformed version of the moving image plus a noise term. As per this model, the likelihood term is equivalent to the sum-of-squared differences image matching metric and is therefore valid only for same-mode image registration. In this paper, we propose a general formalism to quantify Bayesian uncertainty in the registration of multi-modal images through an extended probability model that introduces and then marginalizes out a stochastic transfer function between moving and fixed image intensities.

1 Introduction

1.1 Motivation

Registration is a fundamental tool for many bio-medical image analysis tasks such as longitudinal and population studies, and image guided surgery. However, assuming the physical validity of the deformation mechanism used in the registration procedure, imaging noise and artifacts, such as distortion or bias-field, along with the highly variable presentation of pathology affect the confidence in the optimal solution. This problem is compounded by the high degrees of freedom afforded by non-rigid registration models which introduces the possibility of over-fitting, for example, by through complex warps of regions which have insufficient contrast to guide the registration. This can happen primarily through the use of regularization, which is needed to condition the ill-posed model inversion, but which introduces long range dependencies in the solution. And finally, there is the uncertainty in the specification of model hyper-parameters, such as the mechanical properties of the underlying tissue or the statistics of imaging noise, all of which degrade the validity, sufficiency and accuracy of the deformation obtained through optimization. Therefore, quantifying and conveying the uncertainty in registration is extremely important, especially when clinical decisions are based on registration results.

In the Bayesian approach to non-rigid registration, the registration parameters are random variables and optimization may be used to obtain their *maximum a posteriori*

B.M. Dawant et al. (Eds.): WBIR 2012, LNCS 7359, pp. 50–59, 2012.
© Springer-Verlag Berlin Heidelberg 2012

(MAP) estimates. More importantly, however, the Bayesian approach enables quantification of uncertainty as the posterior distribution over deformations, via measures such as variance, inter-quartile ranges, credibility intervals and entropy [2,9,5]. Here, the likelihood function, corresponding to the data fidelity term, measures the alignment of the two images under a transformation, while the prior corresponds to the regularization term penalizing implausible deformations. While different deformation and regularization combinations – such as freeform deformations with b-splines [9] or finite element (FE) meshes with elastic deformation penalty [2,5] – have been used, the likelihood terms have allowed for only same-modality image registration while assuming additive normal noise.

Specifically, denote the moving image as $M : \Omega_M \to \mathbb{I}_M$ and $F : \Omega_F \to \mathbb{I}_F$, where $\Omega_M \subseteq \mathbb{R}^3$ and $\Omega_F \subseteq \mathbb{R}^3$ are the spatial domain of the fixed and moving images respectively, and $\mathbb{I}_M = \mathbb{I}_F \subseteq \mathbb{R}$ are their equal intensity ranges. The images F and M are treated as random fields and the fixed image is assumed to be generated by applying a transformation $\mathbf{u}$ to the moving image domain as per: $F = M \circ \mathbf{u} + \epsilon$ which also introduces normal noise $\epsilon \sim \mathcal{N}(0, \tau_\epsilon)$. Here, the transform $\mathbf{u}$ too is treated as a random variable with a probability measure, given by the prior distribution. Additionally, the likelihood is assumed to spatially iid.

Therefore, the log-posterior distribution of the transform is:

$$\ln p\left(\mathbf{u} \mid M, F\right) = -\int_{\Omega_F} \frac{|F_\mathbf{x} - M_{\mathbf{u}[\mathbf{x}]}|^2}{2\tau_\epsilon} d\mathbf{x} - \frac{E_{\mathrm{reg}}(\mathbf{u})}{2\tau_{\mathrm{reg}}} + \mathrm{const}, \tag{1}$$

where $E_{\mathrm{reg}}(\mathbf{u})$ is the regularization energy of the transformation. Here, the first term is proportional to the log-likelihood term $\ln p(F, M|\mathbf{u})$ while the second is proportional to the log-prior on the transformations $\ln p(\mathbf{u})$. The temperatures τ_ϵ and τ_{reg} are model hyper-parameters, where τ_ϵ is related to the variance of the image noise, while τ_{reg} controls the variance of the prior on transformations.

This model provides a principled basis for the interpretation of the posterior density as uncertainty in parameter estimates, for setting priors on the model hyper-parameters and as shown in [4], for eliminating the uncertainty due to HPs by marginalizing them out.

1.2   Contribution

One of the main drawbacks, however, of this framework is that it restricts the image similarity term to sum-of-squared differences (SSD) metric and is applicable to only same-mode images. Here, we present an extension for multi-modal image registration through a generalization of the SSD metric that accounts for arbitrary intensity transformations. Specifically, we introduce a latent random process $\eta_{\mathbf{u}[\mathbf{x}]}(m) \in \mathbb{I}_F$ defined on moving image intensities $m \in \mathbb{I}_M$ which serves as a *link function* between the moving image intensity range to that of the fixed image. The posterior density of the link process is directly estimated from the data, and is marginalized out by means of the free-energy equivalence. In this paper, non-parametric kernel density estimation is used, although this framework supports any alternative parametric or non-parametric density estimation method. The new registration model is evaluated on a synthetic T1-to-T2 MR image registration problem with ground-truth. A clinical application (cryoablation) to register pre-operative abdominal MR with an intra-procedural CT image is also demonstrated.

1.3 Related Work

In addition to fixed (known) transfer functions, parametric and non-parametric methods to estimate the intensity transformation from the data are commonly used in multi-modal registration [7]. For example, Guimond *et al.* [3] learn a polynomial mapping between the intensities. Roche *et al.* [6] use the conditional expectation $\mathbb{E}\left\{m \in \mathbb{I}_M | f \in \mathbb{I}_F\right\}$ as the intensity transformation as which leads to the correlation ratio as the image-matching metric. These metrics use point-estimates of the transfer function, in contrast to the full posterior as done here, thereby limiting their ability to deal with non-stationary and noisy intensity mappings.

While image matching based on the joint-histogram of intensities, such as mutual information, generalize to a very wide class of intensity transformations, they do not have an associated probabilistic model and therefore cannot be used to compute a posterior. Zöllei *et al.* [10] present an alternative probabilistic model for image registration using Dirichlet priors on the latent parameters of joint multinomial models on discrete intensities. Marginalization led to objective functions that approximate entropy or likelihood formulations and only MAP estimates were sought.

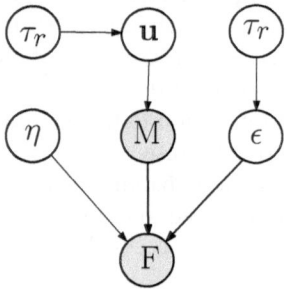

Fig. 1. Proposed probability model for multi-modal image registration. Here, F and M are the fixed and moving images respectively, ϵ is white normal noise with variance τ_ϵ, **u** are the transformation parameters with prior distribution variance controlled by τ_{reg}, and η is the link process that maps moving image intensities to fixed image intensities.

2 Method

2.1 Multi-modal Registration Model

The proposed Bayesian model for the multi-modal registration problem is as follows:

$$F_{\mathbf{x}} = \eta_{\mathbf{u}[\mathbf{x}]}\left(M_{\mathbf{u}[\mathbf{x}]}\right) + \epsilon_{\mathbf{x}}. \tag{2}$$

In this model, the moving and fixed image M and F and additive normal noise ϵ are all spatially iid random processes, while the transformation parameters **u** have a prior distribution specified by the regularization term. The link function η is a stochastic process defined on $\Omega_F \times \mathbb{I}_M$, with $\eta_{\mathbf{u}[\mathbf{x}]}$ defined on the moving image intensity range $\mathbb{I}_M$, such that $\eta_{\mathbf{u}[\mathbf{x}]}\left(M_{\mathbf{u}[\mathbf{x}]}\right) \in \mathbb{I}_F$ maps moving image intensity $M_{\mathbf{u}[\mathbf{x}]} \in \mathbb{I}_M$ to a fixed image intensity. We assume η to be iid in the space dimension (Ω_F) and $\eta_{\mathbf{u}[\mathbf{x}]}$ to be independent in the moving intensity dimension ($\mathbb{I}_M$). In the following discussion, define $f_{\mathbf{u}[\mathbf{x}]} \triangleq \eta_{\mathbf{u}[\mathbf{x}]}(M_{\mathbf{u}[\mathbf{x}]})$. Also, we will drop explicit conditioning on **u**, F and M except when there is ambiguity.

Under the spatial iid assumptions of F and M, and approximating $\epsilon_{\mathbf{x}}$ by its conditional expectation $\mathbb{E}\left\{\epsilon_{\mathbf{x}} \mid M_{\mathbf{u}[\mathbf{x}]}\right\} = 0$, the strong law of large numbers yields that the marginal posterior density of the link process

$$p\left(\eta_{\mathbf{u}[\mathbf{x}]}(M_{\mathbf{u}[\mathbf{x}]}) \mid \mathbf{u}, F, M\right) = p\left(f_{\mathbf{u}[\mathbf{x}]} \mid M_{\mathbf{u}[\mathbf{x}]}\right) \approx \frac{\text{vol}\left\{[F = f_{\mathbf{u}[\mathbf{x}]}] \cap [M \circ \mathbf{u} = M_{\mathbf{u}[\mathbf{x}]}]\right\}}{\text{vol}\left\{[M \circ \mathbf{u} = M_{\mathbf{u}[\mathbf{x}]}]\right\}} \tag{3}$$

We can marginalize out the latent process $\eta_{\mathbf{u}[\mathbf{x}]}$ under its posterior using the free-energy equivalence:

$$\ln p(\mathbf{u} \mid F, M) = \int p(\eta|\mathbf{u}, F, M) \ln p(\mathbf{u}, \eta \mid F, M) d\eta - \int p(\eta|\mathbf{u}, F, M) \ln p(\eta|\mathbf{u}, F, M) d\eta$$

$$= \int p(\eta|\mathbf{u}, F, M) \ln p(\mathbf{u}, \eta \mid F, M) d\eta + \mathbb{H}\{\eta|\mathbf{u}, F, M\}, \tag{4}$$

where $\mathbb{H}\{\eta_{\mathbf{u}[\mathbf{x}]}|\mathbf{u}, F, M\}$ is the differential entropy of $p(\eta_{\mathbf{u}[\mathbf{x}]}|\mathbf{u}, F, M)$. In the case of the model given in eqn. (2), the log-posterior of the deformations is:

$$\ln p(\mathbf{u} \mid F, M) = -\int_{\Omega_F} \int_{\mathbb{I}_F} p\left(\eta_{\mathbf{u}[\mathbf{x}]}(M_{\mathbf{u}[\mathbf{x}]})\right) \frac{\left|F_{\mathbf{x}} - \eta_{\mathbf{u}[\mathbf{x}]}(M_{\mathbf{u}[\mathbf{x}]})\right|^2}{2\tau_\epsilon} d\eta_{\mathbf{u}[\mathbf{x}]}(M_{\mathbf{u}[\mathbf{x}]}) dx$$

$$+ \int_{\Omega_F} \mathbb{H}\left\{\eta_{\mathbf{u}[\mathbf{x}]}(M_{\mathbf{u}[\mathbf{x}]})\right\} dx - \frac{E_{\mathrm{reg}}(\mathbf{u})}{2\tau_{\mathrm{reg}}} + \mathrm{const.}$$

Now, under the spatial iid assumptions of the model, the integral

$$\int_{\Omega_F} \mathbb{H}\left\{\eta_{\mathbf{u}[\mathbf{x}]}(M_{\mathbf{u}[\mathbf{x}]})\right\} dx = \int_{\Omega_F} \int_{\mathbb{I}_F} p\left(f_{\mathbf{u}[\mathbf{x}]} \mid M_{\mathbf{u}[\mathbf{x}]}\right) \ln p\left(f_{\mathbf{u}[\mathbf{x}]} \mid M_{\mathbf{u}[\mathbf{x}]}\right) df_{\mathbf{u}[\mathbf{x}]} dx$$

is equal to $\mathrm{vol}\{\Omega_M\}\mathbb{H}\left\{f_{\mathbf{u}[\mathbf{x}]} \mid m_{\mathbf{x}}\right\}$, where

$$\mathbb{H}\left\{f_{\mathbf{u}[\mathbf{x}]} \mid m_{\mathbf{x}}\right\} = \int_{\mathbb{I}_M} p\left(M_{\mathbf{u}[\mathbf{x}]}\right) \int_{\mathbb{I}_F} p\left(f_{\mathbf{u}[\mathbf{x}]} \mid M_{\mathbf{u}[\mathbf{x}]}\right) \ln p\left(f_{\mathbf{u}[\mathbf{x}]} \mid M_{\mathbf{u}[\mathbf{x}]}\right) df_{\mathbf{u}[\mathbf{x}]} dM_{\mathbf{u}[\mathbf{x}]},$$

is the conditional entropy of the link-process posterior.

Putting it all together, the log-posterior of the deformation model becomes:

$$\ln p(\mathbf{u} \mid F, M) = -\frac{1}{2\tau_\epsilon} \int_{\Omega_F} \int_{\mathbb{I}_F} p\left(f_{\mathbf{u}[\mathbf{x}]} \mid M_{\mathbf{u}[\mathbf{x}]}\right) \left|F_{\mathbf{x}} - f_{\mathbf{u}[\mathbf{x}]}\right|^2 df_{\mathbf{u}[\mathbf{x}]} dx$$

$$+ \mathrm{vol}\{\Omega_F\}\mathbb{H}\left\{f_{\mathbf{u}[\mathbf{x}]} \mid M_{\mathbf{u}[\mathbf{x}]}\right\} - \frac{E_{\mathrm{reg}}(\mathbf{u})}{2\tau_{\mathrm{reg}}} + \mathrm{const.} \tag{5}$$

It can be easily seen that this distribution satisfies an intensity transformation invariance, i.e. $p(\mathbf{u}|F, M) = p(\mathbf{u}|F, \alpha(M))$ where $\alpha : \mathbb{I}_M \to \mathbb{R}$ is a monotonic transfer function on the moving image intensity range such that $\alpha'(m) \neq 0$, at all $m \in \mathbb{I}_M$.

2.2   Estimating the Link Process Posterior

The marginal posterior $p\left(f_{\mathbf{u}[\mathbf{x}]} \mid M_{\mathbf{u}[\mathbf{x}]}\right)$ of the link process $\eta_{\mathbf{u}[\mathbf{x}]}(M_{\mathbf{u}[\mathbf{x}]})$ (§ eqn. (3)), are obtained in non-parametric form using kernel density estimation (KDE) [8]:

$$p\left(f_{\mathbf{u}[\mathbf{x}]} \mid M_{\mathbf{u}[\mathbf{x}]}\right) = \frac{\sum_{i=1}^{N} k_1(f_{\mathbf{u}[\mathbf{x}]} - f_i)k_2(M_{\mathbf{u}[\mathbf{x}]} - m_i)}{\sum_{j=1}^{N} k_2(M_{\mathbf{u}[\mathbf{x}]} - m_j)}, \tag{6}$$

where k_1 and k_2 are two non-negative symmetric kernel functions that integrate to unity, with scales h_1 and h_2 respectively. And, $f_i \triangleq F[\mathbf{x}_i]$ and $m_i \triangleq M_{\mathbf{u}[\mathbf{x}_i]}$ are fixed and moving image values sampled at locations $\mathbf{x}_i$, $i = 1 \ldots N$.

Therefore,

$$\int_{\Omega_F} \int_{\mathbb{I}_F} p\left(f_{\mathbf{u}[\mathbf{x}]} \mid M_{\mathbf{u}[\mathbf{x}]}, \mathbf{u}, F, M\right) \left| F_{\mathbf{x}} - f_{\mathbf{u}[\mathbf{x}]} \right|^2 df_{\mathbf{u}[\mathbf{x}]} d\mathbf{x}$$

$$= \int_{\Omega_F} \frac{\sum_{i=1}^{N} k_2(M_{\mathbf{u}[\mathbf{x}]} - m_i) \left| F_{\mathbf{x}} - f_i \right|^2}{\sum_{j=1}^{N} k_2(M_{\mathbf{u}[\mathbf{x}]} - m_j)} d\mathbf{x} + h_1^2 \text{vol}\{\Omega_F\},$$

and

$$\int_{\mathbb{I}_M} \mathbb{H}\left\{f_{\mathbf{u}[\mathbf{x}]} \mid m\right\} p\left(m \mid \mathbf{u}, F, M\right), dM_{\mathbf{u}[\mathbf{x}]} = -\frac{1}{N} \sum_{i=1}^{N} \ln \frac{\sum_{j=1}^{N} k_1(f_i - f_j) k_2(m_i - m_j)}{\sum_{j=1}^{N} k_2(m_i - m_j)}.$$

As a result, the KDE version of log-posterior of the transformation model is:

$$\ln p(\mathbf{u} \mid F, M) = -\frac{1}{2\tau_\epsilon} \int_{\Omega_F} \frac{\sum_{i=1}^{N} k_2(M_{\mathbf{u}[\mathbf{x}]} - m_i) \left| F_{\mathbf{x}} - f_i \right|^2}{\sum_{j=1}^{N} k_2(M_{\mathbf{u}[\mathbf{x}]} - m_j)} d\mathbf{x}$$

$$- \frac{\text{vol}\{\Omega_F\}}{N} \sum_{i=1}^{N} \ln \frac{\sum_{j=1}^{N} k_1(f_i - f_j) k_2(m_i - m_j)}{\sum_{j=1}^{N} k_2(m_i - m_j)} - \frac{E_{\text{reg}}(\mathbf{u})}{2\tau_{\text{reg}}} + \text{const.}$$

$$(7)$$

3   Results

In this section, we show results registering both synthetic and clinical multi-modal images. A tetrahedral finite-element (FE) model together with a bio-mechanically plausible elastic energy penalty on mesh deformations was used in the experiments. The posterior distribution on deformations was characterized by the Metropolis-Hastings (MH) Markov Chain Monte Carlo (MCMC) method described in [5].

3.1   Synthetic Data

From the BrainWeb[1] database, we acquired simulated T1 and T2 weighted MR images of the brain that are in perfect alignment. The images were resampled to a resolution of $2 \times 2 \times 4$ mm and size $90 \times 108 \times 45$ voxels, and were Gaussian smoothed with 1mm variance. Normally distributed white noise of standard deviation of 0.02 was added to the T1 weighted image which was treated as the fixed image in all the synthetic experiments. Two synthetic moving images were created by applying the same b-spline deformation field (maximum and average displacement of 10.1mm and 4.3mm respectively) to (a) the T1 image; and (b) the T2 image, as shown in Fig. 2.

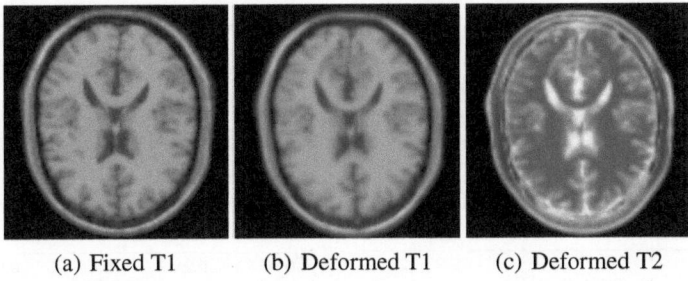

(a) Fixed T1   (b) Deformed T1   (c) Deformed T2

Fig. 2. The three images used in the synthetic experiments. (**a**): The T1-weighted MR image. (**b**): The deformed T1-weighted image. (**c**): The deformed T2-weighted image.

For registration, an FE-based deformation model was employed where the moving image domain containing brain tissue was discretized with 104 tetrahedral elements and 44 FE vertices (giving 3×44 deformation parameters in 3D). The posterior distribution on deformations was characterized by MH-MCMC sampling with a noise temperature of $\tau_\epsilon = 0.04$ and prior temperature of $\tau_{\text{reg}} = 200$. The bandwidths h_1 and h_2 of the kernels k_1 and k_2 were selected using cross-validation. A total of 800×10^3 samples were generated for each MCMC chain, and with burn-in of 300×10^3 samples and a thinning factor of 10, effectively giving 50×10^3 samples from the posterior distribution in each chain.

The posterior mode (MAP), serving as a point estimate, and inter-quartile ranges (IQR), serving as a measure of uncertainty, were computed from the MCMC samples using kernel density estimation for each of the 3×44 components of the deformation field. In Fig. 3(a), the error in the T1-T1 registration versus that in the T1-T2 registration (determined with respect to the ground truth deformations) of the MAP estimate shown. For the T1-T1 experiment, the maximum and median absolute error was 1.6mm and 0.37mm respectively, while for the T1-T2 experiment it was 1.6mm and 0.45mm. Here, we can observe a strong linear relationship between the errors in the estimating same deformation from two different modalities ($r^2 = 0.80$). The T1-T1 registration IQRs are plotted against the T1-T2 registration IQRs in Fig. 3(b). The IQRs are highly correlated across modalities ($r^2 = 0.89$), but the correlation diminishes at higher uncertainties. For the T1-T1 case, the maximum and median IQRs were 0.67mm and 0.34mm respectively, while for the T1-T2 case they were 0.76mm and 0.37mm. These results imply that there is a slight but statistically insignificant decrease in registration accuracy and precision for multi-modal data (one-sided two-sample t-test, no effect for any $p < 0.26$).

For all 3×44 deformation components, the KL-divergence between their posterior distributions from the T1-T1 and T1-T2 cases is graphed in Fig. 4. It can be seen that the posterior distributions over most components are very similar but with a few outliers. Estimating the null distribution of KL-divergences by bootstrapping from the MCMC chain of the T1-T1 registration case, the difference between the posterior distributions of the T1-T1 and T1-T2 cases were not significant at any $p < 0.31$ (false discovery rate corrected).

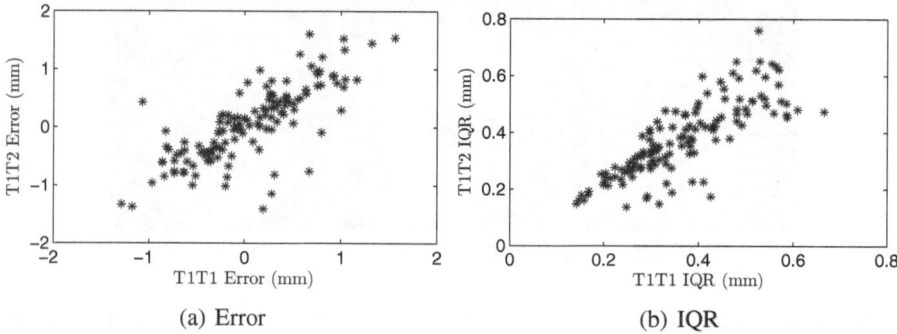

(a) Error   (b) IQR

Fig. 3. (a): Error in MAP estimates of the T1-T1 versus that from T1-T2 registration cases (with respect to ground truth) plotted for each of the 3×44 vertex deformation components. **(b)**: The IQRs posterior distributions of each displacement component for the T1-T1 case versus the T1-T2 case.

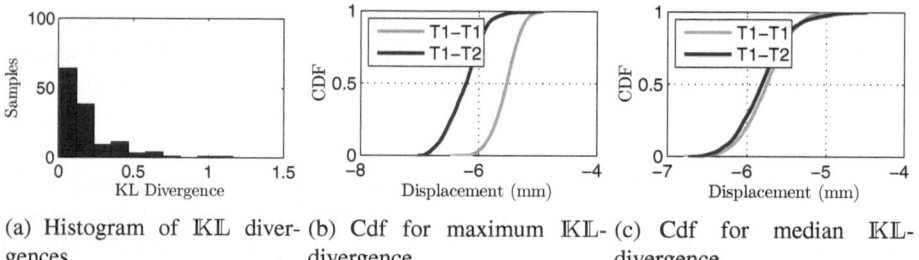

(a) Histogram of KL diver- (b) Cdf for maximum KL- (c) Cdf for median KL-
gences.   divergence.   divergence.

Fig. 4. (a): Histogram of the KL-divergences between the posterior distributions (per displacement component) of the T1-T1 and T1-T2 registration cases. The median and maximum KL-divergences were 0.2 and 1.1 respectively. **(b)** Cumulative distribution function (cdf) of the posterior distribution corresponding to the displacement component with the maximum KL-divergence. **(c)** Cdf of the posterior distribution corresponding to the displacement component with the median KL-divergence.

3.2   Clinical Data

In ablation therapy of liver tumors, the procedure is often planned on pre-operative MR images which provide superior soft-tissue contrast while CT is used for intra-operative guidance. Although registering the pre-operative MR with the intra-operative CT enables real-time guidance of the ablation probe using the enhanced contrast provided by MR, the uncertainty in the results can provide equally important information for the decisions of the surgeon. Next, we demonstrate the quantification of this uncertainty using a data-set obtained during such a procedure (§ Fig. 5). A T1-weighted MR image (size: $512 \times 512 \times 96$, spacing: $0.8 \times 0.8 \times 2.5$ mm) was acquired pre-procedurally, while a CT image (size: $512 \times 512 \times 41$, spacing: $1.0 \times 1.0 \times 5.0$ mm) was acquired intra-procedurally. The MR image was sub-sampled by a factor of 2 in all dimensions, while the CT image was subsampled by a factor of 2 in the x- and y-directions. Both

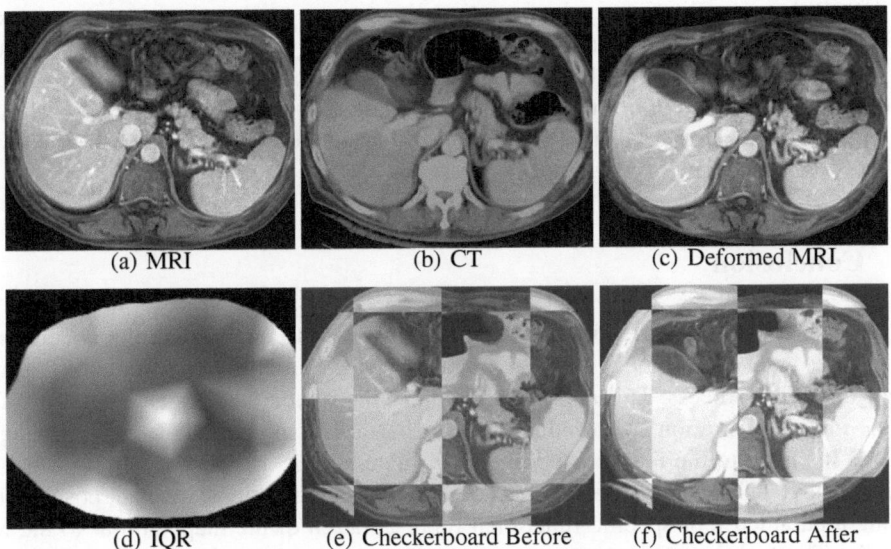

(a) MRI   (b) CT   (c) Deformed MRI

(d) IQR   (e) Checkerboard Before   (f) Checkerboard After

Fig. 5. Registration of pre-operative abdominal MRI in (**a**) with the CT in (**b**) acquired prior to insertion of cryo probe. (**c**): The registered MRI. (**d**): Spatial IQR along the z-direction. The brightest spot in the image has IQR of 3.8mm, while darkest has IQR of 1.0mm. (**e**): Original MR image checker-boarded with CT image. (**f**): Registered MR image checker-boarded with CT image. Notice that the boundaries liver and spleen are well aligned after registration.

images were smoothed with a Gaussian filter of 2.0mm variance and intensities were normalized between the $[0, 1]$ interval. The anatomy in the MR image was fitted with an FE-mesh consisting of 155 vertices and 512 tetrahedra. Starting from a manually determined rigid alignment of the images, 10^6 deformation samples were generated through MH-MCMC, with a burn-in factor of 50% and a thinning factor of 10. The remaining 50×10^3 samples were used to compute the posterior statistics.

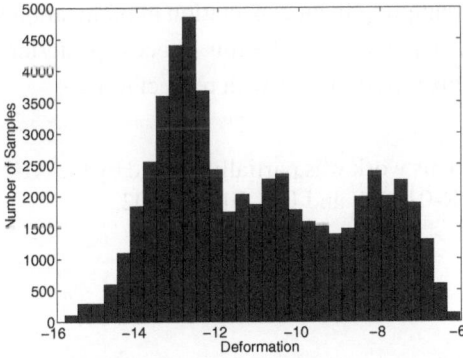

Fig. 6. Marginal probability distribution on displacements (in mm) along the z-direction for the FE-node located in the zone with high uncertainty (IQR)

Fig. 5 shows qualitative results from the alignment as well as corresponding uncertainty estimates. It can be seen that that there is relatively high uncertainty in the center of the slice in the abdominal aortal region. The marginal distribution over displacements in the z-direction of one FE-node in this location of high uncertainty is shown in Fig. 6. It can be observed that it has one distinct mode, but in addition has two two other, smaller, modes.

4   Conclusion

In this paper, we have presented a principled approach to quantifying the uncertainty associated with multi-modal image registration, based on a forward model of the image generation process. This approach augments the standard Bayesian framework for same-mode registration by introducing a stochastic link process that maps moving a image intensity to the fixed image intensity range, and is associated with a probability measure. This can capture a wider range of complex relationships than possible by using a parametric or specific functional representation of the map, similar to the MI metric. The framework furthermore marginalizes out the link-process using the free-energy equivalence. Therefore, in contrast to MI, the fully specified Bayesian model enables measuring the posterior over transformations, without dependencies on the intensity transfer function.

The formulation presented here and by Roche *et al.* [6] are examples of kernel regression. The main difference is that they use kernel regression to estimate the expected value of the fixed image intensity given moving image intensity, while we use kernel regression to estimate the expected difference between the observed and predicted fixed image values. In a regression framework, this is equivalent to the difference between using only the squared bias of the estimator (*i.e.* of the intensity transformation) as in [6] versus using the full mean squared error (MSE) as here, in the image similarity function. Moreover, marginalizing out the link process requires including the entropy of the conditional distribution in the cost function.

The differentiability of the kernel used in eqn. (7) permits computation of gradients of $p(\mathbf{u} \mid F, M)$. Therefore, we can perform direct MAP estimation of the registration parameters, without MCMC sampling in an expectation maximization framework. In the n-th iteration of EM, the E-step computes the link-process posterior $p\left(f_{\mathbf{u}^{(n)}[\mathbf{x}]} \mid M_{\mathbf{u}^{(n)}[\mathbf{x}]}\right)$, while the M-step optimizes $p(\mathbf{u} \mid F, M)$ with respect to $\mathbf{u}$.

Acknowledgements. This work was partially funded by the NIH grants P41EB015898, P41RR019703, P41-RR-013218 and P41-EB-015902.

References

1. Brainweb database, http://www.bic.mni.mcgill.ca/brainweb/ 5
2. Gee, J.C., Bajcsy, R.K.: Elastic matching: Continuum mechanical and probabilistic analysis. In: Brain Warping, p. 183. Academic Press 2

3. Guimond, A., Roche, A., Ayache, N., Meunier, J.: Three-dimensional multimodal brain warping using the demons algorithm and adaptive intensity corrections. IEEE Trans. Med. Imaging 20(1), 58–69 (2001) 3
4. Janoos, F., Risholm, P., Wells, W.M.: Robust non-rigid registration and characterization of uncertainty. In: Zhou, K., Duncan, J.S., Ourselin, S. (eds.) Methods in Biomedical Image Analysis (MMBIA), vol. 1 (2012) 2
5. Risholm, P., Pieper, S., Samset, E., Wells III, W.M.: Summarizing and Visualizing Uncertainty in Non-rigid Registration. In: Jiang, T., Navab, N., Pluim, J.P.W., Viergever, M.A. (eds.) MICCAI 2010, Part II. LNCS, vol. 6362, pp. 554–561. Springer, Heidelberg (2010) 2, 5
6. Roche, A., Malandain, G., Pennec, X., Ayache, N.: The Correlation Ratio as a New Similarity Measure for Multimodal Image Registration. In: Wells, W.M., Colchester, A.C.F., Delp, S.L. (eds.) MICCAI 1998. LNCS, vol. 1496, pp. 1115–1124. Springer, Heidelberg (1998) 3, 9
7. Rogelj, P., Kovačič, S., Gee, J.C.: Point similarity measures for non-rigid registration of multi-modal data. Comput. Vis. Image Underst. 92, 112–140 (2003) 3
8. Silverman, B.: Density Estimation for Statistics and Data Analysis. Chapman & Hall, London (1998) 5
9. Simpson, I.J., Schnabel, J.A., Groves, A.R., Andersson, J.L., Woolrich, M.W.: Probabilistic inference of regularisation in non-rigid registration. NeuroImage (2011) 2
10. Zöllei, L., Jenkinson, M., Timoner, S., Wells, W.: A Marginalized MAP Approach and EM Optimization for Pair-Wise Registration. In: Karssemeijer, N., Lelieveldt, B. (eds.) IPMI 2007. LNCS, vol. 4584, pp. 662–674. Springer, Heidelberg (2007) 3

Hierarchical vs. Simultaneous Multiresolution Strategies for Nonrigid Image Registration

Wei Sun[1], Wiro J. Niessen[1,2], and Stefan Klein[1]

[1] Biomedical Imaging Group Rotterdam,
Departments of Radiology and Medical Informatics, Erasmus MC, Rotterdam, The Netherlands
{w.sun,w.niessen,s.klein}@erasmusmc.nl
[2] Department of Image Science and Technology,
Faculty of Applied Sciences, Delft University of Technology, Delft, The Netherlands

Abstract. Nonrigid image registration algorithms commonly employ multireso-lution strategies, both for the image and the transformation model. Usually a hierarchical approach is chosen: the algorithm starts on a level with reduced complexity, e.g. a smoothed and downsampled version of the input images, and with a limited number of degrees of freedom for the transformation. Gradually the level of complexity is increased until the original, non-smoothed images are used, and the transformation model has the highest degrees of freedom. In this study, we define two alternative approaches in which low- and high-resolution levels are considered simultaneously. An extensive experimental comparison study is performed, evaluating all possible combinations of multiresolution schemes for image data and transformation model. Publicly available CT lung data, with annotated landmarks, are used to quantify registration accuracy. It is shown that simultaneous multiresolution strategies can lead to more accurate registration.

Keywords: Nonrigid Registration, Multiresolution, Hierarchical, Transformation, Scale Space.

1 Introduction

Nonrigid registration can be regarded as a large scale numerical optimization problem, which finds the optimal parameters for a selected transformation model to recover the deformation between images [1, 2, 3]. In practical registration tasks, local minima often exist in the optimization space. How to avoid these local traps, and reach the "correct" minimum, is a major challenge for registration algorithms. To tackle this issue, multiresolution strategies have become popular. Lester and Arridge [4] provided a comprehensive review on multiresolution strategies. They classified the multiresolution strategies into three groups: increasing data complexity, increasing warp complexity, and increasing model complexity. In most existing implementations of nonrigid registration algorithms, one or more of these multiresolution strategies are incorporated. Rueckert *et al.* [5] adopted both increasing data and warp complexities to implement a coarse-to-fine registration with free-form deformations (FFD).

B.M. Dawant et al. (Eds.): WBIR 2012, LNCS 7359, pp. 60–69, 2012.

For registration of lung data, Yin *et al.* [6] applied transformation models at two levels to one image resolution level. Gholipour *et al.* [7] presented several multiresolution approaches that can be used in brain data. Recently, Risser *et al.* [8] proposed a multiresolution strategy for large deformation diffeomorphic metric mapping. Besides the above mentioned works, hierarchical strategies have been widely used in many other registration tasks [9,10,11,12,13,14].

Most current multiresolution approaches adopt a step-by-step approach: the fine-scale registration will not be executed until all of the coarser registrations have been carried out. For example, a common strategy for FFD registration with B-splines is to combine the coarsest B-spline grid with the most blurred image at the beginning of optimization. After the optimization on this combination is complete, a denser B-spline grid and higher resolution image are used for further optimization. So, in these methods both transformation and data complexities are increased *hierarchically*.

Different from these hierarchical methods, several *simultaneous* multiresolution approaches were also presented previously. Stralen and Pluim [15] proposed a simultaneous multiresolution registration approach using a directed acyclic graph (DAG) and dynamic programming (DP). First, they constructed a DAG based on control points at different resolution levels. The DAG cost was defined as the sum of image dissimilarity at multiple scales and the difference between control point displacements in adjacent resolution levels. Then, they applied DP to find the optimum control point displacements. Somayajula *et al.* [16] also proposed a simultaneous multiresolution method for nonrigid registration. They defined corresponding scale-space feature vectors from multiresolution stacks of fixed and moving images at each voxel. Then, they used mutual information to align these feature vectors. In this way, different resolution levels were registered simultaneously, because the elements of each feature vector contained information from different resolution levels.

In this paper, we define three multiresolution concepts, named Hierarchical (H), Simultaneous (S) and Hierarchically Simultaneous (HS) respectively. These strategies can be implemented both for image data (D) and transformation model (T):

- Image data

  - DH = start with most blurred image, then less blurred image, and so on, until original image resolution;
  - DS = use the entire scale stack of different resolutions at once;
  - DHS = start with blurred image, then use blurred and less-blurred, and so on, until the entire scale stack is used.

- Transformation model

  - TH = start with coarsest B-spline grid, next level use finer B-spline grid, and so on, until the finest control point spacing;
  - TS = optimize coarse and fine B-spline deformations simultaneously;
  - THS = start with coarse B-spline, then add finer scale while still optimizing coarse scale, and so on, until all scales are being optimized simultaneously.

Combining these strategies gives 3×3 possibilities, which we implemented and compared in an experiment on publicly available CT lung data with manually anno-tated landmarks. In the following sections a detailed explanation of the proposed mul-tiresolution strategies is given, followed by a description of the evaluation study.

2   Method

2.1   Multiresolution Strategies for Image Data

The N-dimensional moving and fixed images can be denoted by $M(x)$ and $F(y)$, where $x, y \in \mathbb{R}^N$ represent the image coordinates in M and F, respectively. Mov-ing and fixed images on resolution level s can be generated by convolution of the original   images with a Gaussian kernel:

$$\begin{cases} M(x,s) = G(\sigma_s) * M(x) \\ F(y,s) = G(\sigma_s) * F(y) \end{cases}, \tag{1}$$

where $G(\cdot)$ is the Gaussian kernel. σ_s is the variance of the Gaussian filter corres-ponding to resolution level s of the image. For a larger s, σ_s has a smaller value.

Nonrigid image registration is a process which aligns moving image M to fixed image F using a nonrigid transformation model. Mathematically, registration is formulated as an optimization problem, in which the nonrigid transformation $T_{\hat{\mu}}$ is estimated by minimizing the difference C_{diff} between moving and fixed images:

$$\hat{\mu} = \arg \min_{\mu} \left(C_{diff} \left(F, M \circ T_\mu \right) \right), \tag{2}$$

where μ represents the parameters of the transformation T. By making C_{diff} depen-dent on the resolution level we can introduce a multiresolution scheme for the image data. Below, we define the objective functions that correspond to DH, DS, and DHS:

$$\text{DH: } C_{diff}^p = C_{diff} \left(F(y,p), M(x,p) \circ T_\mu \right), \tag{3}$$

$$\text{DS: } C_{diff}^p = \sum_{s=1}^{S} C_{diff} \left(F(y,s), M(x,s) \circ T_\mu \right), \tag{4}$$

$$\text{DHS: } C_{diff}^p = \sum_{s=1}^{p} C_{diff} \left(F(y,s), M(x,s) \circ T_\mu \right), \tag{5}$$

where $p \in [1, S]$ is the current resolution level of the registration, and S denotes the number of resolution levels. Figure 1(a) provides an overview of these three mul-tiresolution strategies, where $S = 3$. Note that the objective function for DS is actual-ly independent of p, since all levels of the image scale stack are taken into account simultaneously.

2.2   Multiresolution Strategies for the Transformation

A classic FFD transformation model based on B-splines [5] can be defined as follows:

$$T_\mu(y) = y + \sum_{y_i \in I_y} c_i \beta^r ((y - y_i)/g), \tag{6}$$

where y_i is a control point of the B-spline grid, and I_y represents the set of control points within a compactly supported region of the B-spline at y. c_i is the B-spline coefficient vector corresponding to control point y_i, and the parameter vector μ is formed by the elements of all c_i. $\beta^r(\cdot)$ is the selected rth order multidimensional B-spline polynomial, and g is the spacing between grid points. By making the definition of the transformation model dependent on the resolution level p, we can define a multiresolution scheme for the transformation complexity. Below, we define the transformation models that correspond to TH, TS, and THS, in which we also introduce a dependence on s, in order to couple the image scale to the transformation complexity:

$$\text{TH: } T_\mu^p(y,s) = y + \sum_{y_i \in I_y^p} c_i^p \beta^r ((y - y_i)/g(p)), \tag{7}$$

$$\text{TS: } T_\mu^p(y,s) = y + \sum_{l=1}^{s} \sum_{y_i \in I_y^l} c_i^l \beta^r ((y - y_i)/g(l)), \tag{8}$$

$$\text{THS: } T_\mu^p(y,s) = y + \sum_{l=1}^{\min(s,p)} \sum_{y_i \in I_y^l} c_i^l \beta^r ((y - y_i)/g(l)), \tag{9}$$

where p is the current resolution level of the registration. $T_\mu^p(y,s)$ represents the transformation at registration level p for a point (y,s) in the scale stack defined by (1). $l \in [1,S]$ denotes the B-spline grid level. c_i^p and c_i^l are the B-spline coefficient vectors at levels p and l, with corresponding grid spacing $g(p)$ and $g(l)$; the grid spacing $g(l)$ reduces with increasing l. Figure 1(b) provides an overview of these three multiresolution strategies for the transformation. With TH, the transformation is upsampled after each resolution (i.e., c_i^p are determined based on c_i^{p-1} such that $T_\mu^p(y,s) = T_\mu^{p-1}(y,s)$ at the start of level p) and only the currently finest level is being optimized, so μ at level p consists of the elements of c_i^p. With TS, the transformation model is independent of p, and formed by a summation of multiple B-spline models with different grid spacings; the parameter vector μ consists of all elements of c_i^l, $\forall l \in [1,S]$. With THS, the model is similar to TS, but the finer B-spline models are only used in the later resolution levels; at resolution level p, the parameter vector μ consists of all elements of c_i^l, $\forall l \in [1,p]$.

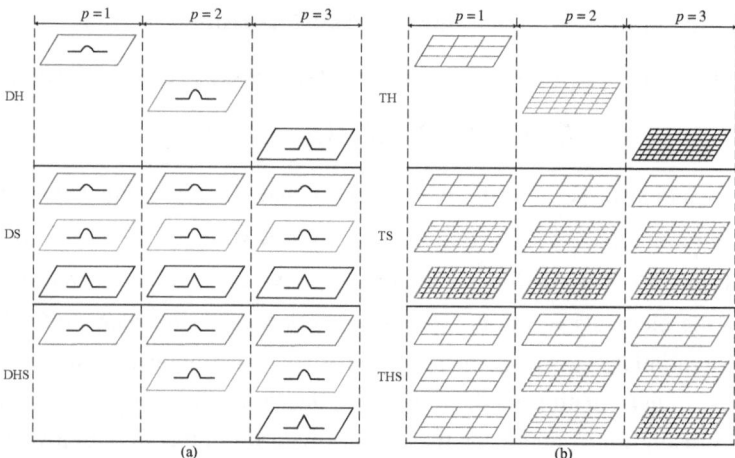

Fig. 1. Multiresolution strategies of data and transformation: (a) Most blurred, less blurred and original images are marked in blue, orange and black, respectively. (b) Coarsest, finer and finest B-spline grid are marked in blue, orange and black, respectively.

2.3 Combinations of Multiresolution Strategies

Because there are three different multiresolution strategies for both data and transformation, we can construct 3×3 combinations for multiresolution registration. Figure 2 presents all possible combinations in which registration processes have three multiresolution levels. In these combinations, the traditional multiresolution strategy is the combination of TH and DH. We impose the restriction that transformation level l (corresponding to the B-spline model with grid spacing $g(l)$) can only be applied to the finer image resolutions $s \in [l, S]$. According to this principle, the combination of TH and DHS becomes equivalent to the traditional multiresolution strategy TH-DH. In addition, TS-DH and TS-DHS are equivalent to THS-DH and THS-DHS, respectively.

2.4 Implementation Details

All experiments were performed with elastix [17], which is an open source package for registration. For C_{diff}, we used the common mean squared difference measure.

Image intensities at non-grid positions were obtained by trilinear interpolation. Third order ($r = 3$) B-splines were adopted for the transformation model. The adaptive stochastic gradient descent optimizer (ASGD) [18] was selected as optimization method. In each iteration of ASGD, a small, randomly selected, subset of samples from the entire image is used. Downsampling the image is not necessary because the computation time is independent of the size of the image. To facilitate the optimization of combined B-spline levels of TS and THS, a diagonal preconditioning matrix $\boldsymbol{B}$ was defined to scale the parameters corresponding to the different transformation levels:

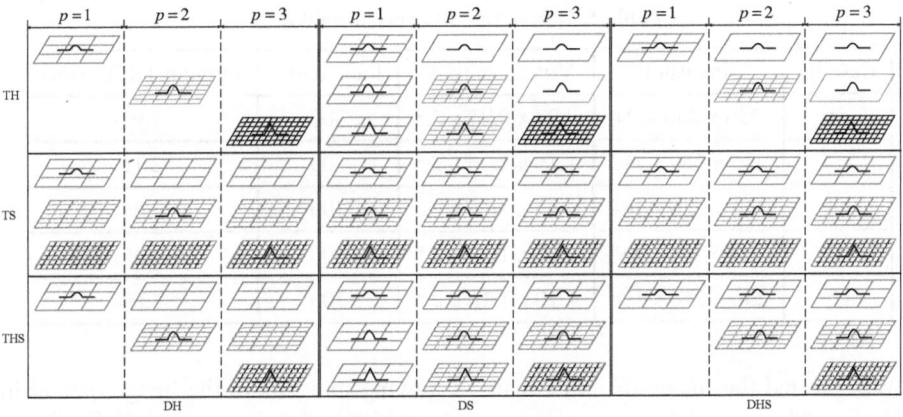

Fig. 2. Different combinations of multiresolution strategies of data and transformation for multiresolution registration

$$\boldsymbol{\mu}_{k+1} = \boldsymbol{\mu}_{k} + \alpha_{k} \boldsymbol{B} \boldsymbol{d} \left(\boldsymbol{\mu}_{k} \right),\tag{10}$$

where k is current iteration number. $\boldsymbol{\mu}_{k+1}$ and $\boldsymbol{\mu}_{k}$ denote the new and current parameter vector, respectively. $\boldsymbol{d}\left(\boldsymbol{\mu}_{k}\right)$ is the derivative of the cost function with respect to $\boldsymbol{\mu}$. α_{k} is a scalar gain factor that determines the step size [18], and $\boldsymbol{B}$ is a diagonal matrix $diag(\ [b_{1,1}\ b_{1,1}\ b_{1,1}\ ...\ b_{l,l}\ b_{l,l}\ b_{l,l}\ ...\ b_{S,S}\ b_{S,S}\ b_{S,S}]\ )$ with $b_{l,l} = \varepsilon^{-(S-l)}$. Based on initial trial-and-error experiments on one of the datasets (c1, described below), we set $\varepsilon = 4$. Here $\boldsymbol{B}$ works as a preconditioning strategy [19], which can enhance the convergence rate.

3   Experiments and Results

3.1   Experimental Data and Settings

To evaluate the performances of different multiresolution combinations, a set of lung data from DIR-lab [20] was used. Table 1 provides a description of these data.

Since manually marked landmarks have been provided in these data, mean of target registration error (mTRE) [21] can be used to evaluate the registration accuracy:

$$\text{mTRE}\left(\boldsymbol{p}^{reg}, \boldsymbol{p}^{gold}\right) = \frac{1}{n}\sum_{i=1}^{n}\left\| \boldsymbol{p}_i^{reg} - \boldsymbol{p}_i^{gold} \right\|,\tag{11}$$

where $\boldsymbol{p}^{reg}$ and $\boldsymbol{p}^{gold}$ represent the registered and ground truth landmarks. $n = 300$ is the number of landmarks in all test cases.

Table 1. Description of experimental data

Case ID	Dimensions	Voxelsize (mm)	Landmarks	Initial mTRE(voxel)
c1	256 x 256 x 94	0.97 x 0.97 x 2.5	300	1.97
c2	256 x 256 x 112	1.16 x 1.16 x 2.5	300	2.12
c3	256 x 256 x 104	1.15 x 1.15 x 2.5	300	3.36
c4	256 x 256 x 99	1.13 x 1.13 x 2.5	300	4.42
c5	256 x 256 x 106	1.10 x 1.10 x 2.5	300	3.69

We selected the image data at exhale as moving image, and the image data at inhale as fixed image. In all test cases, $S = 4$ resolution levels were used. The image scale stacks were generated using $\{\sigma_1,...,\sigma_s\} = \{8, 4, 2, 1\}$. For the transformation, the coarsest grid spacing $g(1)$ was set to 64mm, isotropically. This value is a reasonable choice because it is almost one fourth of the image size. In the experiments the finest grid spacing $g(S)$ was set to 8mm, 10mm, 13mm, or 16mm. So the grid schedule for four transformation levels can be calculated as $\left\{g(1), g(S)(g(1)/g(S))^{2/3}, \; g(S)(g(1)/g(S))^{1/3}, g(S)\right\}$. For example, the grid schedule for $g(S) = 8$mm is $\{64, 32, 16, 8\}$. For each iteration of optimization, the number of random samples was set to 16000 for all combinations. Note that with the DS and DHS approaches these 16000 samples are spread over multiple levels of the image scale stack, whereas with DH all 16000 samples are placed in the current active level $s = p$. The number of iterations was set to 2000 per resolution level.

3.2   Comparison of Different Multiresolution Strategies

The different multiresolution combinations are evaluated using five data pairs with four different finest grid spacings of the B-spline transformation. Figure 3 shows the registration results of all these combinations. As described in Section 2.3, TH-DHS, TS-DH and TS-DHS are actually equivalent to TH-DH, THS-DH and THS-DHS, respectively. So the results of TH-DH, THS-DH and THS-DHS are assigned to their equivalent combinations. In this way we can still make comparison among different multiresolution strategies of data and transformation in a general view. From Figure 3, it can be seen that the differences in most test cases are small, and THS generates better results than TH and TS in most of test cases. In addition, DS generates higher accuracy than DH and DHS. The traditional TH-DH approach has relatively worse performance in most cases. Especially in data pair c4, TH-DH results in unsatisfactory results. As shown in Table 1, c4 has larger average landmarks displacements than the other four data. So this significant deterioration could be caused by too large deformation of data.

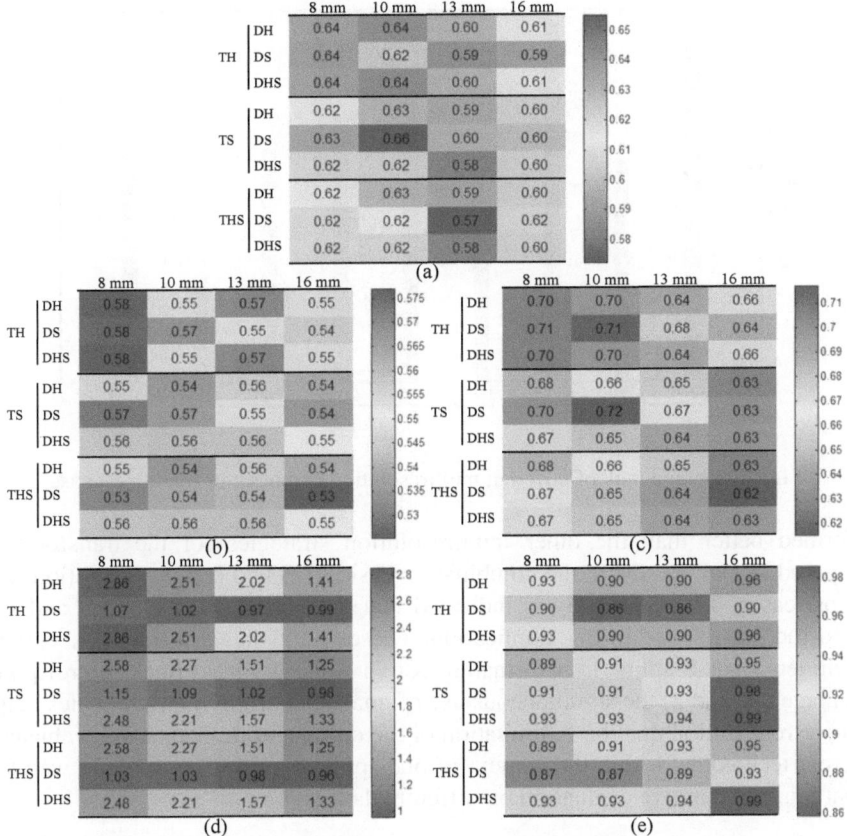

Fig. 3. Performance comparison of different multiresolution combinations. (a)-(e) are the results of lung data c1 to c5. The numbers represent the mTRE in voxels.

To make a further comparison among these combinations, a ranking of the 9 methods was made for each of the 5×4 test cases. The average rank of each method over all 5×4 test cases is presented in Figure 4. We can see that THS-DS has the best registration accuracy. The traditional TH-DH approach has the highest average rank number. It can also be noticed that the combinations with THS have lower rank than the other two multiresolution transformation strategies, when keeping the image resolution strategy the same.

4   Conclusions and Future Work

In this study different multiresolution strategies of data and transformation were compared on a publicly available lung CT dataset. Most observed differences among these combinations were small, and perhaps not statistically significant in this small number of datasets. However, some patterns could be observed. In current test cases, THS

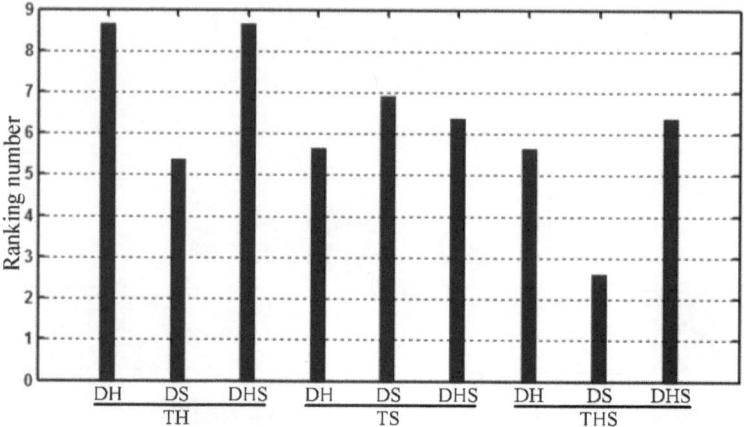

Fig. 4. Average rank of different multiresolution combinations in 20 test cases

performed better than the other multiresolution strategies for the transformation. Compared to DH and DHS, the combinations using DS had better registration results in most cases. The rank analysis indicated that the combination of THS and DS is indeed the best choice in this application. These results suggest that 1) keeping the low-dimensional B-spline transformation active while going to finer control point is advantageous, and 2) the simultaneous use of image data from multiple scales helps to improve registration quality. A limitation of the current work, is that we evaluated the different techniques within the context of one application. In future work, we plan to repeat this comparative evaluation on different data.

References

1. Zitová, B., Flusser, J.: Image registration methods: a survey. Image and Vision Computing 21, 977–1000 (2003)
2. Holden, M.: A review of geometric transformations for nonrigid body registration. IEEE Transactions on Medical Imaging 27, 111–128 (2008)
3. Fischer, B., Modersitzki, J.: Ill-posed medicine - an introduction to image registration. Inverse Problems 24 (2008)
4. Lester, H., Arridge, S.R.: A survey of hierarchical non-linear medical image registration. Pattern Recognition 32, 129–149 (1999)
5. Rueckert, D., Sonoda, L.I., Hayes, C., Hill, D.L.G., Leach, M.O., Hawkes, D.J.: Nonrigid registration using free-form deformations: Application to breast MR images. IEEE Transactions on Medical Imaging 18, 712–721 (1999)
6. Yin, Y., Hoffman, E.A., Ding, K., Reinhardt, J.M., Lin, C.-L.: A cubic B-spline-based hybrid registration of lung CT images for a dynamic airway geometric model with large deformation. Physics in Medicine and Biology 56, 203–218 (2011)
7. Gholipour, A., Kehtarnavaz, N., Briggs, R., Devous, M., Gopinath, K.: Brain functional localization: A survey of image registration techniques. IEEE Transactions on Medical Imaging 26, 427–451 (2007)

8. Risser, L., Vialard, F., Wolz, R., Murgasova, M., Holm, D.D., Rueckert, D.: Simultaneous multi-scale registration using large deformation diffeomorphic metric mapping. IEEE Transactions on Medical Imaging 30, 1746–1759 (2011)
9. Cole-Rhodes, A.A., Johnson, K.L., LeMoigne, J., Zavorin, I.: Multiresolution registration of remote sensing imagery by optimization of mutual information using a stochastic gradient. IEEE Transactions on Image Processing 12, 1495–1511 (2003)
10. Metz, C.T., Klein, S., Schaap, M., van Walsum, T., Niessen, W.J.: Nonrigid registration of dynamic medical imaging data using nD+t B-splines and a groupwise optimization approach. Medical Image Analysis 15, 238–249 (2011)
11. Mattes, D., Haynor, D.R., Vesselle, H., Lewellen, T.K., Eubank, W.: PET-CT image registration in the chest using free-form deformations. IEEE Transactions on Medical Imaging 22, 120–128 (2003)
12. Dinggang, S.: Fast image registration by hierarchical soft correspondence detection. Pattern Recognition 42, 954–961 (2009)
13. Kybic, J., Unser, M.: Fast parametric elastic image registration. IEEE Transactions on Image Processing 12, 1427–1442 (2003)
14. Musse, O., Heitz, F., Armspach, J.P.: Topology preserving deformable image matching using constrained hierarchical parametric models. IEEE Transactions on Image Processing 10, 1081–1093 (2001)
15. van Stralen, M., Pluim, J.P.W.: Optimal discrete multi-resolution deformable image registration. In: 6th IEEE International Symposium on Biomedical Imaging: From Nano to Macro, pp. 947–950 (2009)
16. Somayajula, S., Joshi, A.A., Leahy, R.M.: Mutual information based non-rigid mouse registration using a scale-space approach. In: 5th IEEE International Symposium on Biomedical Imaging: From Nano to Macro, pp. 1147–1150 (2008)
17. Klein, S., Staring, M., Murphy, K., Viergever, M.A., Pluim, J.P.W.: elastix: A toolbox for intensity-based medical image registration. IEEE Transactions on Medical Imaging 29, 196–205 (2010)
18. Klein, S., Pluim, J.P.W., Staring, M., Viergever, M.A.: Adaptive stochastic gradient descent optimisation for image registration. International Journal of Computer Vision 81, 227–239 (2009)
19. Bertsekas, D.P.: Nonlinear Programming. Athena Scientific, Massachusetts (1999)
20. Castillo, R., Castillo, E., Guerra, R., Johnson, V.E., McPhail, T., Garg, A.K., Guerrero, T.: A framework for evaluation of deformable image registration spatial accuracy using large landmark point sets. Physics in Medicine and Biology 54, 1849–1870 (2009)
21. van de Kraats, E.B., Penney, G.P., Tomazevic, D., van Walsum, T., Niessen, W.J.: Standardized evaluation methodology for 2-D-3-D registration. IEEE Transactions on Medical Imaging 24, 1177–1189 (2005)

3D-2D Registration Based on Mesh-Derived Image Bisection

David Thivierge-Gaulin[1], Chen-Rui Chou[2], Atilla P. Kiraly[3],
Christophe Chefd'Hotel[3], Norbert Strobel[4], and Farida Cheriet[1]

[1] École Polytechnique de Montréal, Montreal, QC, Canada
david.thivierge-gaulin@polymtl.ca
[2] University of North Carolina at Chapel Hill, Chapel Hill, NC, USA
[3] Siemens Corporation, Corporate Research and Technology, Princeton, NJ, USA
[4] Siemens AG, Healthcare Sector, Forchheim, Germany

Abstract. Electrophysiology procedures such as catheter ablation for
atrial fibrillation are non-invasive approaches for treating heart arrhyth-
mia. These operations necessitate contrast liquid injections for the left
atrium and pulmonary veins to be visible under fluoroscopy. However,
injections have to be minimized because of their toxicity. To provide visual guidance after the contrast liquid has washed away, it is possible to
overlay a mesh of the left atrium obtained from a pre-operative 3D volume over the intra-operative 2D fluoroscopic images. This paper presents
a novel mesh-based registration algorithm providing such an overlay by
registering the left atrium mesh to fluoroscopic images showing contrast
liquid injection. The registration is based on image bisections generated
by mesh projections, which bypasses the original volumetric data and
digitally reconstructed radiographs generation. The algorithm was validated on 7 clinical datasets and registers with a mean target registration
error of 6.56 ± 2.67mm.

Keywords: Mesh Registration, 3D/2D Registration, 2D/3D Registration, Model-Based Registration, Hybrid Registration, Image-Guided,
Atrial Fibrillation, Catheter Ablation, Electrophysiology.

1 Introduction

Image guidance during electrophysiology (EP) procedures such as catheter ablation (CA) for atrial fibrillation (AF) has been shown to decrease procedure
duration and likelihood of AF recurrence [1]. Since the left atrium (LA) and
pulmonary veins (PV)s are not visible under fluoroscopy without the injection
of contrast liquid [1], the operation is facilitated by overlaying a 3D mesh extracted from pre-operative 3D volume (CT or MRI) over the intra-operative
fluoroscopic images. To provide a correctly aligned overlay, the 3D mesh of the
LA with attached PVs is *registered* at the time on contrast liquid injection to
serve as a visual reference after the contrast liquid has washed away.

It is possible to register the mesh manually, but a quick and automatic registration algorithm is desirable because it allows reducing the number of op-
erative workflow steps, higher reproducibility of results and does not require

B.M. Dawant et al. (Eds.): WBIR 2012, LNCS 7359, pp. 70–78, 2012.
© Springer-Verlag Berlin Heidelberg 2012

a trained professional to be present. Typical automatic 3D-2D registration algorithms transform a 3D pre-operative volumetric image into a 2D digitally reconstructed radiograph (DRR), which is in turn compared to intra-operative fluoroscopic 2D images [2]. The assumption is that since the DRRs simulate fluoroscopic images, they will be resemblant enough so that a well chosen similarity measure between the two will have its global minimum coincide with the registered position of the two (3D-2D) modalities.

An alternative to DRR-based methods is to directly register the mesh to the fluoroscopic images, thus allowing exploitation of the information contained in the mesh's manual segmentation from pre-operative 3D volume. This paper describes such an algorithm that relies on analysis of the image bisection generated by the projection of the mesh. It allows bypassing the production of DRRs as well as not requiring the use of volumetric data. This is useful in EP procedures that do not use the volumetric data as part of their workflow as well as having the potential to be faster than DRR-based registration. The DRR production is usually the main bottleneck to achieve fast registration because it has to be iteratively evaluated in the optimizer inner loop – replacing the DRR by a faster process would greatly enhance registration speed.

The algorithm is described in section 2 and validated on 7 clinical cases (section 3). The potential use, advantages and drawbacks of the solution are outlined in section 4.

2   Methods

This section describes the steps of the mesh-derived registration algorithm:

1. Pre-process the 2D and 3D data (section 2.1).
2. Bisect the fluoroscopic images using mesh-to-mask projection (section 2.2).
3. Compute a cost from the image bisection (section 2.3).
4. Find the registered position using an optimizer (section 2.4).

The four steps are illustrated in figure 1.

2.1   Data Pre-processing

Generating the 2D Subtracted Images. Our source data consists of a bi-plane DICOM sequence of between 15 to 40 fluoroscopic frames of 1024x1024 pixels (2D) showing the injection of contrast liquid in the LA. As can be seen in figure 2 (a), the region of interest (LA and PVs) is not visible under fluoroscopy unless injected with contrast liquid [1]. Contrast liquid cannot be constantly injected during the operation because it is harmful to the patient. It is therefore crucial to process the images taken during the injection in order to get the best approximation of the 2D LA topology. In order to obtain a good delineation of the LA from the background and reduce interference from other image components, a frame that contains contrast liquid is subtracted to a frame that does not. No motion compensation is applied to account for movement between the two time points. The images are downsampled to a resolution of 256x256 pixels in order to speed-up the registration process.

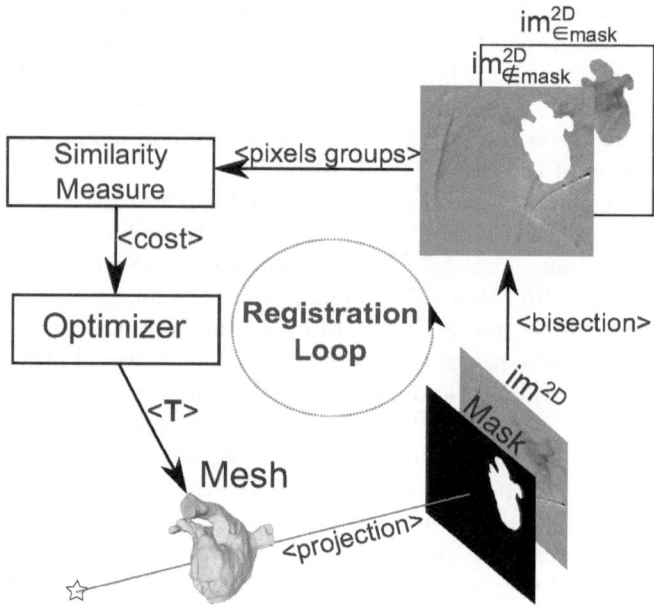

Fig. 1. Overview of the registration algorithm. The mesh is first projected into a mask, which creates a bisection of the 2D image. The cost of the bisection is evaluated by the similarity measure which is fed to the optimizer. The optimizer then iteratively modifies the parameters of the rigid transformation **T** to find the minimum cost.

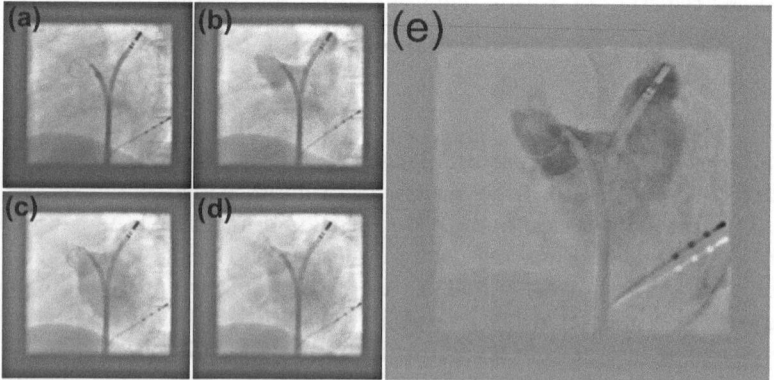

Fig. 2. (a) to (d): Sequence of fluoroscopic images showing the injection of contrast liquid in the LA (frames 0, 10, 19 and 35). (e): Subtracted image (frame 10 - frame 0). Note that the surgical instruments used for EP procedures are present in the images.

Segmentation of the Volumetric Data. In the clinical cases used for this paper, the MRI data was manually segmented into a mesh by a health-care professional.

Mesh Pre-processing. 3D meshes of the LA with attached PVs were used in our experiments. Since the extremities of the small PVs are not visible even during the injection of the contrast liquid, they are manually cut off the mesh before the operation in order to have a better match between the 2D fluoroscopic images and the projected mesh (figure 3).

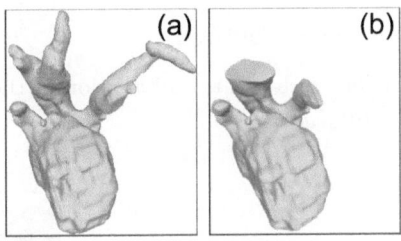

Fig. 3. The LA with PVs mesh, without pre-processing (a) and with shortening of the PVs (b)

2.2   Bisection Using Mesh to Mask Projection

The mesh-derived image bisection method directly uses a mesh extracted from volumetric data to create different *groups* of pixels once projected over a fluoroscopic image. The two groups formed are the pixels that fall under the projection of the mesh ($\in mask$) and the ones that do not ($\notin mask$) (see figure 4). The main insight is that when the mesh is properly *registered*, the grouped pixels will share *common characteristics* because they belong to the same entity (e.g. an organ or a zone that contains contrast liquid).

A projection system is setup in order to transform the mesh into a *mask* that aggregates the pixels in two groups.

$$mask := \mathrm{MaskProjection}(\mathbf{T}, \ \mathbf{P}, \ mesh) \tag{1}$$

where $\mathbf{T} = \{T_x, T_y, T_z, \theta_x, \theta_y, \theta_z\}$ are the extrinsic rigid-body transformation parameter and $\mathbf{P} = \{f, o_x, o_y, s_x, s_y, \theta_y^{biplane}\}$ the intrinsic perspective projection parameters. $\theta_y^{biplane}$ is a rotation parameter centered on the middle of the mesh used to create a second view in cases of biplane registration. The intrinsic parameters $\mathbf{P}$ are determined from the fluoroscopic imaging system and the extrinsic parameters $\mathbf{T}$ are estimated by the registration algorithm. The projection system and the parameters are illustrated in figure 5.

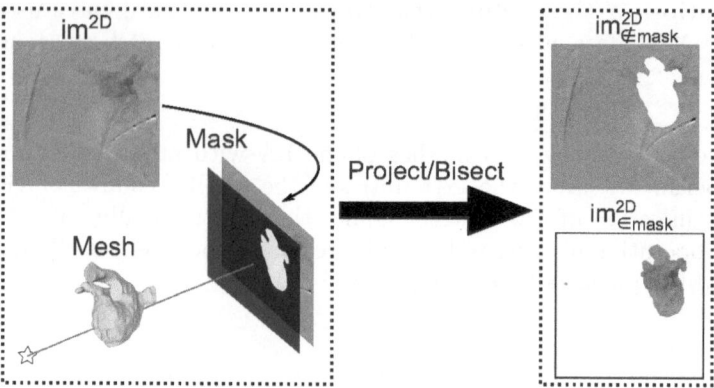

Fig. 4. The projections of the mesh creates a bisection of the image (im^{2D}) into two pixel groups: $im^{2D}_{\in mask}$ and $im^{2D}_{\notin mask}$

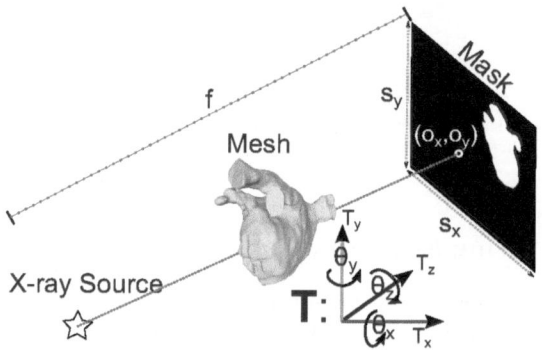

Fig. 5. Projection system used to create the mask from the mesh with extrinsic rigid-body parameters $\mathbf{T} = \{T_x, T_y, T_z, \theta_x, \theta_y, \theta_z\}$ and intrinsic perspective projection parameters $\mathbf{P} = \{f, o_x, o_y, s_x, s_y, \theta_y^{biplane}\}$

2.3   Similarity Measure Driven by Image Bisection

In order to evaluate if the groups of pixels formed by the current mesh pose correspond to a registered mesh, it is necessary to derive a similarity measure that is minimum when the mask is overlaid over the 2D image's target structure and high when over other image regions. The idea to register using pixel groups is inspired by snake methods, where a segmentation is found by iteratively evolving a curve via the minimization of an energy function. The difference in our approach is that the rigid-body parameters $\mathbf{T}$ are iteratively modified instead of the curve's control points, thus *indirectly* changing the contour of the segmentation curve according to the mesh's topology. Another way to see our solution is that it constrains the possible curves to the subset of curves that can be obtained by projecting the mesh.

If one assumes that the target 2D region is relatively homogeneous and markedly different from the other zones of the 2D image, a simple comparison of the average pixel values that fall inside and outside of the mask with the pixels in and out of these groups can be a good indication of the fitness of the position. This is inspired by the cost function of a level-set segmentation approach introduced in [3], which leads to the definition of the following similarity measure:

$$\text{CostFn}(im^{2D}, \ mask) := \sum_{\forall (x,y) \in mask} \left(im_{(x,y)}^{2D} - avg(im_{\in mask}^{2D}) \right)^2$$

$$+ \sum_{\forall (x,y) \notin mask} \left(im_{(x,y)}^{2D} - avg(im_{\notin mask}^{2D}) \right)^2 \qquad (2)$$

where $im_{(x,y)}^{2D}$ is the intensity value of the fluoroscopic image at position (x, y) and $avg(im_{\in mask}^{2D})$, $avg(im_{\notin mask}^{2D})$ are the average intensity values for the *group* of pixels inside and outside the mask respectively.

2.4   Finding the Registered Position Using an Optimizer

The complete registration algorithm, illustrated in figure 1, solves the following equation:

$$\hat{T}_n = \arg \min_{T_n} \ \text{CostFn}\left(im^{2D}, \ mask_{T_n} \right) \qquad (3)$$

where $mask_{T_n}$ is a mask created by the projection of the mesh under transformation T_n (equation 1). The 'arg min' is approximated by a *chain* of two Powell optimizers. The first operates over translation only, followed by an optimization over translation and rotation. The solution of the registration is the rigid transform $\hat{T}_n$ applied to the atrial mesh, generating the grouping of pixels on the 2D image that minimizes equation 2.

3   Results

3.1   Experiment Description

Our dataset contains 7 cases (labeled as 'C#', e.g. C200) of CA for AF, each of which has an atrial mesh that was manually segmented from MRI data along with intra-operative biplane fluoroscopic sequences showing the injection of contrast liquid. The biplane intrinsic perspective projection parameters and the ground truth extrinsic rigid-body transformations that register the meshes to the biplane images are found by careful interactive visual examination of the mesh and subtracted fluoroscopic images. The cost function (equation 2) is adapted for biplane cases by summing the cost for each plane. In order to evaluate the accuracy of the registration algorithm, a deviation of the rigid transformation **T** is applied to the ground truth before registration. The deviation is in millimeters/degrees and contained in the interval: $\Delta\mathbf{T}_{deviation} = \{\Delta T_x, \Delta T_y, \Delta T_z, \Delta\theta_x, \Delta\theta_y, \Delta\theta_z\} = \{-15..15, -15..15, -15..15, -10..10, -10..10, -10..10\}$ where 'A..B' signifies a random number between A and B following a uniform distribution.

Both the mean target registration error (mTRE) and mean projection distance (mPD) [4] are used to assess the accuracy of the algorithm. The mTRE is the mean distance between the registered and ground truth points in 3D space and mPD is similar but *after 3D-2D projection*:

$$\text{mTRE}(P, T_{regist}, T_{truth}) = \frac{1}{k}\sum_{i=1}^{k} \|T_{regist}\mathbf{p}_i - T_{truth}\mathbf{p}_i\| \tag{4}$$

$$\text{mPD}(P, M_{regist}, M_{truth}) = \frac{1}{k}\sum_{i=1}^{k} \|M_{regist}\mathbf{p}_i - M_{truth}\mathbf{p}_i\| \tag{5}$$

where $P = \{\mathbf{p}_1, \ldots, \mathbf{p}_k\}$ are the mesh's vertices (typically $k \approx 15,000$). T_{regist} and T_{truth} are the rigid body transformation found by the registration algorithm and the ground truth; M_{regist} and M_{truth} the *perspective projection* matrixes (the mPD is understood to be calculated after division by the homogeneous coordinate).

3.2   Experiment Results

Using the experiment parameters described in section 3.1, 100 starting positions randomly deviated according to $\Delta\mathbf{T}_{deviation}$ are generated for every case (total 700 starting positions). After registration, the mTRE and mPD error (equations 4 and 5) are measured in millimeters (mm). Table 1 contains the results of the experiment.

Profiling of the mask generation process (implemented in OpenGL) reveals that it takes 0.4 millisecond on a NVIDIA Quadro 2000M to generate a 256x256 mask. This compares favorably to DRR generation implemented on GPU which takes 15 milliseconds to produce a 256x256 image [5].

Figures 6 and 7 show graphical examples of registration results with typical registration errors. Note that the ground truth is not unambiguously *visually* better than the registered result. This is due to the fact that it is very difficult to discern the LA and PVs' frontier under fluoroscopy, even when contrast liquid is injected.

Table 1. mTRE and mPD error after registration initialized with starting positions derived from the ground truth. The variability measure ($\pm\sigma$) is one sample standard deviation.

Case	mTRE (mm$\pm\sigma$)	mPD (mm$\pm\sigma$)
C037	6.76 ± 2.71	6.04 ± 2.11
C129	5.97 ± 2.18	5.83 ± 2.43
C130	6.37 ± 1.96	7.15 ± 2.07
C135	5.59 ± 2.27	4.87 ± 1.84
C137	5.91 ± 1.15	5.49 ± 1.14
C154	9.55 ± 3.42	8.58 ± 3.53
C200	5.76 ± 2.20	6.12 ± 2.23
Average	6.56 ± 2.67	6.30 ± 2.55

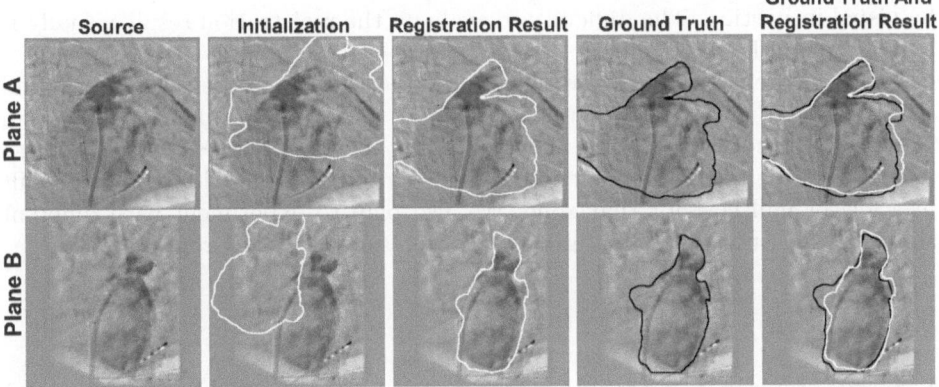

Fig. 6. Case C200 registration result compared with ground truth. The projection distance error for this registration is 7.23mm.

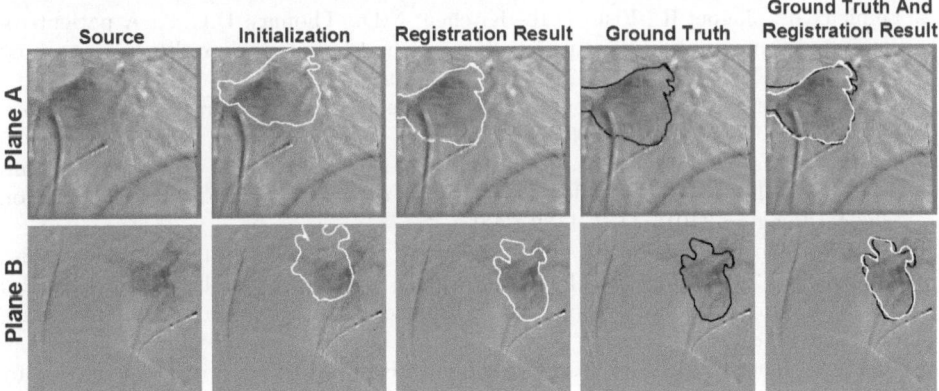

Fig. 7. Case C135 registration result compared with ground truth. The projection distance error for this registration is 4.69mm.

4   Discussion and Conclusion

We presented a mesh-based 2D/3D registration algorithm that can successfully register meshes derived from 3D volumes to fluoroscopic images. The algorithm has the potential to provide near real-time registration. It is especially useful in applications where a 3D mesh is available pre-operatively.

In cases of CA for AF, the fluoroscopic images must contain contrast liquid in order to be used for registration. This means that the algorithm cannot continuously update the registration during the whole operation. However, the registered LA mesh at the time of contrast liquid injection can be used as an initialization for follow-up tracking methods that do not require the presence of contrast liquid [6].

It is not clear if the main source of error is due to the algorithm itself, or to the conditions of the experiment. An important source of error could come from inexact projective geometry and ground truth positions since they were found by visual inspection. The difficulty to evaluate the registration result visually is highlighted in figures 6 and 7.

In the future, we plan to use fully calibrated projection systems and ground truth positions obtained by a medical expert. To get higher precision, we plan to modulate the local cost in function of the mesh's thickness. This will also allow bypassing the manual cutting of the PVs because their thinness will result in a low or null cost for that zone. We also plan to experiment with different similarity measures, including gradient correlation and histogram matching.

References

1. Sra, J., Narayan, G., Krum, D., Malloy, A., Cooley, R., Bhatia, A., Dhala, A., Blanck, Z., Nangia, V., Akhtar, M.: Computed tomography-fluoroscopy image integration-guided catheter ablation of atrial fibrillation. Journal of Cardiovascular Electrophysiology 18, 409–414 (2007)
2. Lemieux, L., Jagoe, R., Fish, D.R., Kitchen, N.D., Thomas, D.G.T.: A patient-to-computed-tomography image registration method based on digitally reconstructed radiographs. Medical Physics 21, 1749–1760 (1994)
3. Chan, T., Vese, L.: Active contours without edges. IEEE Transactions on Image Processing 10(2), 266–277 (2001)
4. van de Kraats, E., Penney, G., Tomazevic, D., van Walsum, T., Niessen, W.: Standardized evaluation methodology for 2-d-3-d registration. IEEE Transactions on Medical Imaging 24(9), 1177–1189 (2005)
5. Miao, S., Liao, R., Zheng, Y.: A hybrid method for 2-d/3-d registration between 3-d volumes and 2-d angiography for transcatheter aortic valve implantation (tavi). In: 2011 IEEE International Symposium on Biomedical Imaging: From Nano to Macro, pp. 1215–1218 (2011)
6. Brost, A., Liao, R., Strobel, N., Hornegger, J.: Respiratory motion compensation by model-based catheter tracking during ep procedures. Medical Image Analysis 14(5), 695–706 (2010)

Inverse-Consistent Symmetric Free Form Deformation

Marc Modat[1], M. Jorge Cardoso[1], Pankaj Daga[1], David Cash[2],
Nick C. Fox[2], and Sébastien Ourselin[1,2]

[1] Centre for Medical Imaging Computing, Department of Medical Physics
and Bioengineering, University College London, UK
[2] Dementia Research Centre, Institute of Neurology,
WC1N 3BG, University College London, UK

Abstract. Bias in image registration has to be accounted for when performing morphometric studies. The presence of bias can lead to unrealistic power estimates and can have an adverse effect in group separation studies. Most image registration algorithms are formulated in an asymmetric fashion and the solution is biased towards the transformation direction. The popular free-form deformation algorithm has been shown to be a robust and accurate method for medical image registration. However, it suffers from the lack of symmetry which could potentially bias the result. This work presents a symmetric and inverse-consistent variant of the free form deformation.

We first assess the proposed framework in the context of segmentation-propagation. We also applied it to longitudinal images to assess regional volume change. In both evaluations, the symmetric algorithm outperformed a non-symmetric formulation of the free-form deformation.

1 Introduction

Non-rigid image registration is a key component of many medical image analysis pipelines. Typically, when performing registration, a floating image is warped into the space of a reference image and the established spatial correspondences can be used to quantify changes through morphometric studies. Tensor-based morphometry, for example, is used to assess differences between different population whereas the Jacobian integration technique [1] aims at quantifying intra-patient longitudinal changes in specific regions of interest. Symmetry in registration is a desired property. Results should be the same when registration is performed from the first image to the second or from the second to the first image. In order to remove bias from the direction of registration, algorithms such as Symmetric Normalization (SyN) [2] from the Advanced Normalization Tools (ANTs[1]) package or the demons-based approaches by Tao et al. [3] or Vercauteren et al. [4] have been proposed. Bias in registration directionality has recently received a lot of attention and shown to generate unrealistic power estimates [5,6,7].

[1] http://picsl.upenn.edu/ANTS

B.M. Dawant et al. (Eds.): WBIR 2012, LNCS 7359, pp. 79–88, 2012.
© Springer-Verlag Berlin Heidelberg 2012

The Free-Form Deformation (FFD) algorithm [8] is a well-known and established method which has been found to perform well for inter-subject registration [9]. It has also been shown to be reliable for longitudinal intra-subject registration [1]. In the last decade, various improvements have been made to the original implementation in order to, for example, ensure one-to-one mapping between the registered scans using either soft constraints on the transformation Jacobian determinants [10] or using hard constraints in the form of boundary conditions [11,12]. The FFD approach is however lacking in symmetry, possibly causing bias towards the registration direction.

Feng *et al.* [13] presented work based on the FFD algorithm where they concurrently optimised a forward and backward transformation in order to minimise the sum of squared differences and a term based on the inverse consistency error [14]. Their implementation however could not be used for morphometric studies as they were only dealing with 2D images and they did not use any regularisation in order to enforce one-to-one correspondences. The proposed work expands the framework in order to obtain a symmetric inverse-consistent registration algorithm. Based on the FFD, we concurrently optimised the forward and backward transformations and penalised both transformations to ensure a one-to-one mapping and generate inverse-consistent and symmetric warping. The normalised mutual information (NMI) is used as a measure of similarity making the algorithm suitable for multi-modal registration.

We assessed our implementation using two datasets. The first part of the validation is based on segmentation-propagation where segmentations were propagated from one subject to another and were compared to manual segmentations that were performed on the same subject. The method was also validated by comparing brain atrophy measurement evaluated in several regions of interest.

2 Method

2.1 Classical Free-Form Deformation Approach

The FFD algorithm is a parametric approach for non-rigid registration of medical images [8]. The transformation $\mathbf{T}$ is parameterised by a regular lattice of control points $\{\boldsymbol{\mu}\}$ and a cubic B-Spline approximation scheme. The normalised mutual information (NMI) is used to assess the alignment between a reference image R and a floating image F after transformation $F(\mathbf{T})$. Maximising the NMI aims at maximising the amount of information that one image has about the other. In order to favor a smooth transformation, one or several penalty terms are added to the objective function. The bending energy (BE) is commonly used but one can also use other penalty terms, for example those based on the divergence of the transformation [15] or on the Jacobian determinant at every voxel position [10], the latter enabling an unfolded and invertible deformation.

2.2 Symmetric Transformation Model

A typical approach is to seek a transformation defined in the space of the reference image that warps the floating image to the reference image space. In order to ensure symmetry, we propose to optimise two transformations: $\mathbf{T}_{Fw}$ and $\mathbf{T}_{Bw}$ where $\mathbf{T}_{Fw}$ is the forward transformation that maps the space of the reference image to the space of the floating image and $\mathbf{T}_{Bw}$ maps the space of the floating image to the space of the reference image. This joint optimisation should reduce directionality bias and increase capture range by using bi-directional gradient in the optimisation procedure.

2.3   Objective Function

In order to ensure inverse-consistency, as in Christensen [14], we used a penalty term based on the inverse-consistency error $\mathcal{P}_{IC}$:

$$\mathcal{P}_{IC} = \sum_{x \forall R} \|\mathbf{T}_{Fw}(\mathbf{T}_{Bw}(\boldsymbol{x}))\|^2 + \sum_{x \forall F} \|\mathbf{T}_{Bw}(\mathbf{T}_{Fw}(\boldsymbol{x}))\|^2 \qquad (1)$$

A $\mathcal{P}_{IC}$ value of zero leads to the following equalities:

$$\mathbf{T}_{Fw} \approx \mathbf{T}_{Bw}^{-1} \text{ and } \mathbf{T}_{Bw} \approx \mathbf{T}_{Fw}^{-1}$$

The computation of the measure of similarity, NMI_{Sym}, also takes advantage of the forward and backward transformation:

$$\text{NMI}_{Sym} = \frac{H(R) + H(F(\mathbf{T}_{Fw}))}{H(R, F(\mathbf{T}_{Fw}))} + \frac{H(R(\mathbf{T}_{Bw})) + H(F)}{H(R(\mathbf{T}_{Bw}), F))}, \qquad (2)$$

where $H(.)$ and $H(.,.)$ denote marginal and joint entropies respectively. Entropies are computed from two joint histograms filled using a Parzen windows approach [16]. The window we used here is a cubic B-Spline kernel.

In order to promote smoothness and to enforce topology conservation we used two other symmetric penalty terms based first on the BE:

$$\begin{aligned}
\mathcal{P}_{BE} = \quad & \sum_{x \forall R} \left\| \frac{\partial^2 \mathbf{T}_{Fw}(\boldsymbol{x})}{\partial x^2} + \frac{\partial^2 \mathbf{T}_{Fw}(\boldsymbol{x})}{\partial y^2} + \frac{\partial^2 \mathbf{T}_{Fw}(\boldsymbol{x})}{\partial z^2} \right. \\
& \left. + 2 \times \left(\frac{\partial^2 \mathbf{T}_{Fw}(\boldsymbol{x})}{\partial xy} + \times \frac{\partial^2 \mathbf{T}_{Fw}(\boldsymbol{x})}{\partial yz} + \times \frac{\partial^2 \mathbf{T}_{Fw}(\boldsymbol{x})}{\partial xz} \right) \right\| \\
+ \quad & \sum_{x \forall F} \left\| \frac{\partial^2 \mathbf{T}_{Bw}(\boldsymbol{x})}{\partial x^2} + \frac{\partial^2 \mathbf{T}_{Bw}(\boldsymbol{x})}{\partial y^2} + \frac{\partial^2 \mathbf{T}_{Bw}(\boldsymbol{x})}{\partial z^2} \right. \\
& \left. + 2 \times \left(\frac{\partial^2 \mathbf{T}_{Bw}(\boldsymbol{x})}{\partial xy} + \times \frac{\partial^2 \mathbf{T}_{Bw}(\boldsymbol{x})}{\partial yz} + \times \frac{\partial^2 \mathbf{T}_{Bw}(\boldsymbol{x})}{\partial xz} \right) \right\|
\end{aligned} \qquad (3)$$

and second on the determinant of the Jacobian matrices of the transformation:

$$\mathcal{P}_{Jac} = \sum_{x \forall R} \log(|\text{Jac}(\mathbf{T}_{Fw}(\boldsymbol{x}))|)^2 + \sum_{x \forall F} \log(|\text{Jac}(\mathbf{T}_{Bw}(\boldsymbol{x}))|)^2 \qquad (4)$$

Note that the penalty term based on the inverse-consistency error does not guarantee folding-free transformations as the inverse-consistency error is minimised but not null.

The final objective function $\mathcal{O}(R, F; \boldsymbol{\mu}_{Fw}, \boldsymbol{\mu}_{Bw})$ to optimise is thus:

$$\mathcal{O}(R, F; \boldsymbol{\mu}_{Fw}, \boldsymbol{\mu}_{Bw}) = (1 - \alpha - \beta - \gamma) \times \text{NMI}_{Sym} \tag{5}$$
$$+ \alpha \times \mathcal{P}_{BE} + \beta \times \mathcal{P}_{Jac} + \gamma \times \mathcal{P}_{IC},$$

where $\{\boldsymbol{\mu}_{Fw}\}$ and $\{\boldsymbol{\mu}_{Bw}\}$ correspond to the control point positions that define the transformation $\mathbf{T}_{Fw}$ and $\mathbf{T}_{Bw}$ respectively and $(\alpha + \beta + \gamma < 1)$

2.4   Optimisation

In order to optimise the objective function value, we used a conjugate gradient ascent approach. It requires the computation of the gradient of $\mathcal{O}$ according to each set of control points:

$$\frac{\partial \mathcal{O}(R, F; \boldsymbol{\mu}_{Fw}, \boldsymbol{\mu}_{Bw})}{\partial \boldsymbol{\mu}_{Fw}} \quad \text{and} \quad \frac{\partial \mathcal{O}(R, F; \boldsymbol{\mu}_{Fw}, \boldsymbol{\mu}_{Bw})}{\partial \boldsymbol{\mu}_{Bw}}.$$

We refer the reader to [17] for an efficient computation of the NMI and BE derivatives and to [18] for the analytical derivative of the Jacobian-based penalty term. The derivatives of the inverse-consistency error penalty term are computed using a voxel-to-node approach where we first compute the derivative of each term at each voxel position and then concatenate the information at each control point position. We perform these computations by first computing four displacement fields through composition:

- $D1_R(\boldsymbol{x}) = \boldsymbol{x} - \mathbf{T}_{Fw}(\mathbf{T}_{Bw}(\boldsymbol{x}))$ where $\boldsymbol{x} \in R$

- $D2_R(\boldsymbol{x}) = \boldsymbol{x} - \mathbf{T}_{Bw}(\mathbf{T}_{Fw}(\boldsymbol{x}))$ where $\boldsymbol{x} \in R$

- $D1_F(\boldsymbol{x}) = \boldsymbol{x} - \mathbf{T}_{Fw}(\mathbf{T}_{Bw}(\boldsymbol{x}))$ where $\boldsymbol{x} \in F$

- $D2_F(\boldsymbol{x}) = \boldsymbol{x} - \mathbf{T}_{Bw}(\mathbf{T}_{Fw}(\boldsymbol{x}))$ where $\boldsymbol{x} \in F$

The residual displacement images $D1_R$ and $D2_R$ are then convolved by a cubic B-Spline kernel in order to reproduce the cubic B-Spline parametrisation of the $\mathbf{T}_{Fw}$ and the residual displacement images $D1_F$ and $D2_F$ are convolved by a kernel that reproduce the cubic B-Spline parametrisation of the $\mathbf{T}_{Bw}$. Using linear interpolation we then extract the gradient information at each control point position $\{\boldsymbol{\mu}_{Fw}\}$ in $D1_R$ and $D2_R$ and at each control point position $\{\boldsymbol{\mu}_{Bw}\}$ in $D1_F$ and $D2_F$

2.5   Implementation

The proposed algorithm has been implemented as part of the NiftyReg package, BSD licence, and can be downloaded from: http://sourceforge.net/projects/niftyreg/. Most symmetric registration implementations require the resampling using a rigid or affine transformation of one image into the space of the other. This enables both images to have the same resolution making the computations easier. It could however bias the registration as different results are obtained depending to which image is interpolated. In the proposed implementation, both transformations $\mathbf{T}_{Fw}$ and $\mathbf{T}_{Bw}$ are defined in the original spaces of the input images and thus no prior resampling is required.

3 Evaluation

3.1 Segmentation Propagation

In order to evaluate the proposed algorithm, we first performed the cross-registration of 40 T1-weighted images from the LPBA40 database[2]. As in Klein *et al.* [9], we quantify the overlap between manually segmented regions of interest and segmentation propagated through registration. This experiment enables direct comparison to the 14 registration algorithms that have been evaluated by Klein *et al.* [9]. The LPBA40 database consists of 40 MRI and their associated brain parcellation into 56 regions of interest. LPBA40 images have been acquired using a 1.5T GE scanner and were used to generate a probabilistic atlas of the human cortical structures [19].

We used a block-matching approach for affine registration in order to initialise every registration [20]. Each non-rigid registration was performed using the proposed symmetric approach as well as using an asymmetric free-form deformation (FFD) implementation in NiftyReg. For every registration, we used a control point spacing of 2.5 millimetres along each axis. This spacing was chosen to replicate the image registration toolkit (IRTK[3]) parameters used in Klein *et al.*, as IRTK is also an FFD implementation. For the proposed approach, FFD-SYM, we set the weights of α ($\mathcal{P}_{BE}$), β ($\mathcal{P}_{Jac}$) and γ ($\mathcal{P}_{IC}$) in equation 5 to 1%, 1% and 10% respectively. The weights for FFD were set to 1% for α ($\mathcal{P}_{BE}$) and β ($\mathcal{P}_{Jac}$). Each registration was performed using a coarse-to-fine approach with 3 levels and the maximum number of iteration for each level was set to 1000.

Figure 1 presents the mean target overlap (TO) defined as:

$$\mathrm{TO} = \frac{1}{N} \sum_{i \forall k} \frac{\mathrm{GS}_k \cap \mathrm{PS}_k}{\mathrm{GS}_k}, \tag{6}$$

where GS_k and PS_k are the gold standard segmentation and the propagated segmentation, respectively, of the kth region of interest and N is the number of regions of interest. The mean (std) target overlap values were 0.650 (0.022), 0.706 (0.025) and 0.714 (0.021) when performing the segmentation propagation using the affine transformation, FFD and the proposed symmetric approach respectively. The symmetric approach yielded significantly higher ($p < 10^{-4}$) target overlap values when compared to the non-symmetric free-form deformation.

---

[2] http://www.loni.ucla.edu/Atlases/LPBA40
[3] http://www.doc.ic.ac.uk/~dr/software/

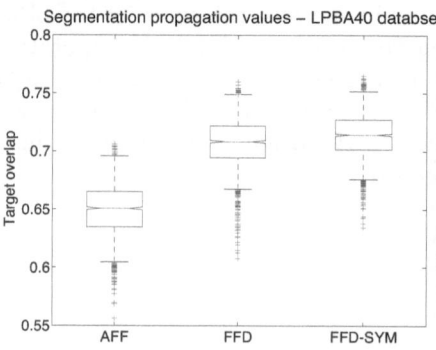
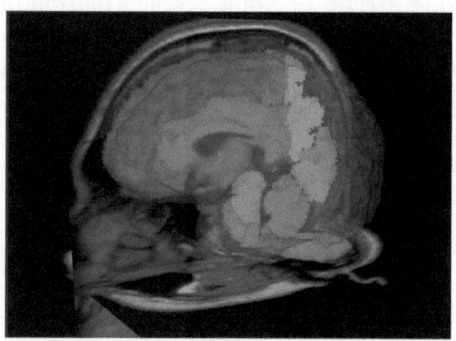

Fig. 1. Left-hand side: Segmentation propagation results. Target overlap are presented after affine registration and two different non-rigid registration approaches, a non-symmetric FFD implementation (FFD) and the proposed symmetric FFD scheme (FFD-SYM).

Right-hand side: Image S01 from the LPBA40 database and its corresponding parcelation.

3.2 Atrophy Measurement

The following experiments are based on a database that consists of T1-weighted MRI scans of 32 subjects with Alzheimer's disease (confirmed with histo-pathology) and 19 age-matched controls. We used three scans for each subject: two back-to-back scans at baseline and one follow-up scan after a year. The data acquisition was performed on a 1.5 T Signa Unit (GE Medical Systems, Milwaukee) with a inversion recovery (IR)-prepared spoiled GRASS sequence: TE 6.4 ms, TI 650 ms, TR 3000 ms, bandwidth 16 kHz, $256 \times 256 \times 128$ matrix with a field of view of $240 \times 240 \times 186$ mm. The first baseline scan and follow-up scan have four manual segmented structures: full brain (white matter plus grey matter), ventricles and left and right hippocampi.

Using the proposed symmetric approach and a non-symmetric FFD implementation, we registered every second baseline scan to its corresponding first baseline scan. As previously, the registrations were initialised using a block-matching technique for affine registration. In order to quantify the amount of deformation, we computed the mean and standard deviation of the Jacobian matrix determinants computed at every voxel position. The Jacobian determinant has the advantage of being unbiased towards any residual error of the initial global registration. The mean (std) in the full brain region of interest for FFD and FFD-SYM were 0.997 (0.006) and 0.998 (0.002) respectively and 0.986 (0.018) and 0.996 (0.011) in the hippocampi regions. Under the assumption that no changes should occur between same day scans, we observed smaller deformations using the proposed symmetric approach when compared to a non-symmetric approach, demonstrating the added value and robustness due to the inverse-consistent constrain.

For the next experiment we registered the first baseline scan of each patient to the corresponding follow-up scan. We also registered the follow-up scan to the first baseline scan. For every registration we assessed the inverse-consistency error and computed the volume change for every region of interest using the integration of the Jacobian map over the regions of interest. We assessed the symmetry of the transformation by comparing the forward transformation from baseline to follow-up with the backward transformation from follow-up to baseline and comparing the backward transformation from baseline to follow-up with the forward transformation from follow-up to baseline. Table 1 presents the inverse-consistency error defined as the euclidean distance between the composition of the forward and backward transformation to the identity transformation.

Table 1. Inverse consistency error. Presented values have been computed from all longitudinal registrations using a non-symmetric (FFD) and a symmetric approach (FFD-SYM).

	IC error (in mm)	Mean values over all subjects		
		mean($\overline{IC}$)	std($\overline{IC}$)	max($\overline{IC}$)
FFD	$\|T_{Fw}(T_{Bw}(x)) - \mathrm{Id}\|$	0.6465	0.1012	0.8991
	$\|T_{Bw}(T_{Fw}(x)) - \mathrm{Id}\|$	0.6498	0.1030	0.9005
FFD-SYM	$\|T_{Fw}(T_{Bw}(x)) - \mathrm{Id}\|$	0.0696	0.0063	0.0864
	$\|T_{Bw}(T_{Fw}(x)) - \mathrm{Id}\|$	0.0698	0.0063	0.0821

Due to order independent construction of the algorithm, no symmetric error was found up to numerical precision, using both single or double floating precision. The proposed method is thus order independent, as for every registration, the forward transformation from follow-up to baseline and backward transformation from baseline to follow-up are identical.

Figure 2 presents the volume changes from baseline to follow-up and follow-up to baseline computed on three regions of interest relevant to Alzheimer's disease: ventricles and hippocampi (left and right hippocampi have been merged into one figure).

In order to assess the symmetry of the method, we performed a one-sample t-test to compare the volume changes computed by registering follow-up to baseline and baseline to follow-up. The confidence intervals and their ranges are shown in table 2.

This confidence intervals show some degree of bias between the values obtained using both the forward and backward Jacobian integrations for every approach. It can however be noticed from the confidence interval that the bias is not only lower but also has a variability range one order of magnitude smaller when using the symmetric approach compared to the non-symmetric approach. Using the proposed symmetric method, the reduced bias towards chosen directionality and the reduced inverse-consistency error lead to an increase in registration robustness, as seen by the reduced number of outliers. It thus results in more realistic group separation estimates. Nonetheless, other sources of bias on both the pre-processing pipeline such as differential bias field and on the manual segmentations still require further investigation.

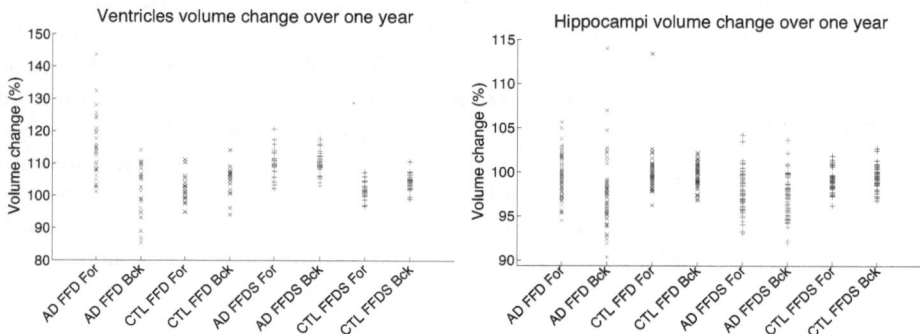

Fig. 2. Regions of interest volume change. The plots presents the volume changes from baseline to follow-up for three regions of interest: ventricles and both hippocampi. The volume changes have been estimated using a non-symmetric (FFD) and a symmetric (FFDS) registration approach and they have been estimated from the registration from follow-up to baseline (FOR) and from baseline to follow-up (BCK). The red and blue crosses correspond to volume change for Alzheimer's disease (AD) patients and for healthy control (CTL) respectively.

Table 2. Confidence intervals of the difference in longitudinal volume changes over the regions of interest estimated through Jacobian integration using both forward and backward transformations

		Ventricles	Hippocampi
FFD	95% CI	[2.2730 11.6473]	[0.6749 2.1020]
	CI range	8.2743	1.4271
FFD-SYM	95% CI	[-1.9593 -1.1673]	[0.0547 0.3497]
	CI range	0.7919	0.2950

4   Conclusion

We presented an extension of the work of Rueckert *et al.* [8] and Feng *et al.* [13] in order to register images without bias towards directionality. Our transformations, forward and backward, are both parameterised using a uniform cubic B-Spline and the normalised mutual information is used as a measure of similarity. The proposed framework has been implemented using a open-source package for registration and is thus available to download under a BSD licence

Using segmentation-propagation to evaluate the proposed method showed the added value of symmetry and inverse-consistency as it leads to increased overlap. We used longitudinal data in order to evaluate atrophy in multiple regions of interest. The proposed approach decreased bias towards the transformation direction when estimating volume changes compared to a non-symmetric approach sharing the same deformation model, regularisation and measure of similarity.

Future work will include a more extensive validation using larger cohort of patients. We also want to apply the proposed algorithm to tensor-based morphometry analysis to quantify the bias towards directionality as in Yushkevich *et al.* [21].

On a more methodological point of view, we will expand the framework to account for multiple time points (more than two) in a common registration framework.

Acknowlegment. The authors would like to thanks Dr Jonathan Schott for his help with the MIRIAD dataset and Tristan Clark for his assistance with the UCL computer science computer cluster. Marc Modat and Sebastien Ourselin were supported by CBRC grant 168. Pankaj Daga was funded by EPSRC-CRUK Comprehensive Cancer Imaging Centre of UCL and KCL (grant number C1519AO). Jorge M. Cardoso was funded by Fundacao para a Ciencia e a Tecnologia, Portugal. Nick C. Fox was employed by University College London Hospitals/University College London, which received a proportion of funding from the Department of Health's National Institute for Health Research Biomedical Research Centres funding scheme. The Dementia Research Centre is an Alzheimer's Research Trust Coordinating Centre and has also received equipment funded by the Alzheimer's Research Trust. Nick C. Fox is a MRC Senior Clinical Fellow and National Institute for Health Research Senior Fellow.

References

1. Boyes, R., Rueckert, D., Aljabar, P., Whitwell, J., Schott, J., Hill, D., Fox, N.: Cerebral atrophy measurements using Jacobian integration: Comparison with the boundary shift integral. Neuroimage 32(1), 159–169 (2006)
2. Avants, B.B., Epstein, C.L., Grossman, M., Gee, J.C.: Symmetric diffeomorphic image registration with cross-correlation: evaluating automated labeling of elderly and neurodegenerative brain. Medical Image Analysis 12(1), 26–41 (2008)
3. Tao, G., He, R., Datta, S., Narayana, P.A.: Symmetric inverse consistent nonlinear registration driven by mutual information. Comput. Meth. Prog. Bio. 95(2), 105–115 (2009)
4. Vercauteren, T., Pennec, X., Perchant, A., Ayache, N.: Symmetric Log-Domain Diffeomorphic Registration: A Demons-Based Approach. In: Metaxas, D., Axel, L., Fichtinger, G., Székely, G. (eds.) MICCAI 2008, Part I. LNCS, vol. 5241, pp. 754–761. Springer, Heidelberg (2008)
5. Thompson, W.K., Holland, D., Initiative, A.D.N.: Bias in tensor based morphometry stat-ROI measures result in unrealistic power estimates. NeuroImage 57(1), 1–4 (2011); discussion 5–14
6. Hua, X., Gutman, B., Boyle, C.P., Rajagopalan, P., Leow, A.D., Yanovsky, I., Kumar, A.R., Toga, A.W., Jack, C.R., Schuff, N., Alexander, G.E., Chen, K., Reiman, E.M., Weiner, M.W., Thompson, P.M.: Accurate measurement of brain changes in longitudinal MRI scans using tensor-based morphometry. NeuroImage 57(1), 5–14 (2011)
7. Fox, N.C., Ridgway, G.R., Schott, J.M.: Algorithms, atrophy and Alzheimer's disease: cautionary tales for clinical trials. NeuroImage 57(1), 15–18 (2011)
8. Rueckert, D., Sonoda, L., Hayes, C., Hill, D., Leach, M., Hawkes, D.: Nonrigid registration using free-form deformations: Application to breast MR images. IEEE Transactions on Medical Imaging 18(8), 712–721 (1999)

9. Klein, A., Andersson, J., Ardekani, B., Ashburner, J., Avants, B., Chiang, M., Christensen, G., Collins, D., Gee, J., Hellier, P., et al.: Evaluation of 14 nonlinear deformation algorithms applied to human brain MRI registration 46(3), 786–802 (July 2009)
10. Rohlfing, T., Maurer Jr., C.R., Bluemke, D.A., Jacobs, M.A.: Volume-preserving nonrigid registration of MR breast images using free-form deformation with an incompressibility constraints. IEEE Transactions on Medical Imaging 22(6), 730–741 (2003)
11. Rueckert, D., Aljabar, P., Heckemann, R.A., Hajnal, J.V., Hammers, A.: Diffeomorphic Registration Using B-Splines. In: Larsen, R., Nielsen, M., Sporring, J. (eds.) MICCAI 2006, Part II. LNCS, vol. 4191, pp. 702–709. Springer, Heidelberg (2006)
12. Sdika, M.: A fast nonrigid image registration with constraints on the Jacobian using large scale constrained optimization. IEEE Transactions on Medical Imaging 27(2), 271–281 (2008)
13. Feng, W., Reeves, S., Denney, T., Lloyd, S., Dell'Italia, L., Gupta, H.: A new consistent image registration formulation with a b-spline deformation model. In: Rosen, B., Brooks, D. (eds.) IEEE International Symposium on Biomedical Imaging: From Nano to Macro, pp. 979–982 (2009)
14. Christensen, G.E., Johnson, H.J.: Consistent image registration. IEEE Transactions on Medical Imaging 20(7), 568–582 (2001)
15. Ashburner, J., Friston, K.J.: Nonlinear spatial normalization using basis functions. Hum. Brain Mapp. 7(4) (June 1999)
16. Mattes, D., Haynor, D.R., Vesselle, H., Lewellen, T.K., Eubank, W.: PET-CT image registration in the chest using free-form deformations. IEEE Transactions on Medical Imaging 22(1), 120–128 (2003)
17. Modat, M., Ridgway, G.R., Taylor, Z.A., Lehmann, M., Barnes, J., Hawkes, D.J., Fox, N.C., Ourselin, S.: Fast free-form deformation using graphics processing units. Comput. Meth. Prog. Bio. 98(3), 278–284 (2010)
18. Modat, M., Ridgway, G.R., Daga, P., Cardoso, M.J., Ashburner, J., Ourselin, S.: Parametric non-rigid registration using a stationary velocity field. In: Zhou, S.K., Duncan, J.S., Ourselin, S. (eds.) IEEE Workshop on Mathematical Methods in Biomedical Image Analysis, MMBIA (2012)
19. Shattuck, D., Mirza, M., Adisetiyo, V., Hojatkashani, C., Salamon, G., Narr, K., Poldrack, R., Bilder, R., Toga, A.: Construction of a 3D probabilistic atlas of human cortical structures 39(3), 1064–1080 (February 2008)
20. Ourselin, S., Roche, A., Subsol, G., Pennec, X., Ayache, N.: Reconstructing a 3D structure from serial histological sections. Image and Vision Computing 19(1-2), 25–31 (2001)
21. Yushkevich, P.A., Avants, B.B., Das, S.R., Pluta, J., Altinay, M., Craige, C., Initiative, A.D.N.: Bias in estimation of hippocampal atrophy using deformation-based morphometry arises from asymmetric global normalization: an illustration in ADNI 3 T MRI data. NeuroImage 50(2), 434–445 (2010)

Fully Automatic Surface-Based Pre- to Intra-operative CT Registration for Cochlear Implant

Fitsum A. Reda[1], Jack H. Noble[1], Robert F. Labadie[2], and Benoît M. Dawant[1]

[1] Dept. of Electrical Engineering and Computer Science
{fitsum.a.reda,jack.h.noble,benoit.dawant}@vanderbilt.edu
[2] Dept. of Otolaryngology-Head & Neck Surgery
Vanderbilt University, Nashville, Tennessee, USA
robert.labadie@vanderbilt.edu

Abstract. Percutaneous cochlear implantation (PCI) is an image-guided surgical approach, where access to the cochlea is achieved by drilling a channel from the outer skull to the cochlea. The PCI requires pre- and intra-operative planning. Computation of a safe drilling trajectory is performed in a pre-operative CT. This trajectory is mapped to intra-operative space using the transformation matrix that registers the pre- and intra-operative CTs. However, the misalignment between the two CTs is too extreme to be recovered by standard registration methods. Thus the registration is initialized manually. In this work we present a method that aligns the scans completely automatically. We compared the performance of this method to the manually initialized registration. There is a maximum difference of 0.19 mm between the entry and target points resulting from the automatic and manually initialized registrations. This suggests that the automatic method is accurate enough to be used in a PCI surgery.

Keywords: Surface registration, feature extraction, level sets, cortical surface, cochlear implant, pre- and intra-operative CT.

1   Introduction

Cochlear implantation (CI) is a procedure in which an electrode array is surgically implanted in the cochlea to treat profound hearing loss. We have recently introduced a minimally-invasive, image-guided CI procedure referred to as percutaneous cochlear implantation (PCI) [1]. In PCI, access to the cochlea is achieved by drilling a linear channel from the outer part of the skull into the cochlea. At present, PCI requires pre-operative and intra-operative planning. In the pre-operative planning phase, a safe drilling trajectory is computed on a high-resolution pre-operative CT scan [2]. This is done a few days before the surgery. In the intra-operative planning phase, the patient is positioned on the operating table in such a way that is convenient for performing the surgery. Then, a CT scan of the head is obtained using an intraoperative CT scanner (e.g. xCAT ENT flat panel volume computerized tomography (Xoran Technologies, Ann Arbor, MI)) and the pre- and intra-operative scans are registered. Finally, the pre-operatively computed drilling trajectory is mapped onto the intra-operative CT

B.M. Dawant et al. (Eds.): WBIR 2012, LNCS 7359, pp. 89–98, 2012.

scan space using the transformation matrix that registers the pre- and intra-operative scans. The pre- and intra-operative scans are registered using intensity-based algorithms after they are manually brought into approximate alignment.

The manual registration initialization is performed by selecting three or more homologous points in each scan. The transformation matrix that registers these points is used to roughly align the scans. We are now working to automate the registration process because: (1) Manually initializing the registration process requires someone who is expert in both temporal bone/inner ear anatomy and in using the planning software to be present at every surgery. (2) The registration step is a time critical process because it must be completed before the next portion of the intervention – creation of a customized microstereotactic frame – can be undertaken. Since this is a critical bottleneck, manual intervention is often stressful. Extra time required to perform this step may prolong the surgical intervention.

Several properties of the intra-operative images obtained with the xCAT scanner complicate automation of the process. While using the xCAT is desirable because it is portable and acquires images with relatively low radiation dose, the images acquired are noisy and suffer from severe intensity inhomogeneity. This diminishes the capture range of standard, gradient descent-based registration techniques. Furthermore, the position, orientation, and field of view of the patient's head in the intra-operative CT are inconsistent. This variation in head orientation alone is larger than the capture range of the image registration algorithm. The inconsistent field of view results in exclusion of regions of the patient's head, which prevents the use of rough orientation matching techniques such as alignment of the pre- and intra-operative images by principal components analysis. Figure 1 shows a typical pre-registered intra-operative image (shown in white and blue) overlaid with a pre-operative image (black and white) in axial, coronal and sagittal views.

We have recently presented a method for coarse registration that is accurate enough to replace the manual initialization process currently used in the intra-operative registration step [3]. This is a feature-based registration method that relies on extracting corresponding features on each image and computes a transformation that best aligns these features. Although this method leads to registration results that are as accurate as the manual initialization-based approach, it cannot be used in the clinical workflow because it still requires some manual intervention and is too slow to be used in the operating room. In this paper, we present a fast and completely automatic approach for pre- to intra-operative CT registration.

2   Methods

2.1   Data

In this study, we analyzed four pairs of pre- and intra-operative CT scans, and one intra-operative reference scan. Typical scan resolutions are $768 \times 768 \times 145$ voxels with $0.2 \times 0.2 \times 0.3$ mm^3 voxel size for the pre-operative images and $700 \times 700 \times 360$ voxels with $0.3 \times 0.3 \times 0.3$ mm^3 voxel size for intra-operative images.

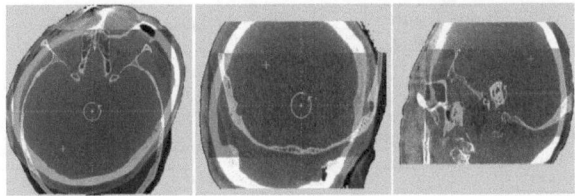

Fig. 1. Intra-operative (blue and white) overlaid on pre-operative (black and white) CT image shown in axial (left panel), coronal (middle panel) and sagittal (right panel) view

2.2 Overview

The approach we follow consists of two main steps. First, we perform a coarse feature-based surface registration using an algorithm that is invariant to initial pose [4]. Next, the registration is refined using a standard intensity-based registration. The coarse registration is performed by matching features computed at the vertices of the cortical surface. This algorithm is sensitive to differences in the field of view of the surfaces, and it is not possible to obtain a full cortical surface from the patient's pre-operative CT because the field of view of these images typically spans only the temporal bone region. Instead of registering the two images directly, we register the intra-operative cortical surface to a reference intra-operative cortical surface, and this reference image is registered offline to the pre-operative CT automatically as described below. Thus, a coarse registration between the pre- and intra-operative CTs can be achieved using the compound transformation. This registration process can replace the manual registration step that is currently performed and, when followed by an intensity-based rigid-body registration to refine the transformation, results in accurate automatic registration of pre- and intra-operative CTs.

A flow chart of the pre- to intra-operative CT scan registration process is shown in Figure 2. In this flow chart, a rectangle represents an operation on images, and a circle represents a transformation matrix when the text is a Greek letter and an image when the text is Roman. P and I are the target pre- and intra-operative images we want to register. IR is another subject's intra-operative scan that we selected to serve as a reference intra-operative image. IR is registered by hand once—offline—to a pre-operative atlas CT A, and A is automatically registered to P in the pre-operative planning stage using standard intensity-based techniques. Thus, using the compound transformation, offline registration between IR and P is achieved automatically prior to surgery. The cortical surface of IR is extracted with a procedure described in section 2.3. In the intra-operative registration step of PCI, the same techniques applied offline on IR for cortical surface extraction are also applied on I to extract the cortical surface. Then, the cortical surface of I is rigidly registered to the cortical surface of IR via a feature-based registration method called spin-image registration [4] described in section 2.4. We combine the transformation matrix obtained from the spin-image registration τ^a and the offline intensity-based registration τ^b. Then, we project I to the

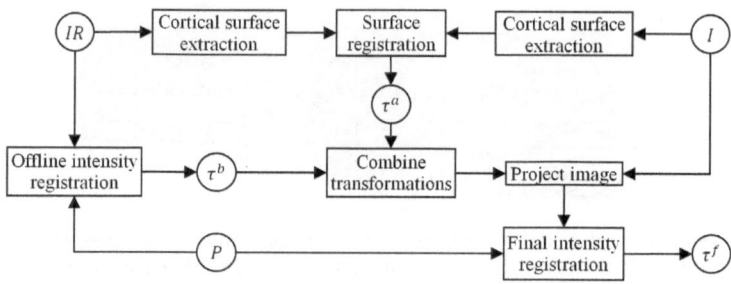

Fig. 2. Registration flow chart

P space using the combined transformation. The final registration of *I* to *P* is obtained by performing an intensity-based rigid registration between the projected *I* and *P*. The full pre- to intra-operative registration transformation matrix is computed as the compounded transformation of τ^a, τ^b and, τ^f.

2.3   Level Set Segmentation of the Cortex

The cortex was chosen as the surface of interest for registration because its surface features are distinct yet similar across subjects. To extract the 3D surface representing the cortex in the intra-operative CT images, we use a level set segmentation method [5]. This method evolves a surface using information from a high dimensional function. The high dimensional time-dependent function, usually defined as a signed distance map, is called the embedding function $\phi(x, t)$, and the zero level set $\Gamma(x, t) = \{\phi(x, t) = 0\}$ represents the evolving surface. The evolution of the surface in time is governed by

$$\frac{\partial \phi}{\partial t} = -|\nabla \phi| \left[\alpha D(I) + (1 - \alpha)\nabla \bullet \frac{\nabla \phi}{|\nabla \phi|}\right].$$

(1)

The term $D(I)$ specifies the speed of evolution at each voxel in *I*, and the mean curvature $\nabla \bullet \nabla \phi / |\nabla \phi|$ is a regularizing term that constrains the evolving surface to be smooth. We designed the speed term that guides the evolution of the surface using the result obtained after applying a "sheetness" filter to *I*, described in the following subsection. The level set method also requires the initial embedding function $\phi(x, t = 0)$ to be defined. We initialize the embedding function automatically with a procedure described below. In the experiments we conducted, α is empirically set to 0.8.

Sheetness Filter. As will be described below, our speed function and our procedure for initialization of the embedding function rely on voxel sheetness scores computed by applying a sheetness filter to *I* [6]. The sheetness filter uses the eigenvalues of the local Hessian matrix to compute a sheetness score that is high for voxels whose underlying iso-intensity surface is sheet-like and low otherwise (for more detailed description on sheetness filter, please see [6]). We limit detection to only include bright sheet-like structures with a darker background. Thus, the sheetness filter will detect

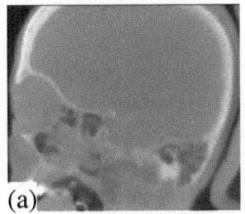 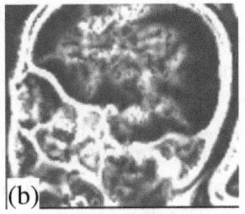

(a)   (b)

Fig. 3. Images used in the level set initialization process. (a) Saggital view of intra-operative C (b) H, the sheetness filter output.

bone as well as some sheet-like soft tissue structures. Figure 3b shows the resulting sheetness score image H of the image I in Figure 3a.

Level Set Initialization. We initialize the embedding function as a signed distance map with zero level inside the cortex and design our speed function to expand until reaching the cortex. Since some parts of the boundary of the cortex have little contrast with surrounding structures, leaking of the level set could occur. To minimize the possibility of leakage, we have designed an approach in which we only propagate the evolving front for a fixed number of iterations (20 in our experiments). We initialize the evolving front such that its distance to the cortex is approximately constant over its surface so that the required number of iterations is consistent.

The procedure we use to identify this initialization surface consists of three main steps that are outlined in Figure 4: (1) A threshold, T_{bone}, that optimally separates the bone from the soft-tissue structures is computed based on the intensity histogram of the image using Reddi's method [7]. However, instead of trying to compute a value for T_{bone} using the histogram of the whole image, which includes several peaks and valleys, we limit the histogram to contain information only from voxels that correspond to bone and sheet-like soft tissue structures, creating a histogram with one distinct valley, and thus simplifying the problem. Specifically, we use the intensity histogram of voxels with: (a) a sheetness score greater than 0.5, which removes information from noisy voxels that don't belong to bright sheet-like structures such as bone and sharpens the histogram so that the valleys are more distinct; and (b) intensity greater than -100, which removes extraneous valleys that exist at lower intensities. The intensity histogram of this set of voxels is shown in Figure 5. As can be seen in the figure, in the limited distribution that we sample, the principal valley is easily identifiable and lies in the middle of the region where the intensity distributions of bone and soft tissue overlap. (2) A rough segmentation of the bone is performed by thresholding the image using T_{bone}. This results in a binary image that contains the skull, some sheet-like soft-tissue structures, and some metal-related artifacts. We filter the segmentation to remove extraneous components inside the cortex. To do so, we

1.	Compute a threshold, T_{bone}, that optimally separates the bone and soft-tissue
2.	Perform a rough segmentation of the skull (bones)
	2.1. Threshold the images using T_{bone} to keep the bones
	2.2. Dilate the resulting image from 2.1
	2.3. Find 8-connected components in a slice by slice fashion
	2.4. Eliminate the components with fewer than 100 pixels
3.	Extract a 3D surface inside the cortex
	3.1. Compute the 3D distance map of the skull segmentation
	3.2. Extract a 3D surface representation of the 6 mm level set
	3.3. Find the second largest connected surface component
	3.4. The result from 3.3 is used to define the position of the evolving front

Fig. 4. Level set initialization process

first dilate the resulting binary image with a spherical structuring element with a diameter of 6 mm. Next, we compute 8-connected components in a slice by slice fashion (we use a 2D rather than a 3D approach to improve computation time). Then, we eliminate the components that have fewer than 100 pixels. (3) A 3D distance map is computed on the resulting binary image. Next, a triangle mesh is obtained by isosurfacing the distance map at 6.0 mm. This mesh contains multiple disconnected surfaces (see Figure 6). The surface with the most triangles corresponds to a distance of 6 mm outside the skull (part of the red contour in the figure). The second largest surface corresponds to a distance of 6 mm inside the skull, and this is used to define the initial position of the evolving front (yellow contour in the figure). Note that the interior portion of the filtered skull segmentation approximates the cortex surface. While this data alone is too noisy to identify and separate the cortex from other structures (see green contour in Figure 6), our technique essentially applies an extreme dilation to the data, which both removes noise and allows a separable surface to be identified that is close enough to the cortex that it can be used to initialize the level set segmentation.

Level Set Segmentation. The speed function is set to $D = 1 - H$, where H is the sheetness score image, which ranges in value from 0 to 1. Instead of defining the speed function using the intensity or intensity gradient type information, which would be very noisy in this application, we use this sheetness score based approach. It consistently assigns low speeds to voxels where there are bones. Thus, the speed function will expand the evolving surface until the zero level set reaches the cortex-bone interface where it will be slowed. Once the speed function is computed, the level set segmentation can be performed. An example segmentation result is shown in Figure 7a, and the 3D surface representation of the segmentation result is shown in Figure 7b.

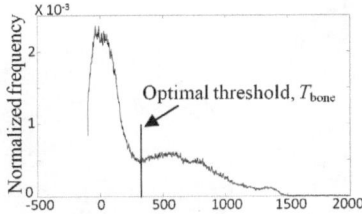 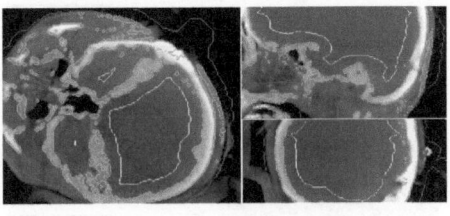

Fig. 5. Intensity histogram of voxels that have both an intensity value greater than -100 and a sheetness value of 0.5. The vertical line is the threshold that optimally separates bone and soft tissue on a global scale.

Fig. 6. Shown in green are the contours of the binary skull segmentation. Contours of the 6 mm level set of the skull distance map are shown in yellow for the second largest surface component and red for all other components.

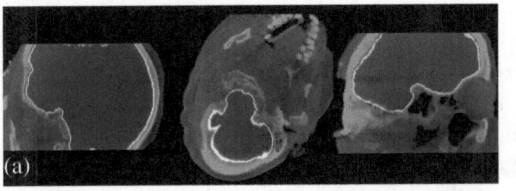 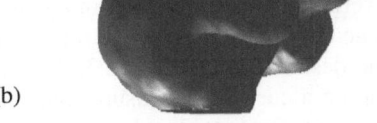

Fig. 7. Result of level set segmentation. Shown in (a) in white are the contours of the cortex level set segmentation result. (b) is a 3D surface representation of the resulting cortex.

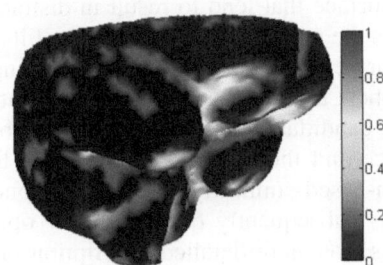

Fig. 8. Reference intra-operative cortical surface. The colors encode the value of curvature on the vertices of the surface.

2.4   Cortical Surface Registration

The first step in feature based registration is feature extraction. We extracted features for each vertex that capture the local shape of the 3D surface using the so-called spin image technique [4]. A spin image describes the organization of neighboring vertices around a vertex in the surface. Given a vertex p in the surface with normal vector $\hat{n}$ and a plane P passing through p and perpendicular to $\hat{n}$, two distances are computed from each other vertex x to the given vertex p: (1) the signed distance in the $\hat{n}$ direction, $\beta = \hat{n} \bullet (x - p)$ and (2) the distance perpendicular to $\hat{n}$, $\alpha = \|x - (p + \beta\hat{n})\|$.

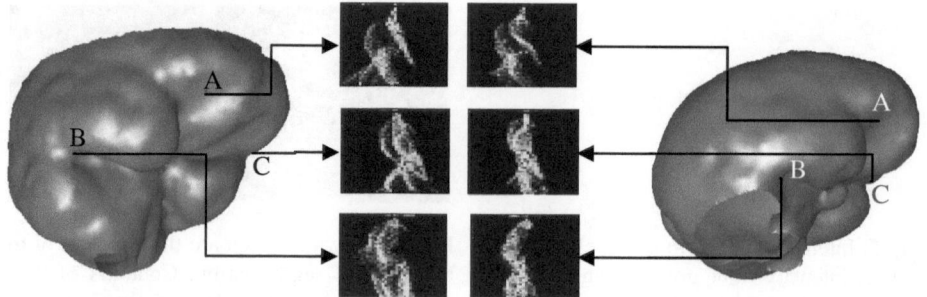

Fig. 9. Cortical surfaces of reference (left) and target (right) intra-operative CT images. Three corresponding points and their associated spin images are shown.

These distances are then used in constructing what are called spin images, one for each vertex. A spin image is a 2D histogram with α on the x-axis and β on the y-axis. Each entry in the histogram represents the number of vertices in a neighborhood of the vertex for which the spin image is computed that belong to that entry.

The cortical surface of the reference intra-operative CT is extracted using the technique described in section 2.3. At each vertex in the extracted reference surface, we compute a curvature measure that ranges from 0 to 1 (see Figure 8) [8]. Then, spin images are computed only at vertices on the reference surface that have curvature value above 0.59. We do this because the regions of the cortex where the curvature is low are those that are flat, and their associated spin images are similar to those of their surrounding vertices. Thus, we increase computational efficiency by using only high curvature regions of the surface that tend to result in distinctive spin images. For the target surface, spin images are computed only for 30% of its vertices (uniformly sampled around the cortical surface) to achieve similar reductions in computation time.

A transformation that best aligns the surfaces is computed by registering corresponding surface points. A candidate correspondence is established between each spin image in the target surface and the set of spin images in the reference surface that satisfy a linear correlation-based similarity constraint. A one-to-one point correspondence between surfaces is subsequently established by optimizing on these sets of candidate correspondences (for more detailed description on spin image registration, please see [4]). Figure 9 shows an example of pairs of corresponding points on a target and reference surfaces and their associated spin images.

3   Results

Each testing pre- and intra-operative image pair was registered with expert initialization or the automatic registration method we propose. Since expert initialization has led to clinically useable results in the clinical trials that have been performed [9], we quantitatively validate our results by comparing transformations computed from our automated technique to those computed using the manual initialization approach. We measured the Euclidean distance between the "entry" (point along the trajectory near critical ear anatomy) and "target" (cochlear implant insertion point) points resulting

Table 1. Distance in millimeters from the entry and target points of the drilling trajectory that is mapped with the proposed registration approach and the previous method [3] which minimize manual intervention to the manually initialized registration

	Patient	1	2	3	4	Average
Proposed	Target point	0.1943	0.0589	0.1215	0.1483	0.1308
approach	Entry point	0.1938	0.0544	0.1234	0.1483	0.1300
Previous	Target point	0.1792	0.0402	0.0211	0.1499	0.0976
approach	Entry point	0.1802	0.0418	0.0209	0.1631	0.1015

from the automatic and manually initialized registration processes. Table 1 presents these distances in millimeters. Table 1 also presents these distances for the registration method we previously developed which minimized manual intervention to one step [3]. The maximum distance for the proposed approach is 0.1943 mm and the average distances at the entry and target points are 0.13 and 0.1308 mm, respectively. These results are comparable to those achieved using our previous approach and suggest that the automatic registration method we propose and the previously presented semi-automatic method are both accurate enough to perform a PCI surgery.

4   Conclusions

PCI surgery requires the registration of the pre- and intra-operative images to map the pre-operatively computed drilling trajectory into the intra-operative space. The field of view and the position and orientation of the patient's head in the intra-operative CT are inconsistent. These differences between the pre- and intra-operative CTs are too extreme to be recovered by standard, gradient descent-based registration methods. In this work, we presented a completely automatic method of pre- to intra-operative CT registration for PCI that is just as accurate as performing the registration using manual initialization. This approach relies on a feature-based registration method that, to the best of our knowledge, has not been used by the medical imaging community. We found this technique to be efficient and accurate.

To quantitatively measure performance, we compared the target and entry points of an automatically registered trajectory to a trajectory mapped using the manual initialization-based approach, which is being clinically validated [9], and we have found a maximum error distance of 0.19 mm. However, since both approaches use the same intensity-based registration approach as the final optimization step and converge to similar results, it is likely that both methods produce equally accurate results. We are currently evaluating the automatic procedure prospectively to confirm this.

We recently presented another method for automating the manual initialization process that also relies on a surface registration component [3]. In that method, feature-based surface registration is performed by matching features on the skull surface. The drawbacks of that method are that the skull surface extraction requires manual intervention and the time required to perform surface extraction is ~20 min. The advantage of the proposed approach is that it eliminates all manual intervention, and it only requires 0.75 min, which is fast enough to be integrated into the PCI workflow since the manual initialization-based approach we currently use typically requires more than 2 min.

One limitation of our proposed registration approach is that it is not invariant to scale. Future work will focus on addressing this issue.

Acknowledgments. This work was supported by NIH grant R01DC010184 from National Institute of Deafness and Other Communication Disorders. The content is solely the responsibility of the authors and does not necessarily represent the official view of this institute.

References

1. Labadie, R.F., Chodhury, P., Cetinkaya, E., Balachandran, R., Haynes, D.S., Fenlon, M.R., Jusczyzck, A.S., Fitzpatrick, J.M.: Minimally invasive, image-guided, facial recess approach to the middle ear: Demonstration of the concept of percutaneous cochlear access in vitro. Otology and Neurotology 26(4), 557–562 (2005)
2. Noble, J.H., Majdani, O., Labadie, R.F., Dawant, B.M., Fitzpatrick, J.M.: Automatic determination of optimal linear drilling trajectories for cochlear access accounting for drill positioning error. Int. J. Med. Robot. Comput. Assist. Surg. 6(3), 281–290 (2010)
3. Reda, F.A., Dawant, B.M., Labadie, R.F., Noble, J.H.: Automatic pre- to intra-operative CT registration for image guided cochlear implant surgery. In: Proc. SPIE, 83161E (2012)
4. Johnson, A.E., Hebert, M.: Surface matching for object recognition in complex three-dimensional scenes. Image and Vision Computing 16(9-10), 635–651 (1998)
5. Sethian, J.: Level Set Methods and Fast Marching Methods, 2nd edn. Cambridge University Press, Cambridge (1999)
6. Descoteaux, M., Audette, M., Chinzei, K., Siddiqi, K.: Bone Enhancement Filtering: Application to Sinus Bone Segmentation and Simulation of Pituitary Surgery. In: Duncan, J.S., Gerig, G. (eds.) MICCAI 2005, Part I. LNCS, vol. 3749, pp. 9–16. Springer, Heidelberg (2005)
7. Reddi, S.S., Rudin, S.F., Keshavan, H.R.: An optimal multiple threshold scheme for image segmentation. IEEE Transactions on Systems, Man and Cybernetics 14, 661–665 (1984)
8. Dong, C., Wang, G.: Curvature estimation on triangular mesh. Journal of Zhejiang University - Science A 6, 128–136 (2005)
9. Labadie, R.F., Mitchell, J., Balachandran, R., Fitzpatrick, J.M.: Customized, rapid production microstereotactic table for surgical targeting: description of concept in vitro validation. Int. J. Med. Robot. Comput. Assist. Surg. 4(3), 273–280 (2009)

Temporally-Dependent Image Similarity Measure for Longitudinal Analysis

Istvan Csapo[1], Brad Davis[2], Yundi Shi[1], Mar Sanchez[3],
Martin Styner[1], and Marc Niethammer[1]

[1] University of North Carolina at Chapel Hill, NC
[2] Kitware, Inc., Carrboro, NC
[3] Emory University, Atlanta, GA
icsapo@cs.unc.edu

Abstract. Current longitudinal image registration methods rely on the assumption that image appearance between time-points remains constant or changes uniformly within intensity classes. This assumption, however, is not valid for magnetic resonance imaging of brain development. Registration methods developed to align images with non-uniform appearance change either (i) locally minimize some global similarity measure, or (ii) iteratively estimate an intensity transformation that makes the images similar. However, these methods treat the individual images as independent static samples and are inadequate for the strong non-uniform appearance changes seen in neurodevelopmental data. Here, we propose a *model-based similarity measure* intended for aligning longitudinal images that locally estimates a temporal model of intensity change. Unlike previous approaches, the model-based formulation is able to capture complex appearance changes between time-points and we demonstrate that it is critical when using a deformable transformation model.

1 Introduction

The analysis of longitudinal images is important in the study of neurodevelopment and its disorders. If global measures are insufficient for analysis, change can be localized by establishing image correspondence via registration. The aim of the registration method is then to find a reasonable geometric transformation between the images according to some similarity measure and a model of spatial transformation. Although longitudinal registration has received some attention in recent years, most of the effort has been focused on the spatial extent of change (various formulations of large-deformation-diffeomorphic-mapping (LDDMM) registration [2,6]) while relying on conservative assumptions about the temporal changes in image appearance.

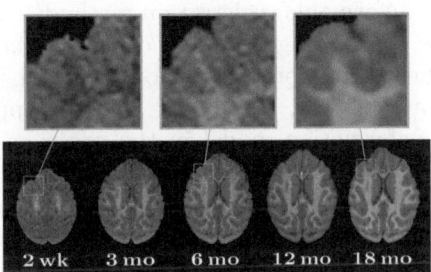

Fig. 1. MR images of the developing monkey brain (2 weeks through 18 months). Unmyelinated white matter in the early stages of development appears darker than the myelinated white matter in later stages.

B.M. Dawant et al. (Eds.): WBIR 2012, LNCS 7359, pp. 99–109, 2012.
© Springer-Verlag Berlin Heidelberg 2012

Commonly used global similarity measures (sum of squared differences (SSD),
normalized cross correlation (NCC), mutual information (MI) [10]), for instance,
expect a one-to-one relationship between the spatially corresponding intensities
(or intensity ranges in the case of mutual information due to histogram binning)
of the different time-points. This is not a valid assumption for certain registration problems. In longitudinal magnetic resonance (MR) imaging studies of brain
development, for example, the biological process of myelination causes a substantial shift in the MR appearance of white matter tissue that is both spatially and
temporally non-uniform [1,8] (Fig. 1 shows MR images of the developing brain).
As a result, deformable registration methods that use global similarity measures
often fail to recover the correct alignment in this setting since inconsistencies
in appearance can be resolved by introducing erroneous local deformations that
are not supported by the underlying structural information [5].

The various approaches that have been proposed for aligning images with non-
uniform appearance change (often for less severe intensity variation arising from
magnetic field inhomogeneities) either (i) locally minimize some global similarity
measure in overlapping subregions that are small enough to have near constant
intensities within tissue types [9,5], or (ii) jointly with registration, estimate an
intensity transformation that makes the images similar [3,7]. While local methods are appropriate for aligning images with spatially smooth and slowly varying
intensity changes within tissue classes, the trade off between registration accuracy and subregion size means that they are inadequate for the strong intensity
gradients seen in myelinating white matter tissue. Intensity transform methods
either have similar spatial limitations due to the slowly varying basis functions
used to approximate the intensity transform [3], or discard spatial information
and therefore cannot capture complex intensity transformations [7].

Here, we formulate a model-based similarity measure (mSM) that estimates
local appearance change over time. Once the temporal model is estimated, existing deformable registration methods can also be used with the model to recover
the correct alignment by changing the appearance of one image to match the
other. After formulating our method in the following section, we first demonstrate in Sect. 3 that MI and our approach both perform well with an affine
transformation model in the presence of non-uniform appearance change, but
then show that using the model-based approach is critical for deformable registration. This method can either (i) estimate the temporal intensity change model
without any prior, or (ii) use a known model for the initial alignment.

2 Modeling Appearance Change

We introduce a spatio-temporal model of appearance change into a general registration framework via a model-based similarity measure. To motivate the model-
based similarity measure consider the standard sum of squared differences (SSD)
similarity term. If a transformation model is involved the SSD can be written as

$$SSD(I_0, I_1) = \int_\Omega (I_0(x) \circ \Phi(x) - I_1(x))^2 \, dx, \tag{1}$$

where $\Phi(x)$ is the transformation that maps the coordinate system of image I_0 to that of image I_1. If we consider the SSD measure a simple model-based registration method, where the image model is simply the given image $I = I_0$, then SSD aims to minimize the squared residuals to this model subject to the sought for transformation. We will therefore consider SSD a special case of a sum of squared residual (SSR) model. With a time-dependent image model and a generalization to multiple images, we can write the corresponding SSR as

$$SSR(\{I_i\}) = \sum_{i=0}^{n-1} \int_{\Omega} (I_i(x, t_i) \circ \Phi_i(x) - \hat{I}(x, t_i))^2 \, dx,$$

where $I_i(\cdot, t_i)$ denotes the measured image at time-point t_i and $\hat{I}(\cdot, t_i)$ the model (estimate) at the same time-point. Note that for two time-points and $\hat{I} = I_1$ the model simplifies to the standard SSD. For simplicity, consider a quadratic (in-time) appearance model

$$\hat{I}(x, t) = \alpha(x)t^2 + \beta(x)t + \gamma(x), \tag{2}$$

where α, β, and γ are spatially varying model coefficients.

2.1 Transformation Model

Assume that we aim to estimate the affine transform of the form $Ax + b$ for each image back to the coordinate system of the model $\hat{I}$ and denote the set of these transformations as $\{A_i, b_i\}$. Then the registration model becomes

$$SSR(\{I_i\}, \{A_i, b_i\}, \alpha, \beta, \gamma) = \sum_{i=0}^{n-1} \int_{\Omega} (I_i(A_i x + b_i, t_i) - \hat{I}(x, t_i))^2 \, dx, \tag{3}$$

resulting in the point-wise linear system

$$\sum_{i=0}^{n-1} \begin{pmatrix} t_i^4 & t_i^3 & t_i^2 \\ t_i^3 & t_i^2 & t_i \\ t_i^2 & t_i & 1 \end{pmatrix} \begin{pmatrix} \alpha(x) \\ \beta(x) \\ \gamma(x) \end{pmatrix} = \sum_{i=0}^{n-1} I_i(A_i x + b_i, t_i) \begin{pmatrix} t_i^2 \\ t_i \\ 1 \end{pmatrix},$$

which amounts to a local fitting of the quadratic model (2) given the current estimate of the affine transformation parameters. Any other model could be substituted here. Note that the image-comparison terms in (3) are strictly with respect to the model (2) which is estimated jointly. Estimation of the model and the affine parameters can then be accomplished by alternating model fitting and transformation parameter estimation steps. In the extreme case one (i) estimates the affine transforms given the current model then (ii) re-estimates the model and then repeats these two steps to convergence. Note also that there is a rotational ambiguity, so one of the coordinate systems should be fixed, e.g., $A_0 = x, b_0 = 0$.

Here, to introduce the decoupled registration and model estimation steps, we started with an affine transformation model. However, the same principle can be applied to more flexible registration methods, such as the deformable elastic registration used for the experiments in Sect. 3.

2.2 Spatial Regularization

Instead of estimating the appearance model parameters independently for each voxel, we can get a more robust estimate by estimating the parameters over subregions of the image, where the subregions are defined on a template (atlas) image. This, however, still leaves the problem of choosing the image subregions. If tissue segmentation is available, one reasonable choice would be to estimate the parameters for each tissue class. Using this approach, for each assumed to be uniform template region R_l the parameter fitting equations for the quadratic case become

$$|R_l| \sum_{i=0}^{n-1} \begin{pmatrix} t_i^4 & t_i^3 & t_i^2 \\ t_i^3 & t_i^2 & t_i \\ t_i^2 & t_i & 1 \end{pmatrix} \begin{pmatrix} \alpha_l \\ \beta_l \\ \gamma_l \end{pmatrix} = \sum_{i=0}^{n-1} \int_{R_l} I_i(A_i x + b_i, t_i)\, dx \begin{pmatrix} t_i^2 \\ t_i \\ 1 \end{pmatrix},$$

everything else stays the same. Here, $|R_l|$ denotes the cardinality of the set R_l and α_l, β_l, and γ_l denote the model parameters valid (constant) on R_l. This approach, however, assumes that the intensity change within a tissue class is spatially uniform.

2.3 Model Parameter Estimation

For the current implementation of the method spatial regularization of the model parameters was achieved by a subregion based approach shown in Fig. 2. Since the intensity change in the white matter occurs dominantly in the posterior-anterior (PA) direction (see Fig. 3) we chose subregions, R_l, that span across the white matter perpendicular to the posterior-anterior direction. So far, this is the same as the subregion method described above. However, instead of estimating the model parameters from R_l only, we use a neighborhood N_l of width w centered on R_l and use robust statistics to estimate the model parameters for R_l. The neighborhoods for

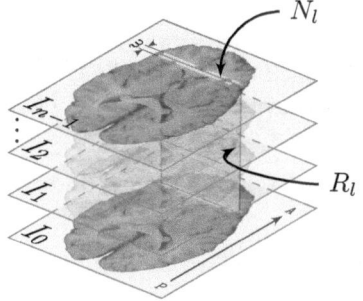

Fig. 2. Subregion based model estimation. Each subregion R_l (red) is defined on the available white matter segmentation (usually at the last-time point). The subregions are perpendicular to the PA direction. The model parameters for R_l are estimated from a neighborhood N_l of width w (yellow).

adjacent R_l are overlapping and therefore encourage spatial regularization in the posterior-anterior direction.

Estimation of the model and affine parameters can be accomplished by alternating the model fitting and transformation parameter estimation steps. In the extreme case we can first estimate the transformation given the model as a separate registration step and then re-estimate the model and repeat these two steps until convergence. In fact, taking this idea even further, one can change the appearance of the estimated image according to the model and use any registration method to estimate the transformation parameters. Here, we use the latter approach which allows the testing of existing registration algorithms with mSM. The algorithm for iterative registration and estimation is is set up as follows:

0) Initialize model $(\hat{I})$ parameters to $\alpha = \alpha_0$, $\beta = \beta_0$, $\gamma = \gamma_0$.
1) Affinely pre-register images $\{I_i\}$ to $\hat{I}$.
2) Estimate the appearance of $\hat{I}$ at times $\{t_i\}$, giving $\{\hat{I}(t_i)\}$.
3) Estimate displacement fields $\{u_i\}$ by registering images $\{I_i\}$ to $\{\hat{I}(t_i)\}$.
4) Estimate model parameters α, β, γ from the registered images $\{I_i \circ u_i\}$
5) Repeat from step 2 until convergence.

Convergence was achieved when the change in the registration energy function between iterations was below tolerance (typically less than 5 iterations).

3   Experimental Results

The similarity measures were tested by registering pairs of 2D synthetic images with a known ground truth transformation between them. The registration accuracy was determined by computing the distance between the ground truth and the recovered transformation. The root mean squared (RMS) error of the voxelwise distance within the mask of the target image then yielded the registration error. All experiments are in 2D, but the method generalizes to 3D.

3.1   White Matter Intensity Distributions from Real Data

An important part of the registration experiments is testing the similarity measures on realistic appearance change while knowing the ground truth deformations. To this end, we calculated the spatial and temporal intensity changes from the MR images of 9 rhesus monkeys during the first 12 months of life. The white matter intensity trajectories acquired from the real monkey data were then used to generate the simulated brain images for Experiment 2 (Sect. 3.3).

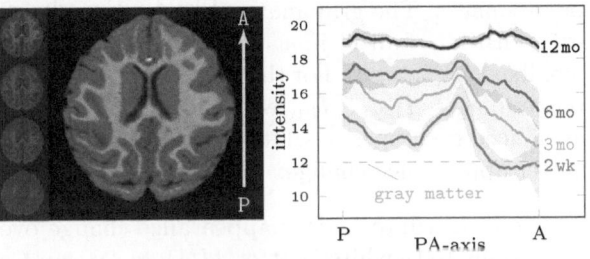

Fig. 3. Spatio-temporal distribution of white matter intensities in 9 monkeys. A single slice from each timepoint is shown in order in the left column (2 week at the bottom), and the white matter segmentation (red) at 12 months is shown in the middle. Plotted, for each timepoint, the mean (line) ± 1 standard deviation (shaded region) of the spatial distribution of the white matter intensities averaged over the whole brain of each monkey in the PA direction. The images were affinely registered and their gray matter intensity distributions matched.

The spatial white matter distributions were calculated for each time-point (2 week, 3, 6, 12 month) of the 9 monkeys. The early time-points have low gray-white matter contrast, therefore the white matter segmentation of the 12 month image was transferred to the earlier time-points (this is often the case for longitudinal studies where good tissue segmentation might only be available at the latest time-point). Due to the few images available at this stage of the study, we averaged the white matter intensity change of the whole brain in a single dimension along the posterior-anterior direction (most of the intensity change is along this direction [4]). Figure 3 shows the mean and variation of the white matter intensity profiles from all four time-points. Myelination starts in the posterior and central regions of the white matter and continues towards the periphery and, dominantly, towards the anterior and posterior regions. These findings agree with existing studies on myelination [4]. Of note is the strong white matter intensity gradient in the early time-points due to the varying onset and speed of the myelination process.

3.2   Experiment 1: Synthetic Data

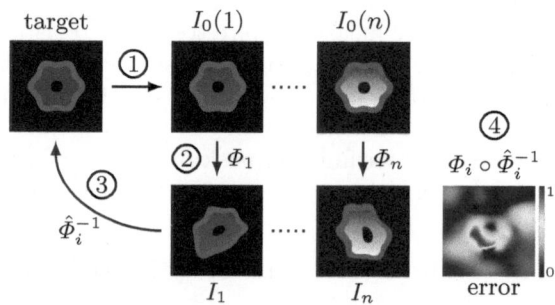

In this experiment, we created sets of 64×64 2D synthetic images. Each set consisted of 11 time-points (I_i, $i = 0, \ldots, 10$). I_0 was designated as the target image and all subsequent time-points as the source images. The gray matter intensities of all 11 images were fixed ($I_i^{gm} = 80$). For the source images, $I_1, \ldots, I_{10}$, we introduced two types of white matter appearance change:

Fig. 4. Experimental setup: 1) Increasing white matter intensity gradient is added to the target, I_0. 2) Adding known random deformations yields the source images, 3) which are registered back to the target. 4) Registration error is calculated from the known (Φ_i) and recovered ($\hat{\Phi}_i^{-1}$) transformations.

i) Uniform white matter appearance change over time, starting as dark (unmyelinated) white matter ($I_1^{wm} = 20$) and gradually brightening (myelinated) white matter ($I_{10}^{wm} = 180$) resulting in contrast inversion between gray and white matter. The target white matter intensity was set to 100.

ii) White matter intensity gradient along the posterior-anterior direction with increasing gradient magnitude over time. The target image had uniform white matter ($I_0^{wm} = 50$). For the source images the intensity gradient magnitude increased from 1 to 7 intensity units per pixel (giving $I_1^{wm} = \{50, \ldots, 70\}$ up to $I_{10}^{wm} = \{50, \ldots, 200\}$). These gradients are of similar magnitude as observed in the real monkey data.

We tested the similarity measures for two types of transformation models: affine; and deformable with elastic regularization. Figure 4 shows the experimental setup with deformable transformation model (for the affine registration experiments Φ_i was an affine transform; for the deformable registration experiment Φ_i was a spline deformation with 20 control points). The aim of the experiment was to recover the ground truth inverse deformation, Φ_i^{-1}, by registering the 10 source images to I_0 (giving $\hat{\Phi}_i^{-1}$) with each of the four similarity measures (SSD, NCC, MI, mSM). We repeated each experiment 100 times for each transformation model with different random deformations giving a total of 16000 registrations (2 white matter change × 2 transformation model × 10 source image × 4 measure × 100 experiment). Significance was calculated with Welch's t-test (assuming normal distributions, but unequal variances) at a significance level of $p < 0.01$.

Note that the synthetic images have longitudinal intensity changes over time, but the random spatial deformations do not have a temporal model. This is intended to be a challenging scenario for the parameter estimation, as true longitudinal data is much less spatially variable, and avoid bias towards any particular longitudinal growth model. Next, we describe the results of the experiments for each transformation model.

Affine Transformation Model. Affine registration is often appropriate for images from the same adult subject. In our case, it is only a preprocessing step to roughly align the images before a more flexible, deformable registration. Nevertheless, the initial alignment can greatly affect the initial model estimation and the subsequent deformable solution. Therefore we first investigate the sensitivity of affine registration to white matter appearance changes separately from deformable registration.

Figure 5 shows the results for registering I_1 through I_{10} to the target image I_0 from multiple sets ($n = 100$, giving 1000 pair-wise registrations for each similarity measure) of longitudinal images with both uniform and gradient spatial white matter intensity profiles. A registration error of less than 1 voxel can be considered good alignment.

With uniform white matter, all four measures performed well when the contrast of the source image was close to the contrast of the target image (near 0 white matter intensity difference in the first plot of the median root means squared registration error). The results for the gradient white matter profiles show that the performance of both SSD and NCC declined as the gradient magnitude increased, while MI and mSM aligned the images well even with the strongest gradient. Overall, mSM significantly outperformed SSD and NCC but not MI, however, for individual time-points mSM did significantly better for $3, \ldots, 10$.

The experiments suggest that affine registration can be reliably achieved by MI or mSM, but for simplicity MI should be used if affine alignment is the only objective.

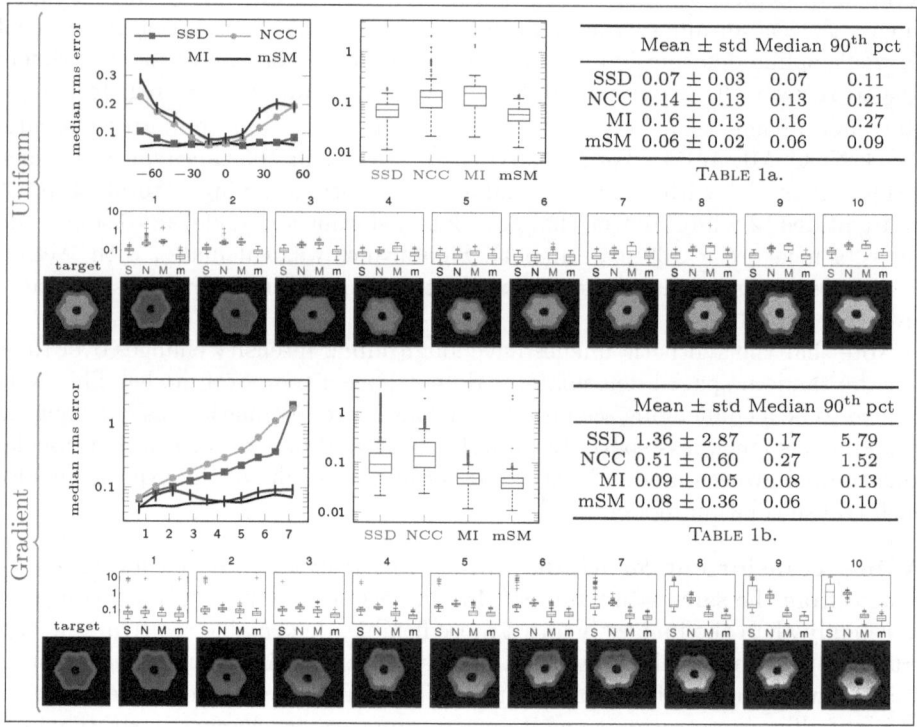

Fig. 5. Results for Experiment 1 with affine transformation, uniform and gradient white matter intensity change. For uniform white matter, the line plot shows the median RMS error vs. the white matter intensity difference between the source and the target images $(I_i^{wm} - I_0^{wm})$ for each time-point (0 means the images have the same contrast). For the gradient white matter, the x-axis of the line plot is the magnitude of the gradient. The boxplots and the tables summarize the aggregate results over all time-points (the box is the 25th and 75th percentile, the red line is the medium, the whiskers are 1.5 × interquartile range, and the red marks are outliers). The small boxplots show results for each time-point (S, N, M, and m are SSD, NCC, MI, and mSM respectively). For each boxplot, the x-label is highlighted in red if mSM performed significantly better than that particular measure. The row of images shows the target and source images for a single trial. Note that all box plots and the bottom line plot have log y scales.

Deformable Registration. Similarly to the affine experiment, Fig. 6 shows the error plots for deformable registrations in the presence of white matter intensity change. For uniform white matter, SSD again produced small registration errors when the contrast difference was small, but fared worse than MI and mSM in the presence of large intensity differences between the target and the source images. mSM performed slightly better than MI for all time-points.

The setup with deformable registration and white matter gradient resembles the real problem closely and therefore is the most relevant. Here, SSD and NCC introduced considerable registration errors with increasing gradient magnitude.

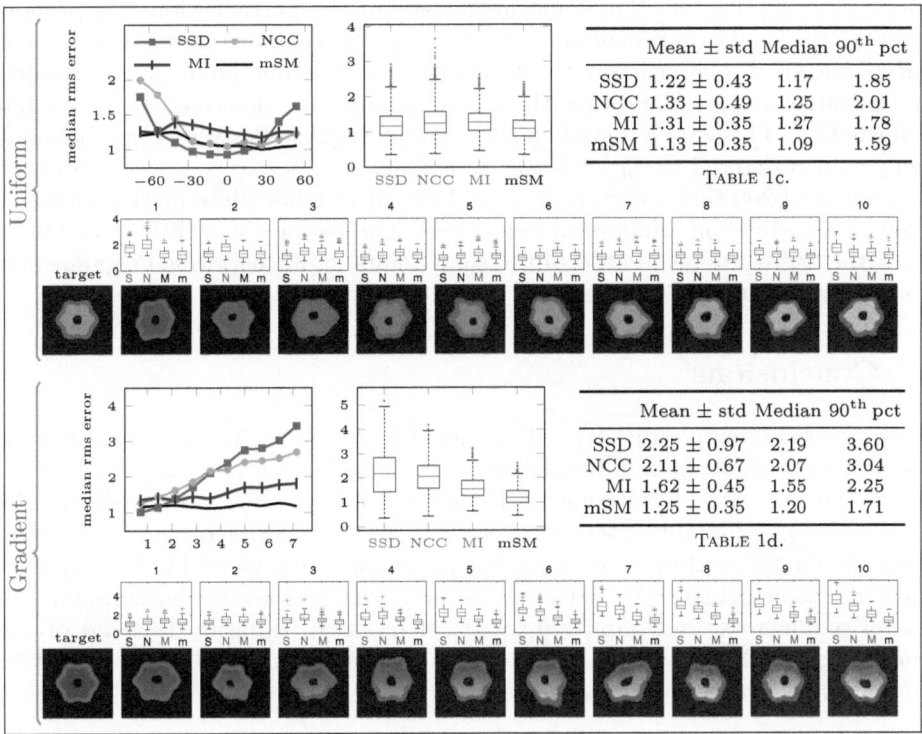

Fig. 6. Experiment 1 results with deformable transformation. The graphs are set up similarly as in Fig. 5 except all plots have linear y scales. The last setup with deformable transformation model and gradient white matter intensity is the most challenging and relevant to the real world problem.

The registration error of MI remained under 2 voxels (mean $= 1.62 \pm 0.45$), while mSM led to significantly less error (mean $= 1.25 \pm 0.35$) for all time-points.

3.3 Experiment 2: Simulated Brain Data

The next set of experiments used simulated brain images with white matter intensity distributions based on the monkey data. Four time-points $I_0, \ldots, I_3$ were generated corresponding to the four time-points of the monkey data. At each time-point, the spatial white

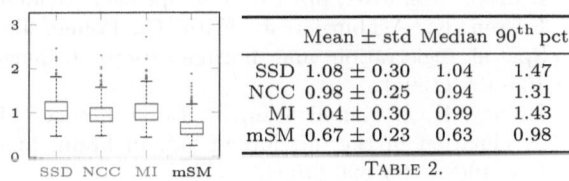

	Mean $\pm$ std	Median	90th pct
SSD	1.08 $\pm$ 0.30	1.04	1.47
NCC	0.98 $\pm$ 0.25	0.94	1.31
MI	1.04 $\pm$ 0.30	0.99	1.43
mSM	0.67 $\pm$ 0.23	0.63	0.98

TABLE 2.

Fig. 7. Experiment 2 results. mSM lead to significantly better alignments than the global measures.

matter intensity distribution of the simulated image was obtained by a random perturbation of the mean monkey white matter distribution for that particular time-point (see Fig. 3). The local magnitude of the perturbation was proportional to the local variation of monkey white matter data, therefore the generated curves had similar variation to the real data. The first time-point was designated as the target image. The other three time-points were deformed by a random deformation. The source images generated this way, similarly to Experiment 1, were then registered to I_0 with the four similarity measures. The experiment was repeated 200 times, each time with different random white matter intensity profiles and different random deformations. The boxplot and Tab. 2 in Fig. 7 show the aggregate results for all the time-points. mSM performed significantly better than SSD, NCC, and MI.

4   Conclusions

We presented a temporally-dependent model-based similarity measure and compared it to three of commonly used measures. mSM performed significantly better in the majority of experiments than the other measures, especially in the presence of considerable intensity gradients. These experiments provide strong evidence for the usefulness of a model based approach. Considerable improvement might be achieved by better model selection, spatial regularization of the model parameters, and improved model of intensity variation (instead of the quadratic model). These improvements and validation on real 3D data will be part of future work.

Acknowledgments. This work was supported by NSF EECS-1148870, NSF EECS-0925875, NIH NIHM 5R01MH091645-02, NIH NIBIB 5P41EB002025-28, U54 EB005149.

References

1. Barkovich, A.J., Kjos, B.O., Jackson, D.E., Norman, D.: Normal maturation of the neonatal and infant brain: MR imaging at 1.5T. Radiology 166, 173–180 (1988)
2. Durrleman, S., Pennec, X., Trouvé, A., Gerig, G., Ayache, N.: Spatiotemporal Atlas Estimation for Developmental Delay Detection in Longitudinal Datasets. In: Yang, G.-Z., Hawkes, D., Rueckert, D., Noble, A., Taylor, C. (eds.) MICCAI 2009, Part I. LNCS, vol. 5761, pp. 297–304. Springer, Heidelberg (2009)
3. Friston, K., Ashburner, J., Frith, C., Poline, J., Heather, J.D., Frackowiak, R.: Spatial registration and normalization of images. Human Brain Mapping 2, 165–189 (1995)
4. Kinney, H.C., Karthigasan, J., Borenshteyn, N.I., Flax, J.D., Kirschner, D.A.: Myelination in the developing human brain: biochemical correlates. Neurochem Res. 19(8), 983–996 (1994)
5. Loeckx, D., Slagmolen, P., Maes, F., Vandermeulen, D., Suetens, P.: Nonrigid image registration using conditional mutual information. IEEE Transactions on Medical Imaging 29(1), 19–29 (2010)
6. Niethammer, M., Huang, Y., Vialard, F.-X.: Geodesic Regression for Image Time-Series. In: Fichtinger, G., Martel, A., Peters, T. (eds.) MICCAI 2011, Part II. LNCS, vol. 6892, pp. 655–662. Springer, Heidelberg (2011)

7. Roche, A., Guimond, A., Ayache, N., Meunier, J.: Multimodal Elastic Matching of Brain Images. In: Vernon, D. (ed.) ECCV 2000, Part II. LNCS, vol. 1843, pp. 511–527. Springer, Heidelberg (2000)
8. Sampaio, R.C., Truwit, C.L.: Myelination in the developing brain. In: Handbook of Developmental Cognitive Neuroscience, pp. 35–44. MIT Press (2001)
9. Studholme, C., Drapaca, C., Iordanova, B., Cardenas, V.: Deformation-based mapping of volume change from serial brain MRI in the presence of local tissue contrast change. IEEE Transactions on Medical Imaging 25(5), 626–639 (2006)
10. Viola, P., Wells III, W.M.: Alignment by maximization of mutual information. In: Proc. Conf. Fifth Int. Computer Vision, pp. 16–23 (1995)

Constant Flow Sampling: A Method to Automatically Select the Regularization Parameter in Image Registration

Benoît Compte[1], Adrien Bartoli[1], and Daniel Pizarro[2]

[1] Université d'Auvergne, ISIT, BP10448, F-63000 Clermont-Ferrand
benoit.compte@u-clermont1.fr, adrien.bartoli@gmail.com
[2] University of Alcala, Alcala de Henares, Spain
pizarro@depeca.uah.es

Abstract. We present a method to automatically select the regularization parameter in the two-term compound cost function used in image registration. Our method is called CFS (Constant Flow Sampling). It samples the regularization parameter using the constraint that the warp-induced image flow be of constant magnitude on average. Compared to other methods, CFS provably provides a global solution at a specified precision and within a finite number of steps. CFS can be embedded within any algorithm minimizing a two-term compound cost function depending on a regularization parameter. We report experimental results on the registration of several datasets of laparoscopic images.

1 Introduction

A warp $\mathcal{W}$ is a parametric function that allows one to register a source to a target image. We here write $\mathbf{q}' = \mathcal{W}(\mathbf{q}; \mathbf{x}) \in \mathbb{R}^2$ the image of a point $\mathbf{q} \in \Omega$ by the warp $\mathcal{W}$ with $\mathbf{x} \in \mathbb{R}^p$ the warp's parameter vector and $\Omega \subset \mathbb{R}^2$ the warp's domain. The optimal warp parameters $\mathbf{x}^* \in \mathbb{R}^p$ are computed by minimizing a cost function containing a data term $\mathcal{E}_d$ and a regularization term $\mathcal{E}_r$ as:

$$\mathbf{x}^*(\lambda) = \arg \min_{\mathbf{x} \in \mathbb{R}^p} \mathcal{E}_d(\mathbf{x}) + \lambda \mathcal{E}_r(\mathbf{x}), \tag{1}$$

where $\lambda \in \mathbb{R}^+$ is the *regularization parameter*, specifying the amount of regularization. Automatically choosing an optimal value for λ is a difficult problem which has not yet received a commonly agreed solution in the scientific community. On the one hand, if the chosen λ is 'too low' the data term will prevail and the warp will overfit the data, including the noise. Consequently, portions of the warp with fewer data will not capture the true deformation. On the other hand, if the chosen λ is 'too large' the warp will be too smooth and will underfit the data.

The general approach to automatically select λ is to construct some test cost function $\mathcal{E}_m : \mathbb{R}^+ \to \mathbb{R}, \lambda \mapsto \mathcal{E}_m(\lambda)$ whose value approximates the difference between the warp estimate at λ and the true image deformation, and minimize:

$$\lambda^* = \arg \min_{\lambda \in \mathbb{R}^+} \mathcal{E}_m(\lambda). \tag{2}$$

B.M. Dawant et al. (Eds.): WBIR 2012, LNCS 7359, pp. 110–119, 2012.

This raises two difficult problems: *(i)* constructing the test cost function from a limited set of data and *(ii)* finding the global minimimum of the test cost function. While problem *(i)* has been well-studied in the literature, problem *(ii)* still lags behind. For instance, the test cost function can be constructed from the paradigm of CV (Cross-Validation) [11] or by combining landmarks and dense intensity-based error measurements [5]. In any case, *the test cost function is always nonlinear and nonconvex*, making problem *(ii)* extremely difficult to solve efficiently and with guarantees of optimality on the estimated solution. Current approaches use general purpose nonlinear optimization methods such as golden-section search and gradient descent, which cannot cope with the extremely nonlinear behaviour of test cost functions such as Ordinary-CV.

We propose CFS (Constant Flow Sampling), a novel approach to the problem of finding λ by optimizing $\mathcal{E}_m$. The key idea is to sample values of λ over the range of admissible values. The difficulties are obviously to find an upper bound λ_{init} and to sample in such a way that the test cost function's global minimum is not overlooked. Defining an a priori sampling scheme, with regular spacing within the space of λ is not relevant, since $\mathcal{E}_m$ is typically almost constant for 'large' values of λ, and may oscillate for 'small' values of λ. CFS proceeds as follows. We first compute an initial value λ_{init} of λ large enough so that the corresponding warp be the $\lambda \to \infty$ asymptotically regularized warp that minimizes the regularization term. We then sample λ between this initial value λ_{init} and 0. Our key contribution is to sample λ regularly with respect to the magnitude of the flow induced by the warp. More specifically, we select the decrease δ such that the average magnitude of the flow between the warp at λ and at $\lambda - \delta$ be some fixed constant $\tau \in \mathbb{R}^+$. The value of τ is expressed in number of pixels and is thus easily fixed. We typically choose $\tau = 1$ pixel. With CFS, λ undergoes large decreases at the early steps since $\mathcal{E}_m$'s graph is typically flat, and smaller decreases around the global minimum of $\mathcal{E}_m$. Our algorithm is thus guaranteed to sample the range of admissible values of λ evenly and in a finite number of steps. The global minimum is found, assuming that the test cost function is convex within a small region, the size of which being related to the chosen flow magnitude constant τ.

Paper Organization. We review the state of the art in §2. We present our CFS method and algorithm in §3. We give experimental results in §4. We finally conclude in §5.

2   State of the Art

The hyperparameter λ is often manually selected by trial and error [3,6]. Here we will describe some methods used to select it automatically.

2.1   Defining the Test Cost Function

The problem of constructing the test cost function $\mathcal{E}_m$ from a limited set of data has been well studied and several criteria have been proposed. The input is a set of n point matches $\{\mathbf{q}_k \leftrightarrow \mathbf{q}_k'\}_{k=1,\ldots,n}$.

The first three criteria are feature-based; they are applicable only when 'enough' point matches are available. The fourth criterion is pixel-based; it uses all the raw information available from the images.

Training/Test Splitting (TTS). TTS is the simplest criterion. It consists in splitting the dataset into a training set used for the optimization of the warp parameters given λ and a test set used for the optimization of λ. It is a classical approach in statistical learning [8]. Let $\{\mathbf{r}_k \leftrightarrow \mathbf{r}'_k\}_{k=1,\ldots,n_{test}}$ be points matches forming the test set (a subset of the input point matches) and $\mathbf{x}^*_{train}(\lambda)$ the warp parameters obtained using the training set. The TTS score $\mathcal{E}^{TTS}_m$ is defined by:

$$\mathcal{E}^{TTS}_m(\lambda) = \frac{1}{n_{test}} \sum_{k=1}^{n_{test}} \left\| \mathbf{r}'_k - \mathcal{W}\left(\mathbf{r}_k; \mathbf{x}^*_{train}(\lambda)\right) \right\|^2. \tag{3}$$

Ordinary-CV (OCV). OCV is also based on a partition of the dataset. Each point is used in turn as a test set while the others form the training set. For a given regularization parameter λ, let $\mathbf{x}^*_{(k)}(\lambda)$ be the warp parameters estimated from the data with the k-th point left out. The OCV score $\mathcal{E}^{OCV}_m$ is defined by:

$$\mathcal{E}^{OCV}_m(\lambda) = \frac{1}{n} \sum_{k=1}^{n} \left\| \mathbf{q}'_k - \mathcal{W}\left(\mathbf{q}_k; \mathbf{x}^*_{(k)}(\lambda)\right) \right\|^2. \tag{4}$$

This score has been used in [1,7]. Its computation time is low thanks to a closed-form solution [11].

V-fold CV (VCV). An alternative to the OCV score is the VCV score. It consists in splitting the dataset into V subsets of nearly equal size, each of them being used alternatively as a test set while the others form the training set. Let $\mathbf{x}^*_{[v]}(\lambda)$ be the warp parameters obtained from the data with the v-th group left out, m_v the number of point correspondences in the v-th group and $\mathbf{q}_{v,k} \leftrightarrow \mathbf{q}'_{v,k}$ the k-th correspondance of the v-th group. The VCV score $\mathcal{E}^{VCV}_m$ is defined by:

$$\mathcal{E}^{VCV}_m(\lambda) = \sum_{v=1}^{V} \frac{m_v}{n} \sum_{k=1}^{m_v} \frac{1}{m_v} \left\| \mathbf{q}'_{v,k} - \mathcal{W}\left(\mathbf{q}_{v,k}; \mathbf{x}^*_{[v]}(\lambda)\right) \right\|^2. \tag{5}$$

This score has been used in [2].

Photometric Error Criterion (PEC). In this criterion, the point correspondences are used as the training set and the photometric information as the test set. Given a regularization parameter λ and the corresponding warp parameters $\mathbf{x}^*(\lambda)$ estimated from the point correspondences, the PEC score $\mathcal{E}^{PEC}_m$ is defined by:

$$\mathcal{E}^{PEC}_m(\lambda) = \frac{1}{B} \sum_{\mathbf{q} \in \mathcal{B}} \left\| \mathcal{S}(\mathbf{q}) - \mathcal{T}\left(\mathcal{W}\left(\mathbf{q}; \mathbf{x}^*(\lambda)\right)\right) \right\|^2, \tag{6}$$

where $\mathcal{B}$ is the set of pixels in the region of interest, $\mathcal{S}$ is the source image and $\mathcal{T}$ is the target image.

2.2   Minimizing the Test Cost Function

The algorithm used to minimize the test cost function is often neglected in the literature. Only a few articles mention the minimization algorithm they use, which can be golden-section search, exhaustive search or downhill simplex [1,5]. We assume that other nonlinear optimization methods, like gradient descent, may have been used. Each of these methods have one or both of the following limitations: the region where to search the minimum is user-defined and the local minimization does not guarantee that the global minimum is found.

3   CFS – Constant Flow Sampling

This section introduces our CFS method and algorithm. We first give general points, then study how to find a constant average flow magnitude decrease δ of λ and how to find an upper bound λ_{init} on λ. We finally discuss some characteristics of CFS.

3.1   General Points and Algorithm

Our CFS is meant to be used with any test cost function $\mathcal{E}_m$ and method to train the warp (or more generally the model) parameters. We thus assume that, given some value of the regularization parameter λ, the corresponding warp parameters $\mathbf{x}^*(\lambda)$ can be found by solving problem (1), and that the test cost function is given. Our goal is here to solve problem (2) with a sampling strategy over λ. The CFS algorithm is as follows:

> **Inputs:** test cost function $\mathcal{E}_m : \mathbb{R}^+ \to \mathbb{R}$, tolerance on the flow $\tau \in \mathbb{R}^+$
> – Choose an upper bound $\lambda_{\text{init}} \in \mathbb{R}^+$ (see §3.3)
> – Set $\lambda \leftarrow \lambda_{\text{init}}$ and $\lambda^* \leftarrow \lambda_{\text{init}}$
> – While $\lambda > 0$ do
> > • Choose the decrease $\delta \in \mathbb{R}^+$ such that the average flow magnitude between the warp with parameters $\mathbf{x}^*(\lambda)$ and $\mathbf{x}^*(\lambda - \delta)$ equals τ (see §3.2)
> > • If $\mathcal{E}_m(\lambda - \delta) < \mathcal{E}_m(\lambda^*)$, Set $\lambda^* \leftarrow \lambda - \delta$
> > • Set $\lambda \leftarrow \lambda - \delta$
> **Outputs:** regularization parameter λ^*, warp parameters $\mathbf{x}^*(\lambda^*)$

3.2   Sampling at a Constant Flow Magnitude

Our algorithm samples λ from its upper bound λ_{init} to 0. For each sample value λ we thus have to compute the next value $\lambda - \delta$ such that the displacement of the warp is constant. We now describe how to compute the flow magnitude at a single point $\mathbf{q} \in \Omega$ between the warps with parameters $\mathbf{x}^*(\lambda)$ and $\mathbf{x}^*(\lambda - \delta_{\mathbf{q}})$. For a decrease $\delta_{\mathbf{q}}$ of the regularization parameter λ, the flow difference constraint between the two parameter vectors is:

$$\|\mathcal{W}(\mathbf{q}, \mathbf{x}^*(\lambda)) - \mathcal{W}(\mathbf{q}, \mathbf{x}^*(\lambda - \delta_{\mathbf{q}}))\| = \tau,$$

where we recall that $\tau \in \mathbb{R}^+$ is the specified tolerance on the flow difference magnitude. We here make the assumption that the warp model being used is linear in its parameter vector (but not necessarily in the point coordinates). This is a common requirement, satisfied by most classical warps such as the Thin-Plate Spline [11], the Free-Form Deformation [10] and others such as Moving Least Squares [9]. The training cost function $\mathcal{E}_d(\mathbf{x}) + \lambda \mathcal{E}_r(\mathbf{x})$ of problem (1) can thus be assumed to be of the form $\mathcal{E}_d(\mathbf{x}) \overset{\text{def}}{=} \|\mathbf{A}\mathbf{x} - \mathbf{b}\|^2$ and $\mathcal{E}_r(\mathbf{x}) \overset{\text{def}}{=} \|\mathbf{K}\mathbf{x}\|^2$. Consequently, we obtain:

$$\mathbf{x}^*(\lambda) = \left(\mathbf{A}^\top \mathbf{A} + \lambda \mathbf{K}^\top \mathbf{K}\right)^{-1} \mathbf{A}^\top \mathbf{b}.$$

We define $\mathbf{a_q} \in \mathbb{R}^p$ to be the lifted coordinates of point $\mathbf{q} \in \Omega$, such that $\mathcal{W}(\mathbf{q}, \mathbf{x}) = \mathbf{a_q}^\top \mathbf{x}$. The flow difference can thus be rewritten as:

$$\left\| \mathbf{a_q}^\top \mathbf{x}^*(\lambda) - \mathbf{a_q}^\top \mathbf{x}^*(\lambda - \delta_\mathbf{q}) \right\| = \tau.$$

This is a high order polynomial in $\delta_\mathbf{q}$. We use Taylor expansion of $\mathbf{x}^*$ around λ to get:

$$\mathbf{x}^*(\lambda - \delta_\mathbf{q}) = \mathbf{x}^*(\lambda) + \sum_{n=1}^{n=\infty} \frac{1}{n!} \frac{\partial^n \mathbf{x}^*(\lambda)}{\partial \lambda^n} \delta_\mathbf{q}^n$$

$$= \mathbf{x}^*(\lambda) + \sum_{n=1}^{n=\infty} \left(\mathbf{A}^\top \mathbf{A} + \lambda \mathbf{K}^\top \mathbf{K}\right)^{-1} \left(\left(\mathbf{K}^\top \mathbf{K}\right) \left(\mathbf{A}^\top \mathbf{A} + \lambda \mathbf{K}^\top \mathbf{K}\right)^{-1}\right)^n \mathbf{A}^\top \mathbf{b}\, \delta_\mathbf{q}^n.$$

An approximate solution is obtained by truncating the above expansion to first order, leading to the following constraint on the flow magnitude difference:

$$\left\| \mathbf{a_q}^\top \left(\mathbf{A}^\top \mathbf{A} + \lambda \mathbf{K}^\top \mathbf{K}\right)^{-1} \left(\mathbf{K}^\top \mathbf{K}\right) \left(\mathbf{A}^\top \mathbf{A} + \lambda \mathbf{K}^\top \mathbf{K}\right)^{-1} \mathbf{A}^\top \mathbf{b}\, \delta_\mathbf{q} \right\| = \tau.$$

This allows us to obtain the following expression for $\delta_\mathbf{q}$ as a function of the current λ and flow magnitude tolerance τ:

$$\tilde{\delta}_\mathbf{q} = \frac{\tau}{\left\| \mathbf{a_q}^\top \left(\mathbf{A}^\top \mathbf{A} + \lambda \mathbf{K}^\top \mathbf{K}\right)^{-1} \left(\mathbf{K}^\top \mathbf{K}\right) \left(\mathbf{A}^\top \mathbf{A} + \lambda \mathbf{K}^\top \mathbf{K}\right)^{-1} \mathbf{A}^\top \mathbf{b} \right\|}.$$

Note that the denominator represents the flow rate with respect to λ. It it of course possible to truncate the Taylor expansion to a higher order. This would lead to a polynomial root-finding problem in a single variable, $\delta_\mathbf{q}$, which can be very easily solved numerically.

In practice, we evaluate the flow for a dense set of points $\mathcal{B} \subset \Omega$ (we use every pixels). Different strategies can be used to select δ. First, the minimum value over all points can be used. This option is the safest by producing a large amount of samples, but still guaranteeing convergence in a finite number of steps. Second, the maximum value over all points can be used. This option will produce fewer samples, and will trade accuracy of the solution for runtime. Third, the average value over all points can be used: this option is a reasonable compromise between accuracy and runtime. Using this third strategy the decrease δ will be:

$$\delta = \frac{1}{\text{size}(\mathcal{B})} \sum_{\mathbf{q} \in \mathcal{B}} \tilde{\delta}_\mathbf{q}.$$

3.3   Finding an Upper Bound

When the algorithm begins, λ generally has a very large value, corresponding to an asymptotic regularization. The corresponding rate of displacement will thus be approximately zero, and will lead to $\delta \gg \lambda$, causing the algorithm to immediately terminate. We thus have to compute an upper bound λ_{init} on λ such that

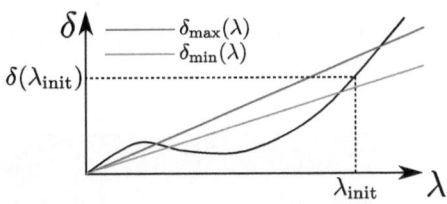

Fig. 1. λ_{init} is chosen so that $\delta_{min} < \delta(\lambda_{init}) < \delta_{max}$

the rate of displacement is large enough to yield a suitable decrease δ in λ. To do this we choose λ_{init} such that $\delta(\lambda_{init})$ lies between two bounds: δ_{min} and δ_{max}. This will ensure that both the rate of displacement of the warp and δ are large enough. We proceed in two steps. First, we start from a high value λ_{max} for λ that we know to be in the asymptotic case (*e.g.* $\lambda_{max} = 10^{10}$). We then iteratively decrease λ by dividing it by 10 and compute δ at each step. We stop when δ is lower than δ_{max} (*e.g.* $\delta_{max} = \frac{\lambda}{2}$). This gives a lower bound λ_{low} for λ_{init}. Second, we check if δ_{low} is greater than δ_{min} (*e.g.* $\delta_{min} = \frac{\lambda}{3}$). If this holds we stop and set $\lambda_{init} \leftarrow \lambda_{low}$. If not, we take $\lambda_{high} = 10\lambda_{low}$ and run a simple bisection search to find λ_{init} such that $\delta_{min} < \delta(\lambda_{init}) < \delta_{max}$, as we can see in figure 1.

3.4   Discussion

CFS has several advantages. First, it guarantees that the estimated λ^* matches the global minimum of $\mathcal{E}_m$ provided that the global minimum is not too sharp for the user defined tolerance τ on the warp-induced flow (*e.g.* $\tau = 1$ pixel). Second, it guarantees that the precision of λ^* with respect to the true global minimum corresponds to the tolerance τ. The trade-off between runtime (less samples) and accuracy (more samples) can be easily specified by changing the value of τ.

4   Experimental Results

4.1   Implementation

In our implementation we use a B-spline warp, also known as the FFD warp [10]. The domain $\Omega \subset \mathbb{R}^2$ of this warp is a rectangle and the warp's shape is controlled by a set of control points which form the warp's parameters.

We present experimental results on two datasets extracted from laparoscopic sequences, with manually-selected point correspondences. For both datasets we tested the TTS and PEC cost functions using the same training set.

4.2 Human Uterus

The first dataset shows a human uterus and has 35 point correspondences, as can be seen in figure 2.

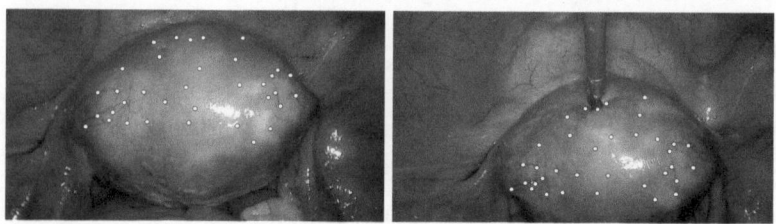

Fig. 2. The uterus image pair with 35 point correspondences

Figure 3 shows the photometric error obtained using PEC. We can see that the photometric error function has several local minima, and that the part corresponding to 'small' values of λ (which is not visible on the linear scale) has many sharp variations that cannot be handled by traditionnal nonlinear optimization methods. Figure 3 also shows the test error obtained using TTS. We found $\lambda^*_{PEC} = 1.256 \times 10^3$ and $\lambda^*_{TTS} = 0.968 \times 10^3$ and the corresponding training errors: $\mathcal{E}^{PEC}_{\text{train}} = 3.787\text{px}$ and $\mathcal{E}^{TTS}_{\text{train}} = 3.657\text{px}$. The average flow difference between the corresponding warps is 1.54 pixels.

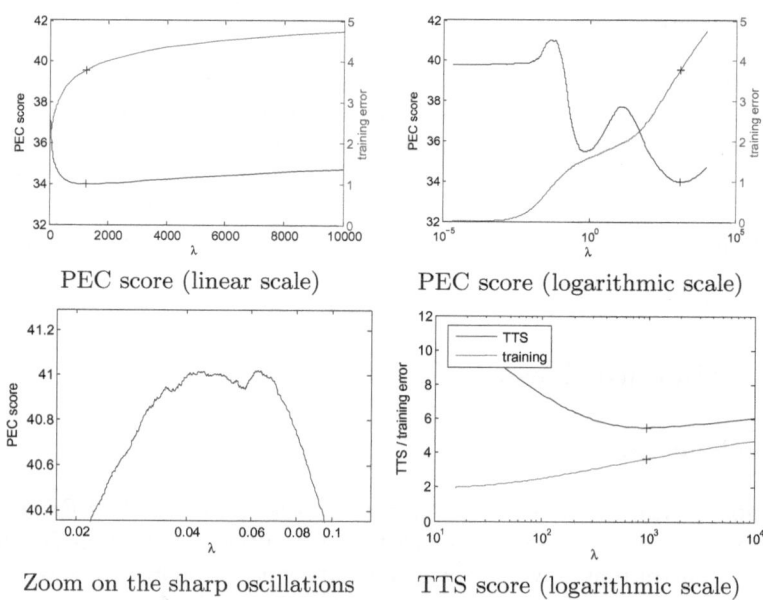

PEC score (linear scale)   PEC score (logarithmic scale)

Zoom on the sharp oscillations   TTS score (logarithmic scale)

Fig. 3. PEC and TTS scores for the uterus dataset

We can see in figure 4 the target points and the warped source points. The difference we can observe is mainly due to the fact that the B-spline warp has difficulties to deal with strong perspective effects like with this couple of images. We could probably obtain better results by using a NURBS warp which has been proved to model perspective better than the B-spline warp [4]. However, the NURBS warp is not linear and would need CFS to be extended to handle that case.

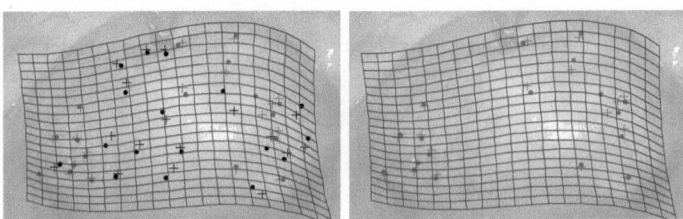

Fig. 4. The deformation grid of the warp, left: TTS criterion, right: PEC criterion, dots: warped source points, crosses: target points, red: training set, black: test set

4.3   Pig Intestines

The second dataset shows pig intestines and has 54 correspondences, as we can see in figure 5. We can see the test error and the photometric error obtained with both tested methods in figure 6. In this particular case, the photometric error seems to be smoother than with the uterus dataset.

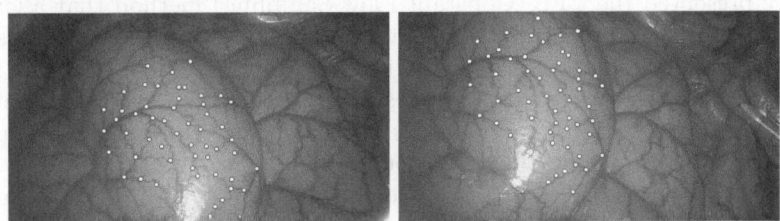

Fig. 5. The intestines image pair with 54 point correspondences

We can see in figure 7 the target points and the warped source points which are really close to each other. On this example we have $\lambda_{PEC}^* = 0.186 \times 10^3$ and $\lambda_{TTS}^* = 0.413 \times 10^3$, with the corresponding training errors: $\mathcal{E}_{train}^{PEC} = 0.3972\text{px}$ and $\mathcal{E}_{train}^{TTS} = 0.379\text{px}$. The difference between these values can be explained by the fact that the photometric error does not vary much near the optimum (optimum: $\lambda_{PEC}^* = 0.413 \times 10^3$, $\mathcal{E}_m^{PEC} = 13.02$; next sample evaluated: $\lambda_{PEC} = 0.141 \times 10^3$, $\mathcal{E}_m^{PEC} = 13.03$).

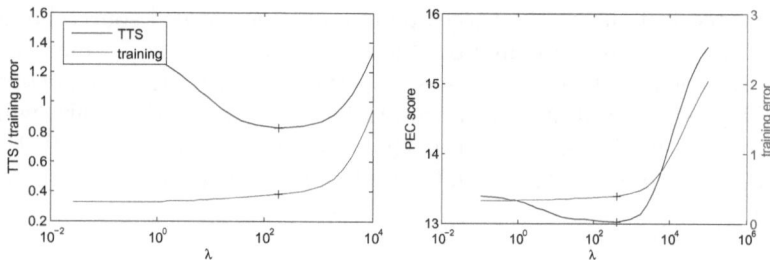

Fig. 6. TTS score (left) and PEC score (right) for the pig intestines dataset

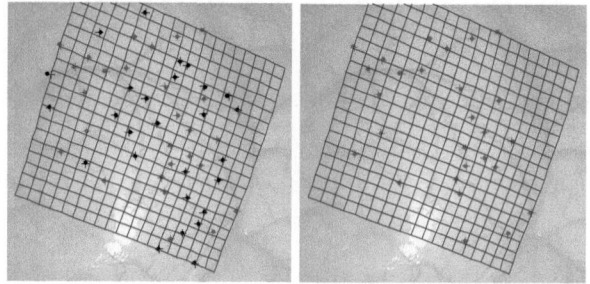

Fig. 7. The deformation grid of the warp, left: TTS criterion, right: PEC criterion, dots: warped source points, crosses: target points, red: training set, black: test set

5   Conclusion

We have presented the CFS (Constant Flow Sampling) method that allows one to find the optimal regularization parameter λ^* of a warp with respect to a given test cost function. It proceeds by sampling the values of λ such that the flow of the warp between two consecutive values is kept approximatively constant. CFS guarantees that the global minimum is found within a user-defined tolerance, under mild constraints on the test cost function. We have successfully tested this method with the photometric error criterion and with the training/test splitting, but it can also be used with any criterion such Ordinary-CV or V-fold CV. A further step will be to implement our method for nonlinear warps, by finding a way to approximate the flow of the warp with respect to λ.

References

1. Bartoli, A.: Maximizing the predictivity of smooth deformable image warps through cross-validation. Journal of Mathematical Imaging and Vision 31(2-3), 135–145 (2008)
2. Brabanter, J.D., Pelckmans, K., Suykens, J., Vandewalle, J., Moor, B.D.: Robust cross-validation score functions with application to weighted least squares support vector machine function estimation. Tech. rep., KU Leuven (2003)

3. Brox, T., Bruhn, A., Papenberg, N., Weickert, J.: High Accuracy Optical Flow Estimation Based on a Theory for Warping. In: Pajdla, T., Matas, J(G.) (eds.) ECCV 2004, Part IV. LNCS, vol. 3024, pp. 25–36. Springer, Heidelberg (2004)
4. Brunet, F., Bartoli, A., Navab, N.: NURBS warps. In: BMVC (2009)
5. Brunet, F., Bartoli, A., Navab, N., Malgouyres, R.: Pixel-based hyperparameter selection for feature-based image registration. In: VMV (2010)
6. Chambolle, A., Darbon, J.: On total variation minimization and surface evolution using parametric maximal flows. International Journal of Computer Vision 84(3) (2009)
7. Farenzena, M., Bartoli, A., Mezouar, Y.: Efficient Camera Smoothing in Sequential Structure-from-Motion Using Approximate Cross-Validation. In: Forsyth, D., Torr, P., Zisserman, A. (eds.) ECCV 2008, Part III. LNCS, vol. 5304, pp. 196–209. Springer, Heidelberg (2008)
8. Hastie, T., Tibshirani, R., Friedman, J.H.: The Elements of Statistical Learning. Springer (2003)
9. Lancaster, P., Salkauskas, K.: Surfaces generated by moving least squares methods. Mathematics of Computation 37(155), 141–158 (1981)
10. Rueckert, D., Sonoda, L.I., Hayes, C., Hill, D.L.G., Leach, M.O., Hawkes, D.J.: Nonrigid registration using free-form deformations: Application to breast MR images. IEEE Transactions on Medical Imaging 18(8), 712–721 (1999)
11. Wahba, G.: Spline Models for Observational Data. Society for Industrial and Applied Mathematics (1990)

Spatial Confidence Regions for Quantifying and Visualizing Registration Uncertainty

Takanori Watanabe and Clayton Scott

Department of Electrical Engineering and Computer Science,
University of Michigan, Ann Arbor, MI 48109, USA
{takanori,clayscot}@umich.edu

Abstract. For image registration to be applicable in a clinical setting, it is important to know the degree of uncertainty in the returned point-correspondences. In this paper, we propose a data-driven method that allows one to visualize and quantify the registration uncertainty through spatially adaptive confidence regions. The method applies to various parametric deformation models and to any choice of the similarity criterion. We adopt the B-spline model and the negative sum of squared differences for concreteness. At the heart of the proposed method is a novel shrinkage-based estimate of the distribution on deformation parameters. We present some empirical evaluations of the method in 2-D using images of the lung and liver, and the method generalizes to 3-D.

1 Introduction

Image registration is the process of finding the spatial transformation that best aligns the coordinates of an image pair. Its ability to combine physiological and anatomical information has led to its adoption in a variety of clinical settings. However, the registration process is complicated by several factors, such as the variation in the appearance of the anatomy, measurement noises, deformation model mismatch, local minima, etc. Thus, registration accuracy is limited in practice, and the degree of uncertainty varies at different image regions. For image registration to be used in clinical practice, it is important to understand its associated uncertainty.

Unfortunately, evaluating the accuracy of a registration result is non-trivial, mainly due to the scarcity of ground-truth data. For rigid-registration, there have been studies where physical landmarks are used to perform error analysis [3]. Statistical performance bounds for simple transformation models have been presented under a Gaussian noise condition [11,13]. However, it is generally difficult or impractical to extend these methods to nonrigid registration, which limits their applicability since many part of the human anatomy cannot be described by a rigid model.

While characterizing the accuracy of a nonrigid registration algorithm is even more challenging, there have been recent works addressing this issue. Christensen et al. initiated a project which aims to allow researchers to perform comparative evaluation of nonrigid registration algorithms on brain images [1]. Kybic used

B.M. Dawant et al. (Eds.): WBIR 2012, LNCS 7359, pp. 120–130, 2012.
© Springer-Verlag Berlin Heidelberg 2012

bootstrap resampling to perform multiple registrations on each bootstrap sample, and used the results to compute the statistics of the deformation parameter [8]. In [6], Hub *et al.* proposed an algorithm and a heuristic measure of local uncertainty to evaluate the fidelity of the registration result. Risholm *et al.* adopted a Bayesian framework in [10], where they proposed a registration uncertainty map based on the inter-quartile range (IQR) of the posterior distribution of the deformation field. Simpson *et al.* also adopted the Bayesian paradigm in [12], where they introduced a probabilistic model that allows inference to take place on both the regularization level and the posterior of the deformation parameters. The mean-field variational Bayesian method was used to approximate the posterior of the deformation parameters, providing an efficient inference scheme.

We view the deformation as a random variable and propose a method that estimates the distribution of the deformation parameters given an image pair and registration algorithm. For illustration purpose, we use the cubic B-spline deformation model and the negative sum of squared differences as the similarity criterion, but the idea is applicable for other forms of parametric model (see [5] for other possible choices) and intensity-based registration algorithms. The estimated distribution will allow us to simulate realizations of registration errors, which can be used to learn spatial confidence regions. To the best of our knowledge, none of the existing methods view the registration uncertainty through spatial confidence regions represented in the pixel-domain. The confidence regions can be used to create an interactive visual interface, which can be used to assess the accuracy of the original registration result. A conceptual depiction of this visual interface is shown in Fig. 1. When a user, such as a radiologist, selects a pixel in the reference image, a confidence region appears around the estimated corresponding pixel in the homologous image. If the prespecified confidence level is, say $\gamma = 0.95$, then the actual corresponding point is located within the confidence region with at least 95% probability. The magnitude and the orientation of the confidence region offers an understanding of the geometrical fidelity of the registration result at different spatial locations.

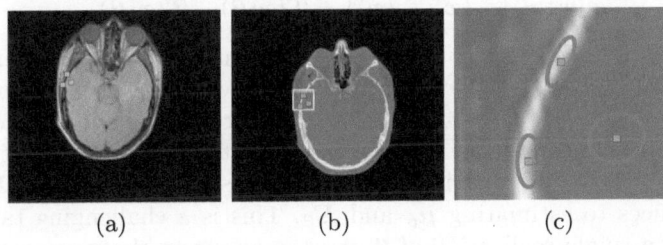

(a)   (b)   (c)

Fig. 1. Conceptual illustration of the proposed method. The marks in (a)-(b) are a few point-correspondences estimated by registration. The confidence regions in (c) offer an understanding of the possible registration error for these pixels. We expect the shape of the confidence regions to reflect the local image structure, as demonstrated in (c).

2   Method

For clarity, the idea is presented in a 2-D setting, but the method generalizes directly to 3-D.

Nonrigid Registration and Deformation Model. When adopting a parametric deformation model, it is common to cast image registration as an optimization problem over a real valued function $\boldsymbol{\Psi}$, a similarity measure quantifying the quality of the overall registration. Formally, this is written

$$\arg\max_{\boldsymbol{\theta}} \boldsymbol{\Psi}\big(\boldsymbol{f_r}(\cdot), \boldsymbol{f_h} \circ \boldsymbol{T}(\cdot\,;\boldsymbol{\theta})\big) \,, \tag{1}$$

where $\boldsymbol{f_r}, \boldsymbol{f_h} : \mathbb{R}^2 \to \mathbb{R}$ are the reference and the homologous images respectively, and $\boldsymbol{T}(\cdot\,;\boldsymbol{\theta}) : \mathbb{R}^2 \to \mathbb{R}^2$ is a transformation parametrized by $\boldsymbol{\theta}$. Letting $\boldsymbol{x} = (x,y)$ denote a pixel location, a nonrigid transformation can be written $T(\boldsymbol{x};\boldsymbol{\theta}) = \boldsymbol{x} + \boldsymbol{d}(\boldsymbol{x};\boldsymbol{\theta})$, where $\boldsymbol{d}(\cdot\,;\boldsymbol{\theta})$ is the deformation. To model the deformation, we adopt the commonly used tensor product of the cubic B-spline basis function β [7], where the deformation for each direction $q \in \{x,y\}$ is described independently by parameter coefficients $\{\boldsymbol{\theta}_q\}$ as follows:

$$d_q(\boldsymbol{x};\boldsymbol{\theta}_q) = \sum_{i,j} \theta_q^{(i,j)}\, \beta\left(\frac{x}{m_x} - i\right) \beta\left(\frac{y}{m_y} - j\right) . \tag{2}$$

The scale of the deformation is controlled by m_q, which is the knot spacing in the q direction. If K knots are placed on the image, the total dimension of the parameter $\boldsymbol{\theta} = \{\boldsymbol{\theta}_x, \boldsymbol{\theta}_y\}$ is $2K$ since $\boldsymbol{\theta}_x, \boldsymbol{\theta}_y \in \mathbb{R}^K$.

Spatial Confidence Regions. Given the image pair $\boldsymbol{f_r}$ and $\boldsymbol{f_h}$, let $\boldsymbol{\Omega}_r \subset \mathbb{R}^2$ and $\boldsymbol{\Omega}_h \subset \mathbb{R}^2$ denote the regions of interest in the reference and homologous image respectively. Also, let $\hat{\boldsymbol{\theta}}$ be the deformation coefficients estimated from registration (1). We will assume that the underlying ground-truth deformation belongs to the adopted deformation class, with deformation parameter $\boldsymbol{\theta}$. Then, the registration error $\boldsymbol{e}$ for pixel $\boldsymbol{x} \in \boldsymbol{\Omega}_r$ is expressed as

$$e(\boldsymbol{x}) = \big(e_x(\boldsymbol{x}), e_y(\boldsymbol{x})\big) = \boldsymbol{T}(\boldsymbol{x};\hat{\boldsymbol{\theta}}) - \boldsymbol{T}(\boldsymbol{x};\boldsymbol{\theta}) . \tag{3}$$

We will view the true deformation $\boldsymbol{\theta}$ as a random variable, which introduces a distribution on $\boldsymbol{e}(\boldsymbol{x})$ for each $\boldsymbol{x}$. The confidence region $\boldsymbol{\Phi}(\boldsymbol{x}) \subseteq \boldsymbol{\Omega}_h$ is a set such that $\Pr\big(\boldsymbol{e}(\boldsymbol{x}) \in \boldsymbol{\Phi}(\boldsymbol{x})\big) \geq \gamma$, where $\gamma \in [0,1]$ is a prespecified confidence level. To estimate the spatial confidence regions, we adopt the following two-step process.

First, we estimate the distribution of $\boldsymbol{\theta}$. We assume $\boldsymbol{\theta} \sim \mathcal{N}(\boldsymbol{\mu_\theta}, \boldsymbol{\Sigma_\theta})$, so the problem reduces to estimating $\boldsymbol{\mu_\theta}$ and $\boldsymbol{\Sigma_\theta}$. This is a challenging task because there is only a single realization of $\boldsymbol{\theta}$, corresponding to the given reference and homologous images, and this realization is not observed.

Second, given the estimates of $\boldsymbol{\mu_\theta}$ and $\boldsymbol{\Sigma_\theta}$, we can then simulate approximate realizations of $\boldsymbol{\theta}$, and thereby simulate spatial errors $\boldsymbol{e}(\boldsymbol{x})$. From this it is straightforward to estimate $\boldsymbol{\Phi}(\boldsymbol{x})$. However, sampling from $\mathcal{N}(\hat{\boldsymbol{\mu}}_\theta, \hat{\boldsymbol{\Sigma}}_\theta)$ is potentially computationally intensive. The total dimension of $\boldsymbol{\theta}$ for the B-spline model is $2K$ in 2-D and $3K$ in 3-D. For a high resolution CT data-set of image size $512 \times 512 \times 480$

with voxel dimensions $1 \times 1 \times 1$ mm^3, B-spline knots placed every 5 mm leads to a dimension on the order of millions. Sampling from a multivariate normal distribution requires a matrix square root of Σ_θ, but this is clearly prohibitive in both computational cost and memory storage. Therefore it is essential that the estimate $\hat{\Sigma}_\theta$ have some structure that facilitates efficient sampling.

Estimation of Deformation Distribution. We use the registration result $\hat{\theta}$ as the estimate for μ_θ, and propose the following convex combination for Σ_θ:

$$\hat{\Sigma}_\theta = (1 - \rho)\Sigma_o + \rho\hat{\theta}\hat{\theta}^T . \tag{4}$$

The first term Σ_o is a positive-definite matrix which is an *a priori* baseline we impose on the covariance structure, and the second term is a rank-1 outer product that serves as the data-driven component. The weighting between the two terms is controlled by $\rho \in [0, 1)$. Note that (4) has a form of a shrinkage estimator reminiscent of the Ledoit-Wolfe type covariance estimate [9], but only using the registration result $\hat{\theta}$.

For the baseline covariance Σ_o, we propose to use a covariance matrix which is motivated from the autoregressive model. Let $\Sigma_{\mathrm{AR}} \in \mathbb{R}_{++}^{K \times K}$ denote the covariance of a first order 2-D autoregressive model, whose entries are given as

$$\Sigma_{\mathrm{AR}}(i, j) = r_x^{|x(i)-x(j)|} r_y^{|y(i)-y(j)|} , \qquad 1 \leq i, j \leq K . \tag{5}$$

Here, $|r_x| < 1$ and $|r_y| < 1$ are parameters that control the smoothness between neighboring knots, and $x(i) = \mod(i - 1, n_x)$, $y(i) = \lfloor (i-1)/n_x \rfloor$ are the mappings from the lexicographic index i to its corresponding (x, y) coordinate, assuming an $(n_x \times n_y)$ grid of knots. A key property of this dense matrix is that its inverse, or the precision matrix $\Theta_{\mathrm{AR}} = \Sigma_{\mathrm{AR}}^{-1}$, is block-tridiagonal with tridiagonal blocks. Specifically, Θ_{AR} has an n_y-by-n_y block matrix structure with each blocks of size $(n_x \times n_x)$, and only the main diagonal and the subdiagonal blocks are non-zero. Furthermore, these non-zero blocks are tridiagonal with the values of the non-zero entries known as a function of r_x and r_y.

Based on Σ_{AR}, we propose to use the following baseline covariance $\Sigma_o \in \mathbb{R}_{++}^{2K \times 2K}$ having a 2-by-2 block matrix structure expressed by the Kronecker product:

$$\Sigma_o = \begin{bmatrix} c_x \Sigma_{\mathrm{AR}} & c_{xy} \Sigma_{\mathrm{AR}} \\ c_{xy} \Sigma_{\mathrm{AR}} & c_y \Sigma_{\mathrm{AR}} \end{bmatrix} = \begin{bmatrix} c_x, c_{xy} \\ c_{xy}, c_y \end{bmatrix} \otimes \Sigma_{\mathrm{AR}} . \tag{6}$$

The coefficients c_x and c_y assign the prior variance level on θ_x and θ_y, whereas c_{xy} assigns the prior cross-covariance level between θ_x and θ_y. The only restriction on these values is $(c_x c_y) > c_{xy}^2$, which ensures Σ_o is positive-definite. It is important to note that the precision matrix Θ_o of this baseline covariance is sparse, also having a 2-by-2 block matrix structure

$$\Theta_o = \Sigma_o^{-1} = \begin{bmatrix} c_x, c_{xy} \\ c_{xy}, c_y \end{bmatrix}^{-1} \otimes \Sigma_{\mathrm{AR}}^{-1} = \begin{bmatrix} p_x, p_{xy} \\ p_{xy}, p_y \end{bmatrix} \otimes \Theta_{\mathrm{AR}} , \tag{7}$$

where $\{p_x, p_y, p_{xy}\}$ are obtained by inverting the 2×2 coefficient matrix. The sparsity structure of Θ_o can be interpreted intuitively under a Gaussian graphical model framework. The conditional dependencies between knots are described

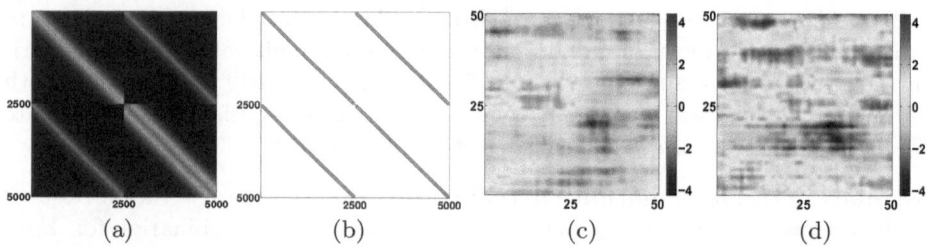

Fig. 2. Illustration of the properties of the baseline covariance $\boldsymbol{\Sigma}_o$. The values used are $(n_x, n_y) = (50, 50)$, $(r_x, r_y) = (0.95, 0.8)$, and $\{c_x, c_y, c_{xy}\} = \{1, 2, 0.5\}$. (a) The baseline covariance $\boldsymbol{\Sigma}_o$, (b) the sparsity structure of $\boldsymbol{\Theta}_o = \boldsymbol{\Sigma}_o^{-1}$, (c)-(d) B-spline coefficients $\boldsymbol{\theta}_x$ and $\boldsymbol{\theta}_y$ obtained from sample $\boldsymbol{\theta} = (\boldsymbol{\theta}_x, \boldsymbol{\theta}_y) \sim \mathcal{N}(0, \boldsymbol{\Sigma}_o)$.

by the non-zero entries in the matrix, which are represented as edges in an undirected graph. For our model, a knot $\theta_x(i, j)$ has 17 edges, 8 connected to its 8-nearest neighbors and the other 9 connected to the corresponding $\theta_y(i, j)$ knot and its 8-nearest neighbors. Fig. 2 provides an illustration of $\boldsymbol{\Sigma}_o$ and the sparsity structure of its inverse $\boldsymbol{\Theta}_o$, along with an example realization of B-spline coefficients $\boldsymbol{\theta} = (\boldsymbol{\theta}_x, \boldsymbol{\theta}_y)$.

Error Simulations and Spatial Confidence Regions. Since the estimate $\hat{\boldsymbol{\Sigma}}_{\boldsymbol{\theta}}$ (4) is a rank-1 updated form of the baseline $\boldsymbol{\Sigma}_o$, we can exploit the sparsity structure of $\boldsymbol{\Theta}_o$ to efficiently draw realizations from $\mathcal{N}(\hat{\boldsymbol{\theta}}, \hat{\boldsymbol{\Sigma}}_{\boldsymbol{\theta}})$ without explicitly storing or computing a matrix square root for the dense matrix $\hat{\boldsymbol{\Sigma}}_{\boldsymbol{\theta}}$. We only need to store the sparse precision matrix $\boldsymbol{\Theta}_o$ and compute its cholesky factor $\boldsymbol{L}_o$, which can be done in $\mathcal{O}(K)$ operations [4]. This allows the sampling procedure to scale gracefully to 3-D.

Using such sampling procedure, we can now generate realizations of registration error $\boldsymbol{e}(\boldsymbol{x})$ as follows:

1. Sample $\boldsymbol{\theta}_i \sim \mathcal{N}(\hat{\boldsymbol{\mu}}_{\boldsymbol{\theta}}, \hat{\boldsymbol{\Sigma}}_{\boldsymbol{\theta}})$.
2. Synthesize reference image $\boldsymbol{f}_r^{(i)}(\boldsymbol{x}) \leftarrow \boldsymbol{f}_h \circ \boldsymbol{T}(\boldsymbol{x}; \boldsymbol{\theta}_i)$.
3. Register $\boldsymbol{f}_h$ on to $\boldsymbol{f}_r^{(i)}$ to get estimate $\hat{\boldsymbol{\theta}}_i$.
4. Compute error $\boldsymbol{e}_i(\boldsymbol{x}) = \boldsymbol{T}(\boldsymbol{x}; \hat{\boldsymbol{\theta}}_i) - \boldsymbol{T}(\boldsymbol{x}; \boldsymbol{\theta}_i)$.

We assume that $\boldsymbol{e}(\boldsymbol{x}) \sim \mathcal{N}(\boldsymbol{\mu}_e(\boldsymbol{x}), \boldsymbol{\Sigma}_e(\boldsymbol{x}))$ for all $\boldsymbol{x}$. Then the spatial confidence region associated with pixel $\boldsymbol{x} \in \boldsymbol{\Omega}_r$ is defined by the ellipsoid

$$\boldsymbol{\Phi}(\boldsymbol{x}) = \{\boldsymbol{x}' : (\boldsymbol{x}' - \boldsymbol{\mu}_e(\boldsymbol{x}))^T \boldsymbol{\Sigma}_e^{-1}(\boldsymbol{x})(\boldsymbol{x}' - \boldsymbol{\mu}_e(\boldsymbol{x})) < \chi_2^2(1 - \gamma)\}, \qquad (8)$$

which is the $100\gamma\%$ level set of the bivariate normal distribution. Under this formulation, confidence region estimation becomes the problem of estimating $\{\boldsymbol{\mu}_e(\boldsymbol{x}), \boldsymbol{\Sigma}_e(\boldsymbol{x})\}$, the mean and covariance of the registration error at pixel location $\boldsymbol{x}$. We estimate these with the sample mean and covariance based on the simulated errors $\{\boldsymbol{e}_i(\boldsymbol{x})\}$. Algorithm 1 outlines the overall spatial confidence region estimation process.

Algorithm 1. Spatial Confidence Regions Generation

Input: f_r, f_h

Output: $\{\hat{\mu}_e(x), \hat{\Sigma}_e(x)\}$ for all $x \in \Omega_r$

$$\hat{\theta} \leftarrow \arg\max_{\theta'} \Psi\left(f_r(\cdot), f_h \circ T(\cdot\,; \theta')\right)$$

$$\hat{\mu}_\theta \leftarrow \hat{\theta}$$
$$\hat{\Sigma}_\theta \leftarrow (1 - \rho)\Sigma_o + \rho\hat{\theta}\hat{\theta}^T$$

for $i = 1, \cdots, N$

    sample $\theta_i \leftarrow \mathcal{N}(\hat{\mu}_\theta, \hat{\Sigma}_\theta)$

    generate $f_r^{(i)}(x) \leftarrow f_h \circ T(x; \theta_i)$

    register $\hat{\theta}_i \leftarrow \arg\max_{\theta'} \Psi\left(f_r^{(i)}(\cdot), f_h \circ T(\cdot\,; \theta')\right)$

    compute $e_i(x) = T(x; \hat{\theta}_i) - T(x; \theta_i)$

end

$$\hat{\mu}_e(x) \leftarrow \tfrac{1}{N}\sum_{i=1}^{N} e_i(x)$$
$$\hat{\Sigma}_e(x) \leftarrow \tfrac{1}{N}\sum_{i=1}^{N} \left(e_i(x) - \hat{\mu}_e(x)\right)\left(e_i(x) - \hat{\mu}_e(x)\right)^T$$

Note that since we are using $\hat{\theta}$ as the estimate for μ_θ, it is important for the original registration to return a sensible result, as severe inaccuracy could negatively impact the quality of the spatial confidence regions.

3 Experiments

We demonstrate an application of the method, and also present preliminary experiments performed in 2-D. For illustration purpose, we used the negative sum of squared differences as the similarity criterion, but other metrics such as mutual information are also appropriate. To encourage the estimated deformation to be topology-preserving, we included the penalty term introduced by Chun *et al.* [2] into the cost function for all experiments.

Application. We first applied the proposed method to two coronal CT slices in the lung region, shown in Fig. 3. Both images are size 256×360, and the exhale-frame served as the homologous image while the inhale-frame served as reference. The notable motion in this data-set is the sliding of the diaphragm with respect to the chest wall. Due to the opposing motion fields at this interface, registration uncertainty is expected to be higher around this region. To model the deformation, we used a knot spacing of $(m_x, m_y) = (3, 8)$, resulting in a parameter dimension of $\theta \in \mathbb{R}^{7650}$. A tighter knot spacing was used for m_x since a finer scale of deformation was needed in the x-direction to model the sliding motion at the chest wall. Since the degree of this slide is relatively small for this data-set, the registration result shown in Fig. 3 looks reasonably accurate based on visual inspection.

Using $\hat{\theta}$ obtained from registering these images, we used the single-shot mean and covariance estimate and the efficient sampling scheme to obtain 100 new realizations of deformations. For the baseline covariance Σ_o, we used values of $(r_x, r_y) = (0.9, 0.9)$ and $\{c_x, c_y, c_{xy}\} = \{2, 4, 0.5\}$. A relatively high value for c_y was used since the magnitude of the overall deformation was higher in the y-direction. Finally, $\rho = 0.1$ was used, as it was found to produce sensible deformation samples. One of the synthesized reference images is shown in Fig. 3. Following Algorithm 1, we obtained a set of spatial confidence regions $\{\Phi(x)\}$ for all x in the region of anatomical interest, using a confidence level of $\gamma = 0.9$. A few of these are displayed in Fig. 3 (a)-(h), along with 100 simulated errors. It is important to note how the shapes of these confidence regions reflect the local image structure. The principal major axes of the ellipses are oriented along the edge, indicating higher uncertainty for those directions. The confidence regions for (c) and (g) take on isotropic shapes due to the absence of well-defined image structures. Finally, notice how the confidence region for (e) is quite large, illustrating how difficult it is to accurately register the sliding diaphragm at the chest wall.

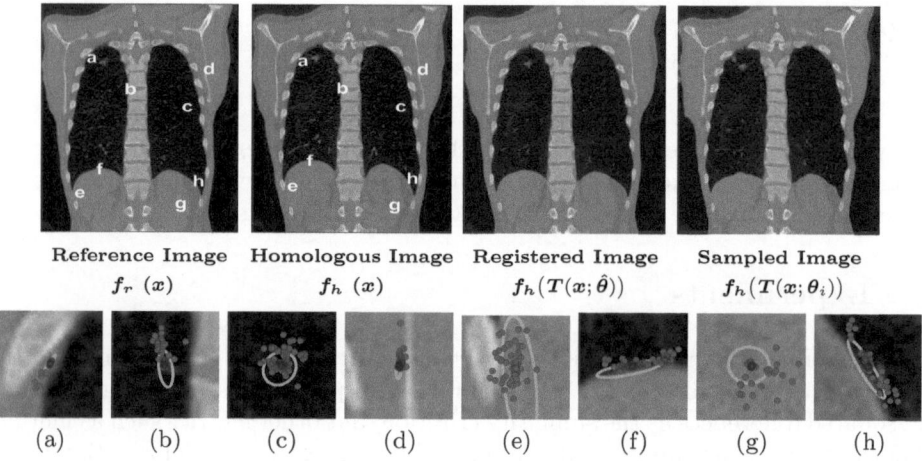

Fig. 3. The top row shows the 2-D data-set used in the first experiment, along with the registration result and an image synthesized using one of the sampled deformations. A few of the confidence regions from $x \in \Omega_r$ are shown in (a)-(h), with the red marks representing 100 realizations of registration error. Note how the confidence regions reflect the local image structure.

Experimental Result. To quantitatively evaluate our method, we manually assigned μ_θ and Σ_θ for the cubic B-spline deformation-generating process. The mean deformation μ_θ was designed to model the exhale to inhale motion in the abdominal area around the liver region, simulated by a contracting motion field. Manually assigning a sensible ground-truth value for the covariance Σ_θ is extremely difficult due to its high dimension and positive-definite constraint. Therefore, we took the shrinkage-based covariance model (4) as the ground-truth, using values of $(r_x, r_y) = (0.95, 0.95)$, $\{c_x, c_y, c_{xy}\} = \{2, 3, 0.5\}$, and $\rho = 0.1$. These values imply that the covariance is smooth with moderate level of correlation in the x and y deformations. We sampled a single instance of deformation θ from this ground-truth distribution, and used it to deform a 2D axial CT slice in the liver region, having image size 512×420. We labeled the original image as the homologous and the deformed image as the reference. This resulting image pair and their difference image are shown in Fig. 4. A knot spacing of $(m_x, m_y) = (8, 8)$ was used to define the scale of the ground-truth deformation, resulting in a parameter dimension of $\theta \in \mathbb{R}^{6656}$.

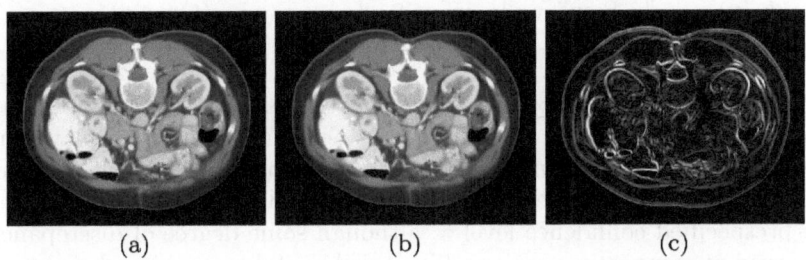

(a)	(b)	(c)

Fig. 4. The data-set used for validation: (a) the homologous image $f_h(x)$, (b) the reference image $f_r(x) = f_h(T(x; \theta))$ generated by a deformation coefficient sampled from the ground-truth distribution $\theta \sim \mathcal{N}(\mu_\theta, \Sigma_\theta)$, (c) the absolute difference image

Next, we generated three classes of spatial confidence regions for this image pair, using confidence levels of $\gamma = 0.9$ and 0.95. The first confidence region $\Phi_1(x)$ corresponds to the case where a correct deformation model is used for registration, and the parameter values for the shrinkage-based covariance estimate $\hat{\Sigma}_\theta$ matches that of the ground truth. The second confidence region $\Phi_2(x)$ corresponds to the case where there is a mismatch in the deformation model. Here, we used a fifth-order B-spline function during registration, with a knot spacing of $(m_x, m_y) = (6, 6)$. In addition, we introduced some discrepancies in the parameter values for $\hat{\Sigma}_\theta$. Finally, the third confidence region $\Phi_3(x)$ corresponds to the ideal case, and is constructed for the purpose of comparison. Here, a correct deformation model is used for registration, and the deformations used to train the spatial confidence regions were sampled from the ground-truth $\mathcal{N}(\mu_\theta, \Sigma_\theta)$ rather than the estimated distribution. The descriptions of these confidence regions are summarized in Table 1. All confidence regions were generated using $N = 200$ simulated errors.

To assess the quality of these spatial confidence regions, we evaluated their *coverage rates* by sampling $M = 500$ additional deformations from the ground-truth distribution $\mathcal{N}(\mu_\theta, \Sigma_\theta)$. Coverage rate for a given pixel x is defined as the percentage of registration errors that are confined within the confidence region $\Phi(x)$, and is written mathematically as

$$\frac{1}{M} \sum_{i=1}^{M} \mathbb{1}\left\{\tilde{e}_i(x) \in \Phi(x)\right\} , \tag{9}$$

where $\mathbb{1}\{\cdot\}$ is the indicator function, and $\tilde{e}_i(x)$ are registration errors generated from deformations sampled from the ground-truth distribution. We computed

Table 1. Spatial Confidence Regions Generated for Validation

	Def. Basis	Def. Scale	Parameter values used for $\hat{\Sigma}_\theta$
Conf. Reg. 1	Cubic	$m_x = 8$	$\rho = 0.1$, $(r_x, r_y) = (0.95, 0.95)$
$\boldsymbol{\Phi}_1(\boldsymbol{x})$	B-spline	$m_y = 8$	$\{c_x, c_y, c_{xy}\} = \{2, 3, 0.5\}$
Conf. Reg. 2	Fifth order	$m_x = 6$	$\rho = 0.15$, $(r_x, r_y) = (0.9, 0.9)$
$\boldsymbol{\Phi}_2(\boldsymbol{x})$	B-spline	$m_y = 6$	$\{c_x, c_y, c_{xy}\} = \{2, 2, 0\}$
Conf. Reg. 3	Cubic	$m_x = 8$	$\hat{\mu}_\theta = \mu_\theta, \hat{\Sigma}_\theta = \Sigma_\theta$
$\boldsymbol{\Phi}_3(\boldsymbol{x})$	B-spline	$m_y = 8$	**(Oracle)**

the coverage rate for the pixels that are located within the region of anatomy. The resulting coverage rates are rendered as heatmaps and are displayed in Fig. 5, along with their corresponding histograms. It can observed that the coverage rates for the first two confidence regions, $\boldsymbol{\Phi}_1(\boldsymbol{x})$ and $\boldsymbol{\Phi}_2(\boldsymbol{x})$, generally come close to the prespecified confidence level γ, although some degree of discrepancy can be observed at some image regions. The third confidence region $\boldsymbol{\Phi}_3(\boldsymbol{x})$ gave the best result as expected; the coverage rate for all pixels comes very close to γ.

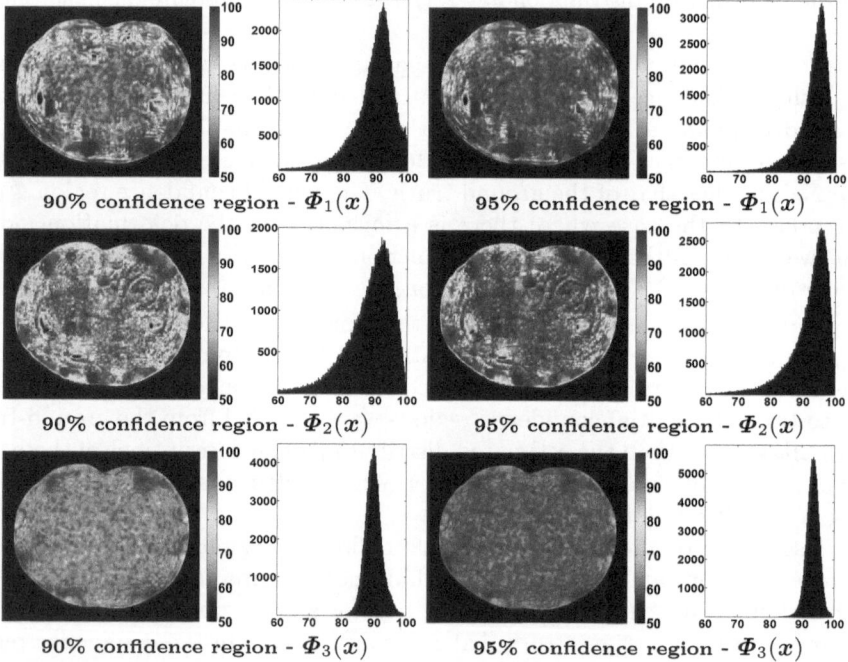

90% confidence region - $\boldsymbol{\Phi}_1(\boldsymbol{x})$ 95% confidence region - $\boldsymbol{\Phi}_1(\boldsymbol{x})$

90% confidence region - $\boldsymbol{\Phi}_2(\boldsymbol{x})$ 95% confidence region - $\boldsymbol{\Phi}_2(\boldsymbol{x})$

90% confidence region - $\boldsymbol{\Phi}_3(\boldsymbol{x})$ 95% confidence region - $\boldsymbol{\Phi}_3(\boldsymbol{x})$

Fig. 5. The coverage rates evaluated for the three classes of spatial confidence regions presented in Table 1, displayed in the form of heatmap and histogram. Note that the performances of $\boldsymbol{\Phi}_1(\boldsymbol{x})$ and $\boldsymbol{\Phi}_2(\boldsymbol{x})$ are fairly comparable to the ideal confidence region $\boldsymbol{\Phi}_3(\boldsymbol{x})$, as the coverage rates for many of the pixels come close to the prespecified confidence level γ.

In summary, the performance of the spatial confidence regions $\Phi_1(\boldsymbol{x})$ and $\Phi_2(\boldsymbol{x})$ turned out to be reasonably close, having results comparable to the ideal case of $\Phi_3(\boldsymbol{x})$. Although further validation studies are required to obtain a more conclusive finding, this is an encouraging preliminary result.

4 Discussion and Conclusion

In this paper, we presented a new method to evaluate the accuracy of a registration algorithm using spatially adaptive confidence regions. Preliminary experimental test results in 2-D suggest the confidence regions are effective based on their coverage rates. However, it is important to note that the computational cost of the proposed method is N times the original registration algorithm, since we must register each of the sampled deformations. Depending on the user's choice, this N can be in the order of hundreds to even thousands, with higher values likely to return more reliable confidence regions. We note that the process is easily parallelizable. Furthermore, in application such as surgical planning and radiation therapy, it may not be necessary to have spatial confidence regions for every voxel in the image volume. Therefore, after completing the original full 3-D registration, we suggest to run the N registrations only within a subregion where the accuracy of the initial registration must be known. This allows one to obtain spatial confidence regions for these locations at a much more reasonable computational expense.

In the future, we will perform more extensive validation studies in 3-D using various similarity criteria and deformation models, and explore a way to quantify the robustness of the method. Furthermore, other choices of *a priori* baseline for the shrinkage-based covariance estimate will be investigated. Finally, we will seek a way to incorporate more data into our model to allow a more sophisticated parameter selection to take place.

Acknowledgments. This work was supported by NIH grant P01CA087634.

The authors would like to thank C. Meyer, A. Hero, and J. Fessler for the valuable discussions and their insightful feedback.

References

1. Christensen, G.E., Geng, X., Kuhl, J.G., Bruss, J., Grabowski, T.J., Pirwani, I.A., Vannier, M.W., Allen, J.S., Damasio, H.: Introduction to the Non-rigid Image Registration Evaluation Project (NIREP). In: Pluim, J.P.W., Likar, B., Gerritsen, F.A. (eds.) WBIR 2006. LNCS, vol. 4057, pp. 128–135. Springer, Heidelberg (2006)
2. Chun, S.Y., Fessler, J.: A simple regularizer for B-spline nonrigid image registration that encourages local invertibility. IEEE J. Sel. Top. Sig. Proc. 3(1), 159–169 (2009); special Issue on Digital Image Processing Techniques for Oncology
3. Fitzpatrick, J.M., West, J.B.: The distribution of target registration error in rigid-body, point-based registration. IEEE Trans. Med. Imaging 20(9), 917–927 (2001)

4. Golub, G.H., Van Loan, C.F.: Matrix computations, 3rd edn. Johns Hopkins University Press (1996)
5. Holden, M.: A review of geometric transformations for nonrigid body registration. IEEE Trans. Med. Imag. 27(1), 111–128 (2008)
6. Hub, M., Kessler, M.L., Karger, C.P.: A stochastic approach to estimate the uncertainty involved in B-spline image registration. IEEE Trans. Med. Imaging 28(11), 1708–1716 (2009)
7. Kybic, J., Unser, M.: Fast parametric elastic image registration. IEEE Transactions on Image Processing 12(11), 1427–1442 (2003)
8. Kybic, J.: Bootstrap resampling for image registration uncertainty estimation without ground truth. IEEE Transactions on Image Processing 19(1), 64–73 (2010)
9. Ledoit, O., Wolf, M.: Improved Estimation of the Covariance Matrix of Stock Returns with an Application to Portfolio Selection. Journal of Empirical Finance 10, 603–621 (2003)
10. Risholm, P., Pieper, S., Samset, E., Wells III, W.M.: Summarizing and Visualizing Uncertainty in Non-rigid Registration. In: Jiang, T., Navab, N., Pluim, J.P.W., Viergever, M.A. (eds.) MICCAI 2010, Part II. LNCS, vol. 6362, pp. 554–561. Springer, Heidelberg (2010)
11. Robinson, M.D., Milanfar, P.: Fundamental performance limits in image registration. IEEE Transactions on Image Processing 13(9), 1185–1199 (2004)
12. Simpson, I.J., Schnabel, J.A., Groves, A.R., Andersson, J.L., Woolrich, M.W.: Probabilistic inference of regularisation in non-rigid registration. NeuroImage 59(3), 2438–2451 (2012)
13. Yetik, I.S., Nehorai, A.: Performance bounds on image registration. IEEE Transactions on Signal Processing 54(5), 1737–1749 (2006)

Registration of Free-Hand Ultrasound and MRI of Carotid Arteries through Combination of Point-Based and Intensity-Based Algorithms

Diego D.B. Carvalho[1], Stefan Klein[1], Zeynettin Akkus[2], Gerrit L. ten Kate[3],
Hui Tang[1,6], Mariana Selwaness[5], Arend F.L. Schinkel[4], Johan G. Bosch[2],
Aad van der Lugt[5], and Wiro J. Niessen[1,6]

[1] Biomedical Imaging Group Rotterdam, Departments of Radiology
and Medical Informatics, Erasmus MC, Rotterdam, The Netherlands
[2] Biomedical Engineering, Erasmus MC, Rotterdam, The Netherlands
[3] Division of Pharmacology, Vascular and Metabolic Diseases,
Department of Internal Medicine, Erasmus MC, Rotterdam, The Netherlands
[4] Department of Cardiology, Thoraxcenter, Erasmus MC, Rotterdam,
The Netherlands
[5] Department of Radiology, Erasmus MC, Rotterdam, The Netherlands
[6] Imaging Science and Technology, Faculty of Applied Sciences,
Delft University of Technology, Delft, The Netherlands

Abstract. We propose a methodology to register medical images of carotid arteries from tracked freehand sweep B-Mode ultrasound (US) and magnetic resonance imaging (MRI) acquisitions. Successful registration of US and MR images will allow a multimodal analysis of atherosclerotic plaque in the carotid artery. The main challenge is the difference in the positions of the patient's neck during the examinations. While in MRI the patient's neck remains in a natural position, in US the neck is slightly bent and rotated. Moreover, the image characteristics of US and MRI around the carotid artery are very different. Our technique uses the estimated centerlines of the common, internal and external carotid arteries in each modality as landmarks for registration. For US, we used an algorithm based on a rough lumen segmentation obtained by robust ellipse fitting to estimate the lumen centerline. In MRI, we extract the centerline using a minimum cost path approach in which the cost is defined by medialness and an intensity based similarity term. The two centerlines are aligned by an iterative closest point (ICP) algorithm, using rigid and thin-plate spline transformation models. The resulting point correspondences are used as a soft constraint in a subsequent intensity-based registration, optimizing a weighted sum of mutual information between the US and MRI and the Euclidean distance between corresponding points. Rigid and B-spline transformation models were used in this stage. Experiments were performed on datasets from five healthy volunteers. We compared different registration approaches, in order to evaluate the necessity of each step, and to establish the optimum algorithm configuration. For the validation, we used the Dice similarity index to measure the overlap between lumen segmentations in US and MRI.

Keywords: Image registration, carotid artery, ultrasound, magnetic resonance imaging, atherosclerosis.

B.M. Dawant et al. (Eds.): WBIR 2012, LNCS 7359, pp. 131–140, 2012.
© Springer-Verlag Berlin Heidelberg 2012

1   Introduction

Medical imaging studies of the carotid artery generally aim to observe the presence of atherosclerotic plaque and the effect on the geometry of the vessel lumen. Both atherosclerotic plaques as well as luminal stenosis are related to cerebrovascular diseases [1]. Various imaging modalities are used to analyze the carotid vessel wall. Magnetic resonance imaging (MRI) has good soft-tissue contrast allowing plaque composition analysis in 3D, but the resolution of the images is often limited, especially in the slice direction. Computed tomography angiography (CTA) visualizes the 3D lumen geometry with high resolution and clearly shows calcifications, but other plaque components (lipids, fibrous tissue, hemorrhage) are hard to distinguish. Ultrasound (US) is less traumatic to the patient, the equipment has a lower cost, it provides a high temporal resolution enabling motion analysis to measure the distensibility of the artery and the images have a higher in-plane resolution. The smaller pixel spacing of US permits accurate measurements of the vessel wall thickness, and allows the observation of bubbles in the vasa vasorum in contrast enhanced examinations, which can be used to study neovascularization in the plaque [2]. However, the US images may present speckle noise, artifacts and a lack of contrast in the direction perpendicular to the beam direction.

In this work, we propose a methodology to register medical images of carotid arteries from free-hand sweep B-Mode US and black-blood proton density weighted (BB-PDw) MRI acquisitions. Co-registration of the US and MR images will facilitate multimodal analysis of atherosclerotic plaque. Because the patient's neck is in a bent position during the US scanning procedure, whereas it is kept straight during MR scanning, a nonrigid transformation is required. Since the US and MR images have rather different characteristics, we choose for a combination of point-based and intensity-based algorithms, using geometrical features that can be extracted reliably in each modality. We investigate the added value of these geometrical features, compared with purely intensity-based registration, in a quantitative evaluation experiment.

Registration of carotid 3D free-hand power Doppler US and Magnetic Resonance Angiography (MRA) has previously been developed by Slomka et al. [3]. Their method is based on maximization of mutual information, using a rigid transformation model. Nanayakkara et al. [4,5] perform the registration of MRI and 3D US with a constrained non-rigid registration, using a 'twisting and bending' transformation model. The 3D US in their work is composed by a sequence of images acquired with a probe moved by a motorized device. Registration of brain vascular structures (not carotid though) from freehand US and MRA has been presented by Reinertsen et al. [6]. The method is based on the alignment of centerlines using the Iterative Closest Point (ICP) Algorithm [7]. Previous research on the registration of free-hand US and MRI of other anatomical regions includes the work by Penney et al., who performed registration on liver images [8]. The US probe's position was estimated with the use of an external optical device and the registration was based on a similarity measure calculated with probabilistic maps generated from training data and features extracted from the images.

Our technique uses the centerlines estimated in the common (CCA), internal (ICA) and external (ECA) carotid arteries in each modality as guides for registration. The MR images provide information such as each slice's 3D position, thickness and distances between neighboring slices, allowing to properly organize the slices in a volumetric representation. On the other hand, the freehand US acquisition is of a 2D nature. In order to represent the US data in a volume, a magnetic positioning device (Flock of Birds - FOB) was attached to the probe. The US machine video output signal is correlated with the FOB data through the publicly available Stradwin software. We applied robust existing algorithms [9,10] to estimate the lumen centerlines in the US and MRI data. To obtain a rough initial alignment, the bifurcation point, together with a set of points at equidistant spacing along the centerline, and one point on the skin, are selected in both modalities. These selected points are matched with a point based rigid registration. After this initial registration, rigid and thin-plate spline ICP registrations are performed using the open source GMMREG software [11]. Finally, the resulting point correspondences are used as prior information in a mutual information based registration, using the open source Elastix software [12].

2   Method

In this section we briefly explain the methods for lumen centerline extraction, after which the registration procedure is described in detail.

2.1   Lumen Centerline Estimation

MRI Centerline. To calculate the carotid centerline in MRI, the algorithm of Tang et al. [10] was used on the BB-PDw sequence. Whereas in [10] a multispectral approach was proposed (using an additional phase-contrast MR sequence to improve robustness), in this work we only used the BB-PDw image, which gave visually satisfactory results.

The method has a pre-processing phase composed by three steps. First, the N3 bias [13] correction is applied on BB-PDw to correct for intensity inhomogeneities. Second, both sequences are denoised with an edge enhancing diffusion filter [14]. The centerline is calculated by a minimum cost path approach, with user defined seed points in the vessel's end points. The lumen intensity similarity term compares the intensities to the distribution in a small neighbourhood within the lumen around the seed points. The total cost function is defined by the reciprocal of a multiplication of the two measures.

The algorithm was evaluated on 152 carotid arteries, and was successful in 148 cases [10], indicating that this centerline can be considered as a robust feature for registration.

US Centerline. To estimate a 3D centerline of the carotid arteries from 2D transversal freehand US acquisitions, the approach described in [9] was implemented. In this approach, the lumen centroid is identified in each 2D image, using an algorithm inspired by Wang's Spoke Ellipse algorithm [15]. The algorithm is robust against missing edge information in parts of the carotid wall, due to the lack of contrast in directions orthogonal to the US beam direction. A magnetic tracking device called Flock of Birds (FOB) (Ascension Technology, Burlington, VT, USA) was attached to the US probe, to register the displacements during the acquisitions. To synchronize the sensor information with the images we used the publicly available Stradwin software (http://mi.eng.cam.ac.uk/rwp/stradwin) [16]. Using the position information, the 2D lumen centroids can be transformed to 3D space.

The algorithm presented in [9] was evaluated on 19 carotids from 15 patients; an average distance of 0.8mm to manual annotations was reported, suggesting that this centerline can also be considered as a robust feature for registration.

Postprocessing of the Centerlines. The MRI algorithm is based on the minimum cost path between an initial point in the CCA and two other points, one in the ICA and other in the ECA; this leads to one centerline connecting the CCA point to the ICA point (line LI), and one centerline connecting the CCA point to the ECA point (line LE). On the other hand, the US algorithm generates three centerlines; one connecting the CCA input point to the bifurcation point, and two others connecting the bifurcation point to the input points in the ECA and the ICA. The MRI centerlines are smoother due to the iterative refinement step. In order to make the US centerline more similar to the MRI counterpart, we connect the CCA to the ICA (LI) and to the ECA (LE), and apply a Gaussian smoothing to both lines, with kernel σ of 5 mm. Subsequently, the MRI and US centerlines are resampled to a resolution of 0.1 mm. Finally, the bifurcation point is automatically determined in both modalities as the point where the Euclidean distance between the centerpoints in LI and LE becomes less than 1 mm. The centerlines are cropped automatically such that the maximum distances before/after the bifurcation in the one modality equal those in the other modality.

2.2   Registration Procedure

Let $U(x)$ represent the reconstructed 3D US volume, $M(x)$ the MRI volume, $\{u\}$ the set of points on the US centerline and $\{m\}$ the set of points on the MRI centerline. The aim of our registration procedure is to find a transformation $T(x)$ that transforms points in $\{u\}$ to the MRI domain, and that can be used to generate a warped MRI image $M(T(x))$, which is registered to $U(x)$.

Centerlines Registration. Initially, eight points are extracted from each centerline to perform a rough rigid registration. These points are: the bifurcation point, a point on the skin of the neck in the same slice as the bifurcation (manually selected), two points in the CCA, two points in the ICA and two points in the ECA. These last six points are at a Euclidean distance δ and $\delta/2$ from their corresponding bifurcation point. In our experiments we used $\delta = 10\,\text{mm}$. The resulting transformation is called $T_0(x)$. An example of the aligned centerlines is shown in Fig. 1a.

An ICP registration is performed on the point sets $\{u\}$ and $\{m\}$, using $T_0(x)$ as initial transformation. The ICP registration is done in two steps. First, a rigid transformation model is used; the result of this stage is called $T_1(x)$. Second, a nonrigid thin-plate spline model is employed to take into account the bending of the patient's neck during the US examination; the result of this stage is denoted $T_2(x)$ and the complete transformation from US to MRI is obtained by composition: $T_2(T_1(T_0(x)))$. We use the publicly available GMMREG [11] implementation for both steps, using the TPS-RPM algorithm developed by Chui&Rangarajan for the thin-plate spline registration [17]. Points at $\Delta = 1\,\text{mm}$ intervals sampled on the MRI centerline are used as thin-plate spline control points. In the rigid registration for the scale parameters of Gaussian mixtures, we used values of σ of 0.5 and 0.1, from coarse to fine. In the non-rigid registration, we used as input parameters: $r = 0.97$ (annealing rate, for the annealing schedule of the energy minimization), and $\lambda = 1$ (regularization parameter). An example of the MR and US centerlines after rigid and non-rigid registration is shown in Fig. 1b and Fig. 1c, respectively.

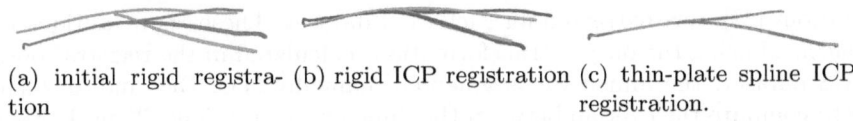

(a) initial rigid registra- (b) rigid ICP registration (c) thin-plate spline ICP
tion   registration.

Fig. 1. Examples of the registration of centerlines after each step, MRI centerline (red), US centerline (green)

Intensity-Based registration. The centerline transformation is used as prior knowledge in a conventional intensity-based registration framework. Image similarity is measured by the mutual information (MI) [18,19]. The point correspondence information is supplied as a soft constraint, i.e., by adding a penalty term to the cost function to be minimized:

$$C(T) = -MI(U, M \circ T) + \omega \frac{1}{N} \sum_u \|T(u) - \tilde{u}\|^2$$

with N the number of points in $\{u\}$, ω a user-defined weighting factor, and $\tilde{u} = T_2(T_1(T_0(u)))$. The transformation T is composed of four sub-transformations, $T(x) = T_4(T_3(T_1(T_0(x))))$, of which T_0 and T_1 are the rigid transformations from previous stages, T_3 is an additional rigid transformation that is optimized in the current stage, and T_4 is a nonrigid B-spline transformation that is optimized subsequently. The thin-plate spline transformation is not directly incorporated in $T(x)$, since it is only meaningful for points on the centerline; it is taken into account via the penalty term.

The registration is implemented using the open source Elastix software [12]. A stochastic gradient descent optimization method [20], using 2000 number of iterations is used to find T_3 and T_4 that minimize the cost function. A 3-level hierarchical strategy is employed to avoid local minima: the amount of image smoothing (Gaussian kernel standard deviation) and the isotropic control point spacing of the B-spline transformation are gradually decreased (by factors of 2). The spacing between control points at the finest level is a user-defined parameter, β. To compute the mutual information, a 256×256 joint histogram is estimated using a Parzen windowing approach [21], based on 2000 image samples randomly selected in every iteration [20]. Linear interpolation is used to evaluate the MR image intensities at non-grid positions.

3   Experiments and Results

US and MR images were acquired in five healthy volunteers. For the US examinations the iU22 Philips machine was used along with the Philips L9-3 probe with a depth of 3cm. For the MRI examination a GE Medical System Signa Excite 1.5 Tesla machine was used. The voxel size in MRI is $0.5 \times 0.5 \times 0.9 \, \mathrm{mm}^3$. The 3D reconstructed US datasets generated by the Stradwin software have a voxel size of $0.16 \times 0.16 \times 0.16 \, \mathrm{mm}^3$. The datasets from volunteers A, B and C are from the left carotid; D and E are from the right carotid.

For validation of the registration method, semi-automated MRI lumen segmentations [22] were extracted for each MRI dataset. These segmentations were transformed using the output transformations calculated in the registrations. In the US dataset, the lumen was segmented manually. The Dice index [23] was used to compute the overlap between the lumen segmentations. A mask was applied such that differences in the length of the segmentation along the arteries do not affect the overlap measure.

We evaluated the registration procedure in seven different configurations: ICP-based rigid ($T = T_1 \circ T_0$), intensity-based rigid ($T = T_3 \circ T_1 \circ T_0$), the complete method with four different values for β (referred to as B-spline β mm), and the complete method with $\beta = 32\,\mathrm{mm}$ and $\omega = 0$ (named B-spline 32 mm*). In the last configuration, the centerline information is largely ignored, and the method boils down to a standard intensity-based nonrigid registration; the centerlines are only used to obtain an initial rigid transformation. The values for β that were tested are 8, 16, 24, and 32 mm.

The results are reported in Table 1. It can be seen that the intensity-based rigid approach is as good as or better than the ICP-based rigid registration in all cases. It must be noted though that the intensity-based rigid registration is largely based on the result of the ICP-based rigid method. Our second observation is that the method with $\omega = 0$ fails in all cases, even though its initial rigid transformation (namely, ICP-rigid) is reasonable, which suggests that the centerline prior is essential to keep the intensity-based registration 'well-behaved'. Based on the average Dice index, the complete method with B-spline control point spacing of 32 mm performs the best. With smaller values of β the

Table 1. Overlap between the carotid lumen segmentations after various registration procedures, for volunteers A, B, C, D, and E

Description	Settings	A	B	C	D	E	Average
ICP rigid	$T = T_1 \circ T_0$	0.76	0.54	0.68	0.68	0.67	0.67
Intensity rigid	$T = T_3 \circ T_1 \circ T_0, \omega = 1$	0.77	0.56	0.68	0.74	0.73	0.69
B-spline 8mm	$T = T_4 \circ T_3 \circ T_1 \circ T_0, \omega = 1, \beta = 8$	0.70	0.56	0.38	0.76	0.72	0.62
B-spline 16mm	$T = T_4 \circ T_3 \circ T_1 \circ T_0, \omega = 1, \beta = 16$	0.77	0.54	0.40	0.79	0.77	0.65
B-spline 24mm	$T = T_4 \circ T_3 \circ T_1 \circ T_0, \omega = 1, \beta = 24$	0.77	0.54	0.64	0.78	0.75	0.69
B-spline 32mm	$T = T_4 \circ T_3 \circ T_1 \circ T_0, \omega = 1, \beta = 32$	0.77	0.54	0.72	0.77	0.74	0.71
B-spline 32mm*	$T = T_4 \circ T_3 \circ T_1 \circ T_0, \omega = 0, \beta = 32$	0.00	0.00	0.00	0.25	0.00	0.05

performance drops, which suggests that the transformation has too many degrees of freedom, given the large differences in image characteristics between US and MRI. Figure 2 shows volume renderings of the lumen segmentations after B-spline 32 mm registration.

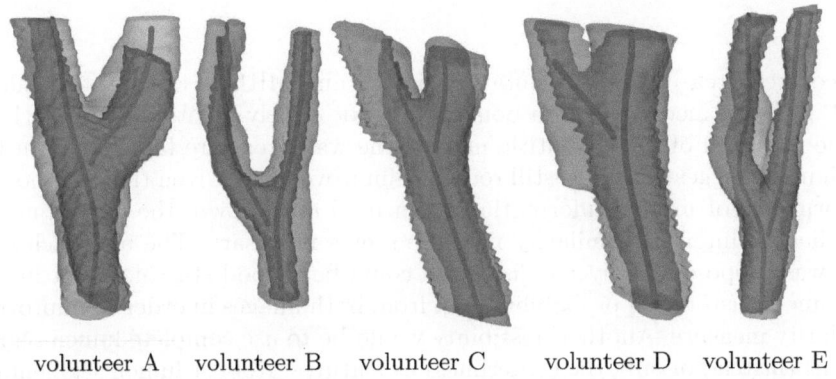

volunteer A   volunteer B   volunteer C   volunteer D   volunteer E

Fig. 2. Isosurfaces of the lumen segmentations after B-spline registration ($\beta = 32$mm). Green: US segmentation; red: transformed MRI segmentation; blue: US centerline.

4   Conclusion and Discussion

A method for the alignment of freehand US and MRI scans of the carotid artery was proposed and evaluated. The method starts by robust semi-automated extraction of lumen centerlines in both modalities, followed by a point-based registration and a subsequent intensity-based registration. Initial results on five volunteers' data sets show the beneficial effect of the use of centerlines as landmarks. The use of the mutual information metric as a single metric led to complete misalignments. In Fig. 3 it is possible to observe the large difference between the US and MR image characteristics., which apparently lead to misinterpretations when using only the mutual information. There might be a difference between

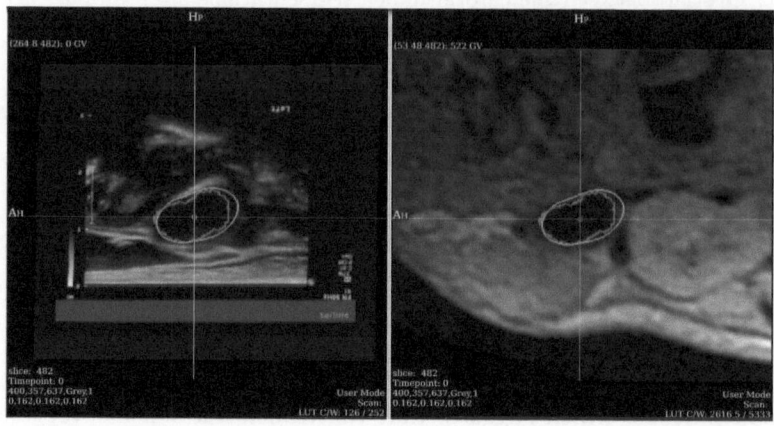

Fig. 3. US slice(left) and MRI slice (right) after registration. Volunteer A, after B-spline 32 mm registration. The areas delineated by the red line represent the MRI segmentation after the transformation. The areas in green represent the US manual segmentation.

the covered area in the segmentations in US and MRI. According to Underhill et al. [24], the media-adventia boundary is not clearly identifiable in MRI. Due to the inclusion of the adventitia in MRI the wall areas are larger than in US.

Figure 2 suggests there is still room for improvement. Given the disappointing performance of mutual information when used on its own, the development of a dedicated intensity similarity measure seems necessary. The approach by [8] that was proposed for liver registration could be a good starting point in order to define a customized probability map from both images in order to improve the similarity measure. Another possibility would be to use complete lumen segmentations (instead of only the centerlines) as features. Robust lumen segmentation in US is a challenge though, because of the missing edge information at boundaries parallel to the US beam direction, the high noise level, and the presence of shadowing artifacts behind calcified plaque.

In the current setup, the US scanning still requires an external magnetic sensor to allow 3D reconstruction. An approach that directly performs a 2D-3D registration, simulating US slices from the MRI data could remove the need for a tracking device.

The MRI and US scans have very different image characteristics, and the tissue is deformed due to bending of the neck and compression of the skin during the US examination. These conditions make the registration a difficult task. Our approach that combines the carotids centerlines and the images intensities resulted in an average Dice similarity index of 0.71 in the best configuration.

Acknowledgements. This research was performed within the framework of CTMM, the Center for Translational Molecular Medicine (www.ctmm.nl), project PARISk (grant 01C-202), and supported by the Netherlands Heart Foundation.

References

1. McCarthy, M.J., Loftus, I.M., Thompson, M.M., Jones, L., London, N.J.M., Bell, P.R.F., Naylor, A.R., Brindle, N.P.J.: Angiogenesis and the atherosclerotic carotid plaque: An association between symptomatology and plaque morphology. Journal of Vascular Surgery 30, 261–268 (1999)
2. Feinstein, S.B.: Contrast ultrasound imaging of the carotid artery vasa vasorum and atherosclerotic plaque neovascularization. Journal of the American College of Cardiology 48, 236–243 (2006)
3. Slomka, P.J., Mandel, J., Downey, D., Fenster, A.: Evaluation of voxel-based registration of 3-D power Doppler ultrasound and 3-D magnetic resonance angiographic images of carotid arteries. Ultrasound in Medicine & Biology 27, 945–955 (2001)
4. Nanayakkara, N.D., Chiu, B., Samani, A., Spence, J.D., Samarabandu, J., Fenster, A.: A "twisting and bending" model-based nonrigid image registration technique for 3-D ultrasound carotid images. IEEE Transactions on Medical Imaging 27, 1378–1388 (2008)
5. Nanayakkara, N.D., Chiu, B., Samani, A., Spence, J.D., Samarabandu, J., Parraga, G., Fenster, A.: Nonrigid registration of three-dimensional ultrasound and magnetic resonance images of the carotid arteries. Medical Physics 36, 373–385 (2009)
6. Reinertsen, I., Descoteaux, M., Siddiqi, K., Collins, D.L.: Validation of vessel-based registration for correction of brain shift. Medical Image Analysis 11, 374–388 (2007)
7. Besl, P.J., McKay, N.D.: A method for registration of 3-d shapes. IEEE Trans. Pattern Anal. Mach. Intell. 14, 239–256 (1992)
8. Penney, G.P., Blackall, J.M., Hamady, M.S., Sabharwal, T., Adam, A., Hawkes, D.J.: Registration of freehand 3D ultrasound and magnetic resonance liver images. Medical Image Analysis 8, 81–91 (2004)
9. Carvalho, D.D.B., Klein, S., Akkus, Z., ten Kate, G.L., Schinkel, A.F.L., Bosch, J.G., van der Lugt, A., Niessen, W.J.: Estimating 3d lumen centerlines of carotid arteries in free-hand acquisition ultrasound. International Journal of Computer Assisted Radiology and Surgery 7, 207–215 (2012)
10. Tang, H., van Walsum, T., van Onkelen, R.S., Klein, S., Hameeteman, K., Schaap, M., van den Bouwhuijsen, Q.J.A., Witteman, J.C.M., van der Lugt, A., van Vliet, L.J., Niessen, W.J.: Multispectral MRI centerline tracking in carotid arteries. In: SPIE: Medical Imaging (2011)
11. Jian, B., Vemuri, B.C.: Robust Point Set Registration Using Gaussian Mixture Models. IEEE Transactions on Pattern Analysis and Machine Intelligence 33, 1633–1645 (2011)
12. Klein, S., Staring, M., Murphy, K., Viergever, M.A., Pluim, J.P.W.: elastix: a toolbox for intensity-based medical image registration. IEEE Transactions on Medical Imaging 29, 196–205 (2010)
13. Sled, J.G., Zijdenbos, A.P., Evans, A.C.: A nonparametric method for automatic correction of intensity nonuniformity in MRI data. IEEE Transactions on Medical Imaging 17, 87–97 (1998)
14. Perona, P., Malik, J.: Scale-space and edge detection using anisotropic diffusion. IEEE Transactions on Pattern Analysis and Machine Intelligence 12, 629–639 (1990)
15. Wang, D., Klatzky, R.L., Amesur, N., Stetten, G.: Carotid Artery and Jugular Vein Tracking and Differentiation Using Spatiotemporal Analysis. In: Larsen, R., Nielsen, M., Sporring, J. (eds.) MICCAI 2006, Part I. LNCS, vol. 4190, pp. 654–661. Springer, Heidelberg (2006)

16. Gee, A., Prager, R., Treece, G., Berman, L.: Engineering a freehand 3D ultrasound system. Pattern Recognition Letters 24, 757–777 (2003)
17. Chui, H., Rangarajan, A.: A new point matching algorithm for non-rigid registration. Computer Vision and Image Understanding 89, 114–141 (2003)
18. Maes, F., Collignon, A., Vandermeulen, D., Marchal, G., Suetens, P.: Multimodality image registration by maximization of mutual information. IEEE Transactions on Medical Imaging 16, 187–198 (1997)
19. Viola, P., Wells III, W.M.: Alignment by maximization of mutual information. Int. J. Comput. Vision 24, 137–154 (1997)
20. Klein, S., Pluim, J.P.W., Staring, M., Viergever, M.A.: Adaptive Stochastic Gradient Descent Optimisation for Image Registration. Int. J. Comput. Vision 81, 227–239 (2009)
21. Thevenaz, P., Unser, M.: Optimization of mutual information for multiresolution image registration. IEEE Transactions on Image Processing 9, 2083–2099 (2000)
22. Tang, H., van Onkelen, R.S., van Walsum, T., Hameeteman, R., Schaap, M., Tori, F.L., van den Bouwhuijsen, Q.J.A., Witteman, J.C.M., van der Lugt, A., van Vliet, L.J., Niessen, W.J.: A Semi-automatic Method for Segmentation of the Carotid Bifurcation and Bifurcation Angle Quantification on Black Blood MRA. In: Jiang, T., Navab, N., Pluim, J.P.W., Viergever, M.A. (eds.) MICCAI 2010, Part III. LNCS, vol. 6363, pp. 97–104. Springer, Heidelberg (2010)
23. Dice, L.R.: Measures of the amount of ecologic association between species. Ecology 26, 297–302 (1945)
24. Underhill, H.R., Kerwin, W.S., Hatsukami, T.S., Yuan, C.: Automated measurement of mean wall thickness in the common carotid artery by MRI: a comparison to intima-media thickness by B-mode ultrasound. Journal of Magnetic Resonance Imaging: JMRI 24, 379–387 (2006)

IVUS-Histology Image Registration

Amin Katouzian[1,2], Athanasios Karamalis[1], Jennifer Lisauskas[4],
Abouzar Eslami[1,3], and Nassir Navab[1]

[1] Computer Aided Medical Procedures (CAMP), Technical University of Munich, Germany
[2] Biomedical Engineering Department, Columbia University, New York, USA
[3] Institut für Biomathematik und Biometrie, Helmholtz Zentrum München
[4] Infraredx® Inc., Burlington, MA, USA
amin.katouzian@cs.tum.edu

Abstract. In this paper, for the first time, we present a systematic framework to register intravascular ultrasound (IVUS) images with histology correspondences. We deployed intermediate representations of images, generating segmentation masks corresponding to lumen and media-adventitia borders for both histology and IVUS images, incorporated into a non-rigid registration framework using discrete multi-labeling and approximate curvature penalty for smoothness regularization. The resulting deformation field was then applied to the original histology image to transfer it to IVUS coordinate system. Finally, the results were quantified on 14 cross sections of interest. The main contribution of this work is that the registered results could be used for systematic labeling of tissues, which ultimately will lead to reliable construction of training dataset for feature extraction and supervised classification of atherosclerotic tissues.

Keywords: Intravascular Ultrasound (IVUS), Atherosclerosis, Histology, Registration.

1   Introduction

The importance of atherosclerotic disease in coronary artery has been a subject of study for many researchers in the past decade. In brief, the aim is to understand progression of such a chronic disease, detect plaques at risks (vulnerable plaques [1]), and treat them selectively to prevent mortality and immobility. In general, the ultimate goal is to provide interventional cardiologists with reliable clinical tools so they can identify these plaques, make decisions confidently, choose the most appropriate drugs or implant devices (*i.e.* stent), and stabilize them during catheterization procedures with minimal risk. This has motivated researchers to employ intravascular ultrasound (IVUS) technology, in addition to angiogram that is routinely used, because it provides real-time cross-sectional images of arterial wall structures with useful information about tissues microstructures. Hence, different IVUS-derived atherosclerotic tissue characterization algorithms have been developed [2].

The key steps in designing supervised plaque classification algorithm is labeling and construction of a reliable training dataset. Traditionally, histopathologists manually label the most visually recognizable homogenous regions for each tissue on

B.M. Dawant et al. (Eds.): WBIR 2012, LNCS 7359, pp. 141–149, 2012.
© Springer-Verlag Berlin Heidelberg 2012

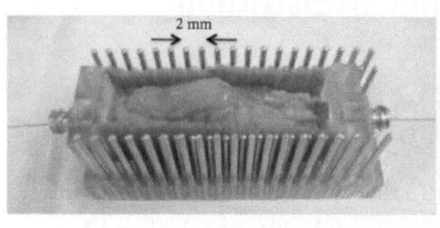 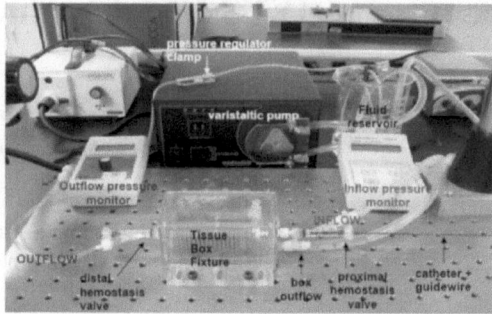

Fig. 1. Tissue cage fixture (left), *in vitro* experiment set-up (right). (Developed by Jennifer Lisauskas at InfrareDx (Burlington, MA))

histology images and they are somewhat require to be transformed onto IVUS grayscale images prior to feature extraction (*i.e.* spectral or textural). Most of existing radiofrequency (RF)- or textural-based atherosclerotic tissue characterization algorithms have not described how this crucial step has been taken into account [3-5]. In fact, the challenge has been implicitly pointed in [6,7]. Authors in [7] deployed an intuitive registration methodology and visually annotated IVUS images. To the best of our knowledge, Nair *et al.* [8] was the only group who claimed to register IVUS and histology images through the thin plate spline (TPS) deformation technique [9], however, neither qualitative nor quantitative results was provided.

In this paper, we present a systematic method to register and superimpose IVUS and histology images via a non-rigid registration framework. The proposed approach would ensure the accuracy of labeling process, enhance the reliability of training dataset, increase the consistency among extracted features, and ultimately improve atherosclerotic tissue classification results. The quantification of classification results is out of scope of this paper and the main focus is registration process.

2   Data Collection and Histology Preparation Methodologies

The IVUS-histology matching problem is challenging due to: 1) presence of curvatures in coronary arteries especially in the left circumflex (LCX); 2) misalignment between IVUS imaging plane and slicing plane of microtome, and 3) shrinkage of arteries after formaldehyde fixation. Therefore, a precise data collection method is necessary to obtain the most accurate IVUS-histology dataset. At Infraredx® (Burlington, MA), researchers developed a systematic *in vitro* acquisition protocol to collect IVUS data from coronary arteries using single-element 40 MHz transducer. In this methodology, the arteries were dissected from cadaver hearts (24 hours postmortem), placed in tissue cage fixture and attached to a circulating fluid flow system, **Figure 1**. Average length of the arterial segments attached to the fluid system could be up to 50mm. The arterial segments were perfused with saline at body temperature (37°C) and pulsatile flow (60 bpm, 135mL/min) at physiologic

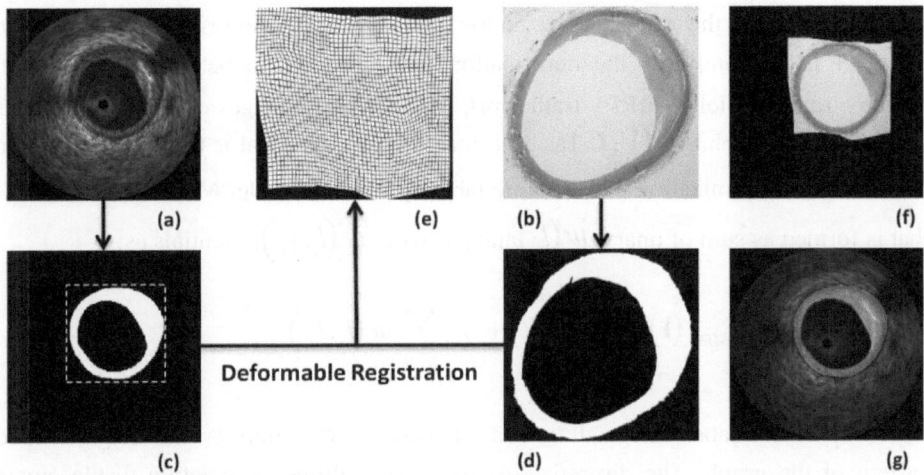

Fig. 2. Example of deformable registration process. Image a) IVUS, b) histology, c) segmentation of IVUS, d) segmentation of histology, e) deformation field from histology to IVUS, f) deformation applied to histology, g) visual overlap of deformed histology to IVUS.

pressure (80-120 mmHg). Then, an IVUS catheter was advanced on a 0.014" guide wire and a complete automatic pullback was taken from distal to proximal side. The acquired data was then saved onto an external hard disk.

After imaging, the arteries were pressure fixed with 10% buffered formaldehyde followed by decalcification. The histology blocks were prepared for every 2mm (corresponding to 120 frames of the IVUS pullback) using the sidebars. All blocks were embedded in paraffin and sectioned for histological staining. Two 5μm thick histologic cross sections were stained with hematoxilin and eosin (H&E) and Russell-Movat Pentachrome.

The main advantage of this methodology is the fact that the orientation of artery is not changed throughout the whole procedure. Therefore, more reliable IVUS-histology pairs could be obtained and the number of cross sections of interest (CSIs) per vessel is significantly increased (average of 25 regions).

3   Non-rigid Registration Framework through MRF Discrete Multi-labeling

The registration between IUVS, I_{IVUS} (Figure 2(a)), and histology, I_{hist} (Figure 2(b)), images is performed through minimization of a matching function $\Im$ that expresses underlying non-rigid deformation, T, along with regularization R as follows:

$$\hat{T} = \arg\min_{T} \Im\left(I_{IVUS}, I_{hist} \circ T\right) + \lambda R(T) \tag{1}$$

where λ controls the effects of regularization term. The non-rigid transformation $T = \mathbf{x} + D(\mathbf{x})$ comprises the deformation field D and can be estimated through Markov random field (MRF) framework and forming images as discrete objects represented in graph $g = (V, C)$ as described in [10]. The goal is to find deformation field through minimization of a discrete labeling of a first-order MRF function f_{MRF} that is formed as sum of unary $\psi(l_i)$ and pairwise $\psi(l_i, l_j)$ potentials as:

$$f_{MRF}(\mathbf{l}) = \sum_{i \in g} \psi(l_i) + \sum_{i \in g} \sum_{j \in N_i} \psi(l_i, l_j) \qquad (2)$$

where l_i is the label assigned to node i and $N_i \subset g$ defines the neighborhood system of the graph. The discretized search space allows associating displacement $\mathbf{d}^{l_i}$ to each label l so one can encode the matching and regularizations terms in Eq. (1) by unary and pairwise terms, respectively, in an iterative process as follows:

$$\psi_i(l_i) = \left| I_{IVUS}(\mathbf{x}_i) - I_{hist}\left(\mathbf{x}_i + D^{t-1}(\mathbf{x}_i) + \mathbf{d}^{l_i}\right) \right| \qquad (3)$$

$$\psi_{ij}(l_i, l_j) = \lambda \left\| \left(D^{t-1}(\mathbf{x}_i) + \mathbf{d}^{l_i}\right) - \left(D^{t-1}(\mathbf{x}_j) + \mathbf{d}^{l_j}\right) \right\| \qquad (4)$$

The main advantage of this technique is that it can be implemented in an efficient fashion by introducing a transformation model through sparse set of M control points in combination with interpolation strategy (ex. cubic B-spline) [10] and define the dense displacement field as:

$$D(\mathbf{x}) = \sum_{i=1}^{M} \eta_i(\mathbf{x}) \mathbf{d}_i \qquad (5)$$

where η_i is a weighting function, determining the contribution of control point displacement $\mathbf{d}_i$ to the displacement of histology image point $\mathbf{x}$. Now, the unary and pairwise terms can be reformulated as follows:

$$\psi_i(l_i) = \sum_{\mathbf{x} \in \Omega_i} \left| I_{IVUS}(\mathbf{x}_i) - I_{hist}\left(\mathbf{x}_i + D^{t-1}(\mathbf{x}_i) + \mathbf{d}^{l_i}\right) \right| \qquad (6)$$

$$\psi_{ij}(l_i, l_j) = \lambda \left\| \left(\mathbf{d}_i^{t-1} + \mathbf{d}^{l_i}\right) - \left(\mathbf{d}_j^{t-1} + \mathbf{d}^{l_j}\right) \right\| \qquad (7)$$

where Ω_i is local image patch centered at i-th control point. Ultimately, the MRF objective function in Eq. (2) can be written as:

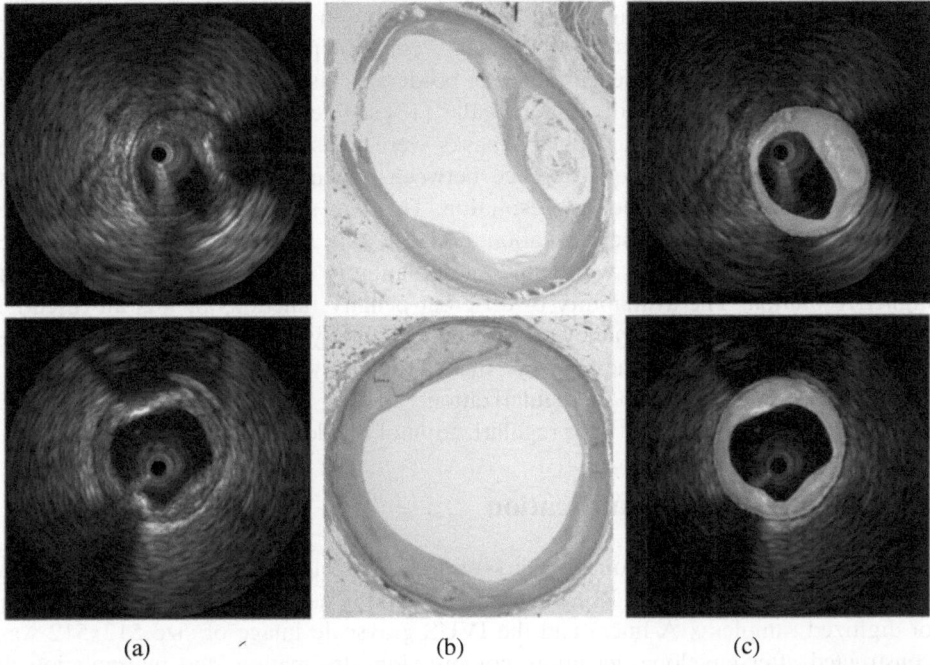

Fig. 3. IVUS grayscale image (a), corresponding histology image (b), and resulting deformed histology image imposed on IVUS frame (c)

$$f_{MRF}(\mathbf{l}) = \sum_i^M \psi_i(l_i) + \sum_i^M \sum_{j \in N_i} \psi_{ij}$$

$$= \underbrace{\sum_i^M \sum_{x \in \Omega_i} \left| I_{IVUS}(\mathbf{x}) - I_{hist}\left(\mathbf{x} + D^{t-1}(\mathbf{x}) + \mathbf{d}^{l_i}\right) \right|}_{\approx \mathfrak{S}(I_{IVUS}, I_{hist} \circ T)} +$$

$$\underbrace{\sum_i^M \sum_{j \in N_i} \lambda \left\| \left(\mathbf{d}_i^{t-1} + \mathbf{d}^{l_i}\right) - \left(\mathbf{d}_j^{t-1} + \mathbf{d}^{l_j}\right) \right\|}_{\approx \lambda R(T)}$$

(8)

This registration methodology supports any similarity measure and can be incorporated with wide range of smoothing penalty functions. Consequently, we performed intensity-based registration on an intermediate representation of both IVUS and histology images, which were binary segmentation of stenosis regions in both modalities, as shown in Figure 2. The segmentation of lumen [11] and media-adventitia (MA) [12] borders in IVUS images could be performed automatically with manual refinement. We retrieved the same borders in histology images via the robust and supervised semi-automatic random walks [13] segmentation approach.

Subsequently, the extracted binary masks were registered as described above. In order to compensate for the difference between resolutions, the IVUS image was upsampled to match the histology resolution. This was simply done by detecting the bounding box of the IVUS segmentation, dotted-box in Figure 2 (c), and resizing the content of the bounding-box with cubic interpolation to match the histology image of higher resolution. The availability of different penalty functions in was an essential criterion for choosing this framework. More specifically, the lack of image structure and information inside the binary mask region would result in unrealistic deformations without proper regularization. In our approach we utilized the approximate curvature penalty for regularization of the deformation field [10].

4   Results and Quantification

We applied our algorithm on 14 pairs of IVUS-histology images. For each cross section of interest (CSI), the RF signals were stored in a matrix of 2048x256 (number of digitized samples x A-lines) and the IVUS grayscale image of size 512x512 was constructed after envelope detection, compression, decimation, and interpolation in axial and lateral directions, respectively. On the other hand, the sizes of histology images were varied since a histopathologist cropped the plaques using rectangles of different sizes.

Figure 3 demonstrates two distinct IVUS grayscale images along with their histology image correspondences and the final superimposed results after registration. The results are of particular interest since the shrinkage of artery, because of formaldehyde fixation, is well compensated by proposed registration framework. As we can see, the lumen and MA borders in both IVUS and histology images are perfectly aligned, Figure 4. The Dice similarity that measures the overlapping among areas enclosed by borders was 96.21±0.63 (≥95.26%). We also measured the line distances including Hausdorff and mean distance errors among delineated borders in IVUS and histology, after transformation, and found them to be 2.73±0.51 (≤3.6 pixels) and 0.65±0.05 (0.76 pixels), respectively. This confirmed the reliability of registration framework as well as the robustness of designed experimental set-up, obtaining the most reliable IVUS-histology matched database.

Existing supervised classification algorithms extract features and construct training datasets by looking at histology images and labeling tissues on IVUS images. In this method, the registration process is performed visually. However, finding the most homogenous region in histology image that represent a singular tissue type and therefore corresponding region in IVUS image is a very tedious and challenging task if not impossible. To validate the accuracy and reliability of such approach, we asked the histopathologist to identify the most recognizable regions, mainly consist of calcified regions, in both IVUS and histology images. The reason was the fact that calcified tissues are very well exhibited in histology images and there is an apparent

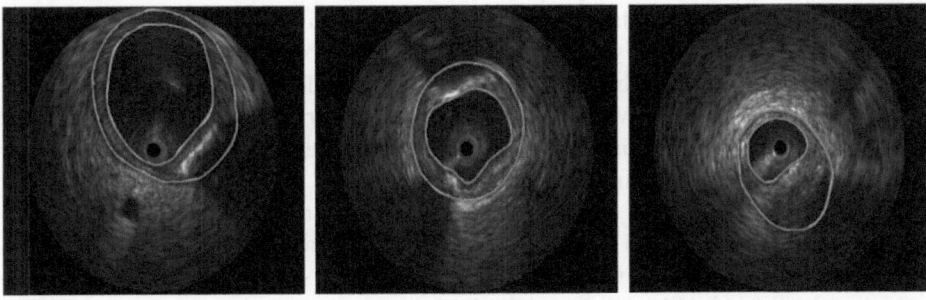

Fig. 4. Lumen and MA borders traced on IVUS images (yellow) and resulting borders drawn on corresponding histology images after registration (red)

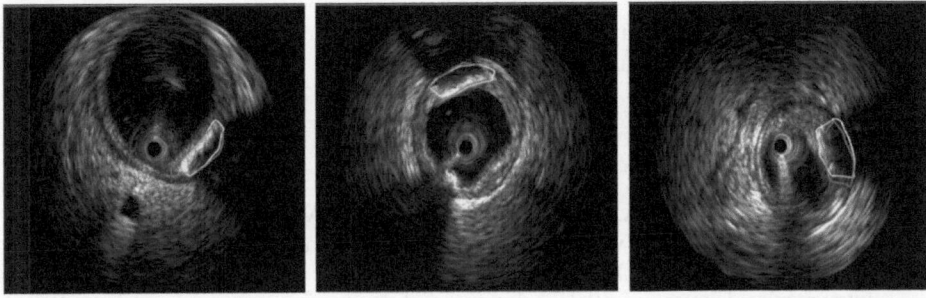

Fig. 5. Labeled tissues on three distinct IVUS images by the histopathologist (yellow) and resulting corresponding labeled tissues on histology images after registration (red)

shadowing behind arc of calcified plaques in IVUS images due to severe attenuation of IVUS signals. Figure 5 shows resulting manual labeled tissues driven from histology images after registration imposed along with corresponding labels on IVUS grayscale frames. We quantified the results using abovementioned similarity metrics and found Dice, Hausdorff, and mean distance errors as 54.86±13.41 (≥41.14%), 35.33±21.36 (≤86.56 pixels). As it is observed, the quantitative and qualitative results indicate that the precision of manual/visual labeling is not adequately high as it is expected. The main reason could be the ambiguity in segmentation of tissues in the IVUS image due to shadowing and lack of sufficient contrast or resolution. From atherosclerotic tissue classification point of view, this may result in inconsistency among extracted features and hamper the reliability of training dataset [7].

5   Discussion and Conclusion

In this paper, for the first time, we presented a registration framework for IVUS and histology images and provided quantitative as well as qualitative results. We observed that traditional manual/visual atherosclerotic tissue labeling, usually employed for classification, would lead to improper results. Therefore, a systematic robust registration is a must for atherosclerotic plaque characterization where tissues exhibit highly stringent characteristics. Although the current registration framework may not be seen novel, its application certainly is. Nevertheless, further improvement is needed.

The data collection and histology preparation methodologies helped considerably, achieving good registered IVUS-histology results. To further improve the registration results, additional regularization is required for the internal plaque deformations to preserve as much textural information as possible so a histolpathologist can toggle between images and then confidently label tissues on superimposed histo-IVUS images, Figure 3(c). As an alternative, a biomechanical model of the histology is advantageous in order to restrict possible deformations similar to what proposed for modeling brain-shift [14]. However, to the best of our knowledge, a mapping from histology image intensities to biomechanical is not available and seems elusive to acquire.

Acknowledgement. Authors would like to thank Dr. Stephane Carlier for his invaluable help collecting data and clinical feedbacks.

References

[1] Virmani, R., Burke, A.P., Kolodgie, F.D., Farb, A.: Pathology of the thin-cap fibroatheroma: A type of vulnerable plaque. J. Inteven. Cardiol. 16(3), 267–272 (2003)

[2] Katouzian, A., Laine, A.F.: Methods in Atherosclerotic Plaque Characterization Using Intravascular Ultrasound (IVUS) Images and Backscattered Signals. Atherosclerosis Disease Management Book, pp. 121–152. Springer (2010)

[3] Kawasaki, M., Takatsu, H., Noda, T., Sano, K., Ito, Y., Hayakawa, K., Tsuchiya, K., Arai, M., Nishigaki, K., Takemura, G., Minatoguchi, S., Fujiwara, T., Fujiwara, H.: In: Vivo Quantitative Tissue Characterization of Human Coronary Arterial Plaques by Use of Integrated Backscatter Intravascular Ultrasound and Comparison With Angioscopic Findings. Circulation, 2487- 2492 (May 2002)

[4] Taki, A., Roodaki, A., Pauly, O., Setarehdan, S., Unal, G., Navab, N.: A new method for characterization of coronary plaque composition via ivus images. In: IEEE International Symposium on Biomedical Imaging: From Nano to Macro, ISBI (2009)

[5] Escalera, S., Pujol, O., Mauri, J., Radeva, P.: Intravascular Ultrasound Tissue Characterization with Sub-class Error-Correcting Output Codes. J. Sign. Process. Syst. 55(1-3), 35–47 (2009)

[6] Seabra, J., Ciompi, F., Pujol, O., Mauri, J., Radeva, P., Sanchez, J.: Rayleigh Mixture Model for Plaque Characterization in Intravascular Ultrasound. IEEE Tran. Bio. Med. Eng. 58(5) (2011)

[7] Katouzian, A., Sathyanarayana, S., Baseri, B., Konofagou, E.E., Carlier, S.G.: Challenges in Atherosclerotic Plaque Characterization with Intravascular Ultrasound (IVUS): From Data Collection to Classification. IEEE Trans. on Information Technology in Biomedicine 12(3), 315–327

[8] Nair, A., Kuban, B.D., Obuchowski, N., Vince, D.G.: Assessing spectral algorithms to predict atherosclerotic plaque composition with normalized and raw intravascular ultrasound data. Ultrasound Med. Biol. 27(10), 1319–1331 (2001)

[9] Bookstein, F.L.: Principal warps: Thin-plate splines and the decomposition of deformations. IEEE Trans. Patt. Anal. Mach. Intell. 2(6), 567–585 (1989)

[10] Glocker, B., Komodakis, N., Paragios, N., Navab, N.: Approximated curvature penalty in non-rigid registration using pairwise MRFs. In: Advances in Visual Computing, pp. 1101–1109 (2009)

[11] Katouzian, A., Angelini, E.D., Sturm, B., Laine, A.F.: Automatic Detection of Luminal Borders in IVUS Images by Magnitude-Phase Histograms of Complex Brushlet Coefficients. In: IEEE Proceeding of EMBC, Buenos Aires, Argentina (2010)

[12] Unal, G., Bucher, S., Carlier, S., Slabaugh, G., Fang, T., Tanaka, K.: Shape-Driven Segmentation of the Arterial Wall in Intravascular Ultrasound Images. IEEE Trans. Info. Tech. Biomed. 12(3), 335–347 (2008)

[13] Grady, L.: Random walks for image segmentation. IEEE Transactions on Pattern Analysis and Machine Intelligence 28(11), 1768–1783 (2006)

[14] Ferrant, M., Warfield, S.K., Nabavi, A., Jolesz, F.A., Kikinis, R.: Registration of 3D Intraoperative MR Images of the Brain Using a Finite Element Biomechanical Model. In: Delp, S.L., DiGoia, A.M., Jaramaz, B. (eds.) MICCAI 2000. LNCS, vol. 1935, pp. 19–28. Springer, Heidelberg (2000)

Optimization over Random and Gradient Probabilistic Pixel Sampling for Fast, Robust Multi-resolution Image Registration

Boris N. Oreshkin and Tal Arbel

McGill University, Center of Intelligent Machines,
3480 University Street, Montreal, Quebec, Canada, H3A 2A7
`boris.oreshkin@mail.mcgill.ca`, `arbel@cim.mcgill.ca`

Abstract. This paper presents an approach to fast image registration through probabilistic pixel sampling. We propose a practical scheme to leverage the benefits of two state-of-the-art pixel sampling approaches: gradient magnitude based pixel sampling and uniformly random sampling. Our framework involves learning the optimal balance between the two sampling schemes off-line during training, based on a small training dataset, using particle swarm optimization. We then test the proposed sampling approach on 3D rigid registration against two state-of-the-art approaches based on the popular, publicly available, Vanderbilt RIRE dataset. Our results indicate that the proposed sampling approach yields much faster, accurate and robust registration results when compared against the state-of-the-art.

Keywords: image registration, pixel selection, sampling.

1 Introduction

Image registration is one of the critical problems in the field of medical imaging. It transcends wide range of applications from image-guided interventions to building anatomical atlases from patient data. Typically, the evaluation of the similarity measure and its derivatives are required to perform the optimization over transformation parameters. However, performing these computations based on all the available image pixels can be prohibitively costly. The expense is mainly due to the large number of pixel intensity values involved in the calculations. Time-sensitive applications, like image guided intervention, generally benefit from techniques to speed up direct image registration by utilizing only a subset of available pixels during registration. In these contexts, several percent of accuracy decrease could be tolerated and traded for preservation of robustness and significant decrease in registration time. However, significant speedups attained via *aggressive* reduction in the number of selected pixels (less than 1% of the total number of pixels) often result in deterioration of robustness (increase in failure rate) and relatively rapid increase of registration error.

Many pixel sampling schemes have been suggested in the literature. Uniformly random pixel selection (URS), in which a random subset of all pixels sampled

B.M. Dawant et al. (Eds.): WBIR 2012, LNCS 7359, pp. 150–159, 2012.
© Springer-Verlag Berlin Heidelberg 2012

with uniform probabilities is used to drive the optimization, gained popularity due to its simplicity and robustness [9, 13]. Other techniques strived to improve registration accuracy by optimizing the pixel selection process. The deterministic pixel selection strategy [10] consists in calculating a selection criterion for each pixel (e.g. based on Jacobian of the cost function [4]) and comparing it to the threshold. The subset of pixels whose selection criterion values transcend a predefined threshold are used for registration. This led to a clustering phenomenon, as pointed out by Dallaert and Collins [4], who attempted to overcome this effect and proposed a probabilistic pixel selection strategy that uniformly samples from subset of pixels having top twenty percent values of selection criterion pixels. Brooks and Arbel [2] extend the approach of Dellaert and Collins [4] by proposing an information theoretic selection criterion and by addressing the issue of Jacobian scale inherent to the gradient descent type optimization algorithms. Benhimane et al. [1] proposed a criterion to speed up the convergence of the optimization by selecting only the pixels that closely verify the approximation made by the optimization. Sabuncu and Ramadge used information theoretical approach to demonstrate the fact that the pixel sampling scheme should emphasize pixels with high spatial gradient magnitude [11]. Here the moving image is probabilistically subsampled using non-uniform grid generated based on the probabilities proportional to the gradient magnitude. This approach allows to diversify and spread subsampled pixels while still giving attention to image details. This approach alleviates the effects of selected pixel clustering inherent to deterministic pixel selection strategy discussed e.g. by Reeves and Hezar [10] while still allowing to focus on the more useful pixels. Finally, curvlet based sampling, recently proposed by Freiman et al. [6] tested on Vanderbilt RIRE dataset [5] revealed approximately the same level of accuracy as the gradient subsampling approach [11].

Exploring the method of Sabuncu and Ramadge, one notices that the strategy works well for relatively large pixel sampling rates (1 to 10%). However, as the number of selected pixels decreases, it tends to concentrate exclusively on pixels with the highest gradient magnitude, which limits its exploratory capability and leads to deterioration of robustness and accuracy. The uniformly random sampling strategy, on the other hand, has very good exploratory behaviour as any pixel has equal probability to be used in the similarity metric calculations. At the same time, the uniformly random sampling lacks attention to image structural details that often aid in achieving easier and more accurate registration results. Thus the URS often provides better robustness, but fails to produce the same accuracy levels as the gradient magnitude based approach.

In this paper, we propose to combine the virtues of the two techniques to obtain faster and more robust image registration. We introduce a new multi-scale sampling scheme, whereby the sampling probabilities are based on the convex combination of the uniformly random sampling probabilities [9, 13] and the gradient based sampling probabilities [11]. We further propose to learn the value of the convex combination parameter off-line by optimizing the empirical target registration error obtained from a small training dataset via particle swarm optimization [7]. Our approach effectively serves to improve the performance of one of the best existing state-of-the-art sampling methods and achieve the greatest reduction in the number of pixels used for the evaluation of the similarity metric under the constraint of preserving the accuracy and robustness at reasonable levels. We test the proposed approach on the Vanderbilt RIRE dataset [5]. Our results indicate that the proposed approach allows to significantly reduce the number of pixels used in the evaluation of the similarity metric and hence accelerate the registration procedure while improving robustness and preserving accuracy of the gradient based sampling technique.

2   Problem Statement

The direct image registration problem can be formulated for the reference $I(\mathbf{x})$ and the moving $J(\mathrm{T}_\theta(\mathbf{x}))$ images defined by their pixel intensity values I_i, J_i : $\mathcal{X} \to \mathcal{I}, i = 1 \ldots N$ seen as mappings from the coordinate space $\mathcal{X} \subseteq \mathbb{R}^d$ to the intensity space $\mathcal{I} \subseteq \mathbb{R}$, where d is the dimensionality of coordinate space and N is the number of pixels (here we assume, without loss of generality, that the number of pixels in the images is equal). The problem is solved by finding the parameters $\theta \in \Theta$ of the warp $\mathrm{T}_\theta : \mathcal{X} \to \mathcal{X}$ that maximize the similarity metric $D_N : \mathcal{I}^{N \times 2} \to \mathbb{R}$ that maps N intensity values of the reference and N intensity values of the moving images into a number characterizing the degree of similarity between these images for a given value of the warp parameters:

$$\theta_{\mathrm{opt}} = \arg \max_{\theta \in \Theta} D_N[I(\mathbf{x}), J(\mathrm{T}_\theta(\mathbf{x}))]. \tag{1}$$

Widely used similarity metrics are mutual information [13] and normalized mutual information (NMI) [12]. The pixel selection process can be viewed as the approximate solution using the calculation of the similarity metric based on only M pixels of each of the images:

$$\theta_{\mathrm{opt}} = \arg \max_{\theta \in \Theta} D_M[I(\mathbf{x}), J(\mathrm{T}_\theta(\mathbf{x}))], \tag{2}$$

Since this solution is based on $M < N$ pixels it is less computationally expensive. As was indicated in Section 1, the deterioration of robustness and accuracy of the existing pixel subsampling methods, and gradient based sampling in particular, is a major problem when the number of pixels used to calculate the similarity metric is small, $M \ll N$. At the same time, the small sampling rate condition $M/N \ll 1$ ensures that significant computational gain results from the pixel selection. In this paper we strive to solve the problem of robustness and accuracy deterioration for small M. To this end, we propose the approach to combine the uniformly random sampling with the gradient based sampling within the multi-scale framework that we discuss in detail in the next section.

3   Proposed Algorithm

Sabuncu and Ramadge used information theoretical approach to demonstrate the fact that the pixel sampling scheme should emphasize pixels with high spatial gradient magnitude [11]. Based on this observation they proposed the sampling strategy where pixel i is sampled with the probability $q_i = \alpha \|\nabla J_i\|_2$, where $\|\nabla J_i\|_2$ is the magnitude of spatial intensity gradient of pixel i and α is the normalization factor that determines the average number of subsampled pixels. The URS sampling approach attaches equal sampling probability to each pixel. The gradient magnitude based sampling puts more emphasis on the image gradient details that provide for more accurate registration. However, this often reduces registration robustness by reducing image exploration. URS explores images well via extensive uniform sampling, but lack of attention to image details reduces its accuracy.

We propose to combine the positive properties of the two techniques just described and to obtain a better multi-scale sampling scheme designed for fast image registration. In our algorithm we combine the probabilities of the gradient magnitude based sampling approach and the URS approach such that the sampling probability of the proposed algorithm is the convex combination of the probabilities defined by the two corresponding component approaches. The optimal value of the convex combination parameter is learned off-line by optimizing the empirical target registration error (ETRE) obtained from a training dataset. In the remainder of this section we describe the details of the proposed algorithm.

Assume that there are R resolution levels in the registration scheme, r is the resolution level number and N_r is the number of pixels at level r. Assume that $r = 1$ corresponds to the highest resolution level (original images) and hence $N_1 = N$. Denote $\mathbf{q}^r = [q_1^r, \ldots, q_{N_r}^r]$ the vector of sampling probabilities for the gradient magnitude sampling method at level r and assume that the normalization factor α^r at this level is chosen so that the average number of pixels equals M_r. Similarly, for the URS method the vector of sampling probabilities is $\mathbf{u}^r = [M_r/N_r, \ldots, M_r/N_r]$ resulting in the average number of pixels sampled being equal to M_r. The vector of sampling probabilities for the proposed approach, $\mathbf{r}^r$, is the convex combination of the two previously defined vectors:

$$\mathbf{r}^r = (1 - \beta^r)\mathbf{q}^r + \beta^r \mathbf{u}^r, \tag{3}$$

where $\beta^r \in [0,1]$ is the mixing parameter. Greater values of β^r emphasize the exploration brought about by the URS and lower values of this parameter emphasize prominent image features that could facilitate more accurate registration. In a general situation we expect that at every level r and for every pixel sampling rate M_r/N_r there is an optimal value of β^r that compromises image exploration and exploitation of prominent image features.

It is hard (if at all possible) to analytically formulate and solve the problem of optimizing β^r based on statistical models of the images. At the same time, if a small, but representative training dataset is available for the registration problem at hand, the value of this parameter could be learned empirically off-line. The learned value of this parameter could then be used upon each subsequent application of the proposed algorithm. The proposed algorithm could be retrained whenever there is a need to solve a new registration problem with significantly different image specifics. This is not an unreasonable assumption since in the application domain the specifics of particular registration problem often affect e.g. the choice of similarity metric, optimization strategy and interpolation scheme. This implies that at least some training information in the form of the small set of exemplar image pairs from the problem-specific modalities using certain acquisition and post-processing protocols must always be available to the registration algorithm designer to guide the algorithm development.

Based on the assumption that we have a training data set and the gold standard registration parameters for the image pairs in this dataset we formulate the empirical learning criterion $Q^r(\beta^r)$. We define the ETRE as the average over V image pairs in the training dataset and U Monte-Carlo trials:

$$Q^r(\beta^r) = \frac{1}{V}\frac{1}{U}\sum_{v=1}^{V}\sum_{u=1}^{U}\|\mathbf{X}_v - \widehat{\mathbf{X}}_{u,v}^r(\beta^r)\|_2^2. \tag{4}$$

Here $\mathbf{X}_v$ is the set of transformed coordinates obtained using gold standard registration parameters for image pair v and $\widehat{\mathbf{X}}_{u,v}^r(\beta^r)$ is the set of transformed coordinates for image pair v and Monte-Carlo trial u found using the empirical estimate of the registration parameters obtained via the optimization of the similarity metric at resolution scale r using the proposed pixel sampling algorithm with a given value of mixing parameter β^r. As the pixel sampling algorithm is randomized, some degree of Monte-Carlo averaging could be beneficial if V is relatively small ($3\ldots5$ images). Thus we repeat the registration procedure for the same candidate value β^r, level r and image pair v U times and calculate $\widehat{\mathbf{X}}_{u,v}^r(\beta^r)$ based on the new registration parameter estimate each time.

We propose to learn the value of β^r by minimizing the ETRE $Q^r(\beta^r)$:

$$\widehat{\beta}^r = \arg\min_{\beta^r\in[0;1]} Q^r(\beta^r). \tag{5}$$

The function $Q^r(\cdot)$ is generally extremely irregular and non-smooth, because of the possible registration failures and because of complex dependence of the ETRE on the value of β^r. At the same time, the domain of this function is well defined and restricted. Thus any optimizer capable of performing global or quasi-global search on a restricted interval using only the objective function values will suffice to solve this problem. We propose to use the particle swarm optimization (PSO) [7] in order to find $\widehat{\beta}^r$. Our algorithm proceeds by finding $\widehat{\beta}^R$, the value of the mixing parameter for the scale with the lowest resolution using PSO. The multi-scale registration algorithm proceeds from the lowest resolution level to the highest resolution level sequentially utilizing the registration parameters obtained at the lower resolution level as an initialization for the current resolution level. Our learning algorithm thus uses the identified value of $\widehat{\beta}^R$ to find the estimate of the registration parameters at resolution level R. Then the optimal value $\widehat{\beta}^{R-1}$ for the next higher-resolution level is found using the registration parameters identified at level R as initialization. This procedure iterates until the values of mixing parameter for all resolution levels $R, R-1, \ldots, 1$ are identified.

4   Experiments with the RIRE Vanderbilt Dataset

4.1   Dataset Description

To test the proposed algorithm we made use of the real clinical data available in RIRE Vanderbilt dataset [5]. The performance of algorithms was evaluated by registering 3D volumes corresponding to CT images to geometrically corrected MR images. MR image set included images acquired using T1, T2 and PD acquisition protocols. The total number of different image pairs used was 19. Those pairs were taken from patients 001, 002, 003, 004, 005, 006, 007 for which geometrically corrected images are available. Patients 003 and 006 did not have geometrically corrected PD and MR-T1 images respectively. According to the data exchange protocol established by the RIRE Vanderbilt project, registration results obtained via algorithms under the test were uploaded to the RIRE Vanderbilt web-site. Algorithm evaluation results were calculated by the RIRE Vanderbilt remote computer using the gold standard transformation not available to us and published on their web-site in the form of tables containing registration errors calculated over 6 to 10 volumes of interest (VOIs) for each image pair. For patient 000 geometrically corrected MR-T1, MR-T2, MR-PD images and corresponding CT image are available along with the set of transformed coordinates obtained using gold standard registration parameters. Three image pairs from patient 000 were used to learn the values of mixing parameters according to the algorithm described in Section 3.

4.2   Experimental Setup

All images were first resampled to a common 1mm grid using bicubic interpolation. We used 4-scale registration based on the low-pass filtered and downsampled image pyramid. Resolution level number four had grid spacing 4 mm along each axis and resolution level number one had grid spacing 1mm along each axis. The estimate of the registration parameters obtained at a lower resolution level was used as a starting point for the registration at the next higher resolution level; level 4 had all its parameters initialized to zero values. We concentrated on recovering 6 rigid registration parameters (3 translations and 3 rotations) using the NMI similarity metric [12]. Histogram for the evaluation of the similarity metric was calculated using the partial volume approach with Hanning windowed sinc kernel function [8]. Similarity metric was optimized using the trust region Gauss-Newton approach [3]. We implemented the most calculation intensive part of the code (calculation of the cost function and its derivatives) in C and benchmarked the algorithms within the MATLAB environment.

We evaluated the performance of following pixel sampling approaches. The uniformly random sampling (**URS**) technique consists of randomly selecting pixels with equal probabilities at every iteration [13]. At a given resolution level r all pixels have equal probability of being selected, M/N_r if $M < N_r$ and 1 if $M \geq N_r$; the average number of selected pixels is thus equal to M

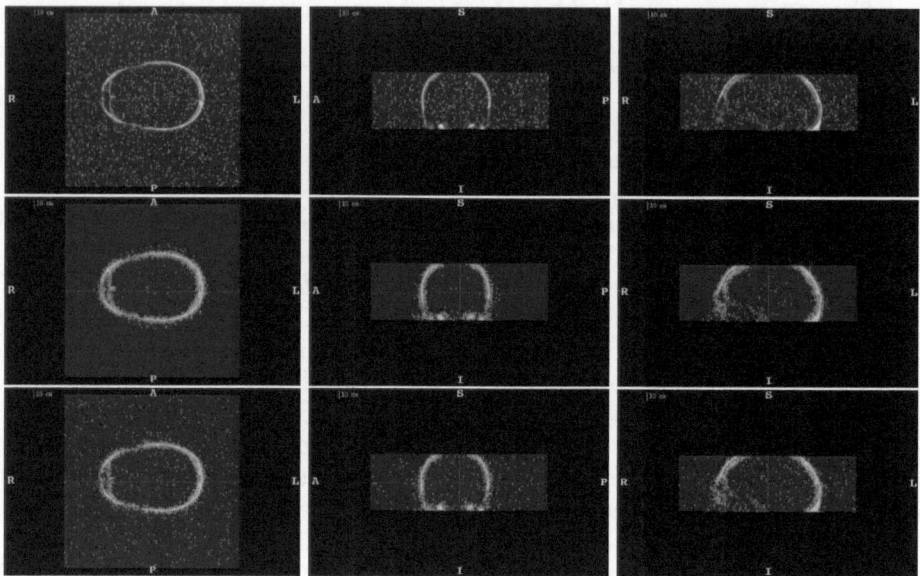

Fig. 1. Pixel selection masks generated using different approaches at the highest resolution level for sampling rate 0.5%. (FIRST ROW) **URS**; (SECOND ROW) **GMS**; (THIRD ROW) proposed approach with learned value of the mixing parameter $\widehat{\beta}^1 = 0.2$. First column axial slice, second column sagittal slice, third column coronal slice. All images are obtained using ITK-SNAP [14].

at each resolution level. Note that we used equal number of selected pixels for all resolution scales. Gradient magnitude sampling (**GMS**), a slight modification of gradient based subsampling originally proposed by Subuncu and Ramadge [11], consists in calculating spatial gradient magnitude $\|\nabla J_i\|_2 = \sqrt{(\partial J_i/\partial x_i)^2 + (\partial J_i/\partial y_i)^2 + (\partial J_i/\partial z_i)^2}$ and sampling pixels at every optimization iteration according to the probabilities proportional to it, where the proportionality coefficient is chosen so that the average number of pixels selected at every resolution scale is equal to M. Proposed method described in Section 3 (**Proposed**) consists of mixing the probabilities obtained from URS and GMS methods and learning the value of the mixing parameter using the training dataset constructed from image pairs of patient 000. We evaluate these three algorithms for the following values of pixel sampling rates (given in %): $M/N \in \{0.02, 0.04, 0.065, 0.1, 0.5, 1\}$ (sampling rate is calculated with respect to the image size at the highest resolution level, N).

4.3 Results

Figure 1 shows the examples of pixel selection masks generated using tested approaches at the highest resolution level for pixel sampling rate 0.5%. It is obvious that the samples generated with the URS approach are extremely spread,

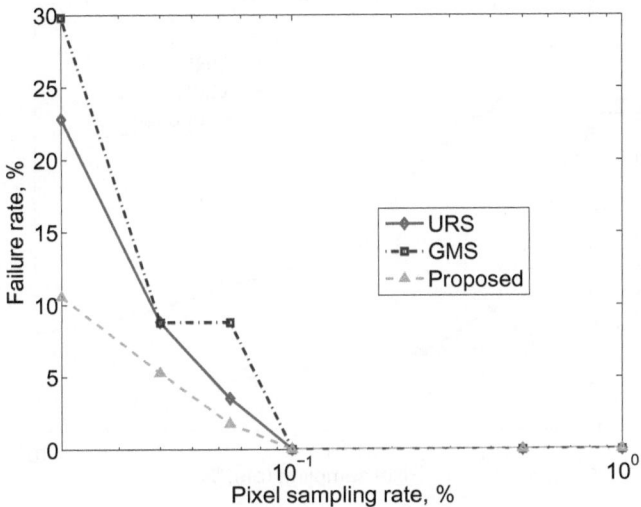

Fig. 2. Failure rate for different pixel sampling mechanisms: gradient magnitude sampling (GMS), uniformly random sampling (URS), Proposed. Note that the proposed approach consistently outperforms in terms of robustness.

whereas the samples generated with the GMS approach are overly concentrated along the gradient magnitude structures present in the image. The proposed approach produces samples that balance those two extremities.

Figure 2 shows registration failure rate for the following set of pixel sampling rates (in %): $\{0.02, 0.04, 0.065, 0.1, 0.5, 1\}$. We define a failure as any case with error exceeding 10mm in any of the VOIs. We can see that the proposed approach consistently outperforms other approaches in terms of robustness.

Figure 3 shows the trimmed mean target registration error (mTRE). We compute the trimmed mTRE as the mTRE of the successful (non-failed) cases. The mTRE is minimal for the proposed approach compared to other methods. The proposed approach retains high level of accuracy and robustness even with low pixel sampling rates. This allows to significantly reduce computational time in a practical system without exploding the failure rate or reducing accuracy.

Such results support our conjecture that balancing image exploration induced by URS and the exploitation of the prominent image features induced by GMS using a small problem specific training dataset can significantly improve and accelerate the performance of the registration algorithm. Overall, the proposed technique at 0.1% pixel sampling rate is better than other techniques at 1% pixel sampling rate, simultaneously maintaining zero failure rate and 1.15 mm accuracy. Thus on average our approach can use 10 times less pixels for registration, achieve 0 failure rate and improve accuracy over the other two techniques. This is significant improvement over both alternative methods and it allows to reduce the time from 210 seconds per registration for 1% pixel sampling rate to 32 seconds per registration for 0.1% pixel sampling rate in our implementation.

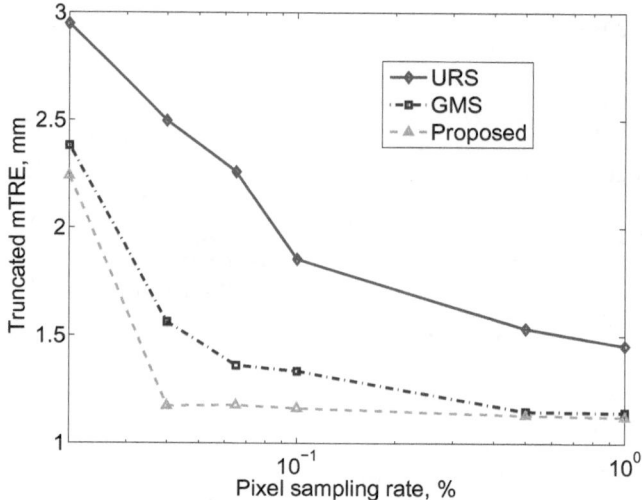

Fig. 3. Trimmed average registration error for different pixel sampling mechanisms: gradient magnitude sampling (GMS), uniformly random sampling (URS), Proposed. Note that the proposed approach consistently outperforms in terms of accuracy.

5   Conclusions and Discussion

In this paper we presented a novel approach to pixel sampling for faster and more accurate registration. Our approach mixes the uniformly random sampling probabilities with those obtained using the gradient magnitude based sampling approach. The mixing parameter that balances image exploration induced by uniform probabilities and the exploitation of image features via gradient magnitude based sampling is learned off-line from a small training dataset. Our experiments with the Vanderbilt RIRE dataset demonstrate that the proposed approach works much faster and produces much more accurate and robust registration results. We conjecture that the concept of mixing the sampling probabilities can be further generalized to obtain even better results. In this case rather than mixing only two sampling methods we could mix three, four or more methods and learn the optimal problem specific mixing coefficients using a small training dataset and a suitable mixing parameter optimization scheme. Exploring this venue based on the experiments with Vanderbilt RIRE dataset and other available datasets as well as testing it on non-rigid registration problems to study the generalizability of the proposed approach seems to be an attractive venue for future research.

References

1. Benhimane, S., Ladikos, A., Lepetit, V., Navab, N.: Linear and quadratic subsets for template-based tracking. In: Proc. IEEE CVPR, Minneapolis, MN, USA (June 2007)

2. Brooks, R., Arbel, T.: The importance of scale when selecting pixels for image registration. In: Proc. CRV, Paris, France, pp. 235–242 (May 2007)
3. Brooks, R.: Efficient and Reliable Methods for Direct Parameterized Image Registration. Ph.D. thesis, McGill University (2008)
4. Dellaert, F., Collins, R.: Fast image-based tracking by selective pixel integration. In: Proc. ICCV, Kerkyra, Greece (September 1999)
5. Fitzpatrick, J., West, J., Maurer, C.: Predicting error in rigid-body point-based registration. IEEE TMI 17(5), 694–702 (1998)
6. Freiman, M., Werman, M., Joskowicz, L.: A curvelet-based patient-specific prior for accurate multi-modal brain image rigid registration. Med. Imag. Anal. 15(1), 125–132 (2010)
7. Kennedy, J., Eberhart, R.: Particle swarm optimization. In: Proc. IEEE Int. Conf. Neural Networks, vol. 4, pp. 1942–1948 (November 1995)
8. Lu, X., Zhang, S., Su, H., Chen, Y.: Mutual information-based multimodal image registration using a novel joint histogram estimation. Computerized Medical Imaging and Graphics 32(3), 202–209 (2008)
9. Mattes, D., Haynor, D., Vesselle, H., Lewellen, T., Eubank, W.: PET-CT image registration in the chest using free-form deformations. IEEE TMI 22(1), 120–128 (2003)
10. Reeves, S.J., Hezar, R.: Selection of observations in magnetic resonance spectroscopic imaging. In: Proc. ICIP, vol. 1, pp. 641–644 (October 1995)
11. Sabuncu, M.R., Ramadge, P.J.: Gradient based nonuniform subsampling for information-theoretic alignment methods. In: Proc. IEEE IEMBS., vol. 1, pp. 1683–1686 (September 2004)
12. Studholme, C., Hill, D.L.G., Hawkes, D.J.: An overlap invariant entropy measure of 3D medical image alignment. Pattern Recognition 32(1), 71–86 (1999)
13. Viola, P., Wells, W.M.: Alignment by maximization of mutual information. IJCV 24(2), 137–154 (1997)
14. Yushkevich, P.A., Piven, J., Hazlett, C.H., Smith, G.R., Ho, S., Gee, J.C., Gerig, G.: User-guided 3D active contour segmentation of anatomical structures: Significantly improved efficiency and reliability. Neuroimage 31(3), 1116–1128 (2006)

Quad-tree Based Entropy Estimator
for Fast and Robust Brain Image Registration

Žiga Špiclin, Boštjan Likar, and Franjo Pernuš

Faculty of Electrical Engineering, Laboratory of Imaging Technologies,
University of Ljubljana, Tržaška 25, 1000 Ljubljana, Slovenia
{ziga.spiclin,bostjan.likar,franjo.pernus}@fe.uni-lj.si

Abstract. The performances of information-theoretic multi-modality image registration methods crucially depend on the model representing the joint density function of the co-occurring image intensities and on the implementation of the entropy estimator. We proposed an entropy estimator for image registration based on quad-tree (QT) that is essentially an entropic graph entropy estimator, but can be adapted to work as a plug-in entropy estimator. This duality was achieved by incorporating the Hilbert kernel density estimator. Results of 3-D rigid-body registration of multi-modal brain volumes indicate that the proposed methods achieve similar accuracies as the registration method based on minimal spanning tree (MST), but have a higher success rate and a higher capture range. Although the MST and QT have similar computational complexities, the QT-based methods had about 50% shorter registration times.

Keywords: brain image registration, multi-modality, entropic graph, Rényi entropy, Hilbert kernel, minimal spanning tree, quad-tree.

1 Introduction

Multi-modality imaging is a commonplace in medical studies and image-based diagnosis and follow-up of patients. Imaging modalities that are typically used to observe structural and/or functional information include computed tomography (CT) and magnetic resonance imaging (MRI), positron emission tomography (PET) and ultrasound (US). Applications that employ multiple modalities are automated image analysis, information fusion and correlation detection, biomarker extraction, image-based prediction, etc. A critical requirement in these applications is that the multi-modal images are in good spatial alignment, which can be achieved through image registration.

Registering medical images presents a challenging problem, especially due to the high variety of the physical imaging modalities. The multi-modality medical images undergoing registration frequently exhibit highly nonlinear relationships between the co-occurring image intensities. A common approach to registering such multi-modality images is to evaluate the statistical dependency between the co-occurring image intensities using information-theoretic criteria. The statistical dependency is represented by a joint density function (JDF) of the co-occurring image intensities and quantified by the information-theoretic criteria,

B.M. Dawant et al. (Eds.): WBIR 2012, LNCS 7359, pp. 160–169, 2012.

which in general represent a measure of divergence of the observed JDF from the JDF that would be obtained if the co-occurring image intensities were independent [11]. The representation model of the JDF of the co-occurring image intensities plays a central role and typically defines the class of estimators for the information-theoretic criteria [5,14,4,6]. Among all the information-theoretic criteria, mutual information has been studied and applied most extensively [10]. The critical component of mutual information, and the related f-information criteria [11], is the approach to estimating the entropy of the observed JDF. Hence, the choice of the model representing the JDF and the particular implementation of the entropy estimator crucially define the overall performances of the image registration method [10].

A common approach to representing the JDF is to compute the histogram of the co-occurring intensities or to apply the Parzen kernel density method [13]. Such explicit representations of the JDF lead to the so-called *plug-in* entropy estimators, which have been used extensively for multi-modal image registration [14,5,10]. Some approaches use the implicit JDF representation, given by the partitioning of the scatter space of the co-occurring image intensities to derive the entropy estimators. Miller [6] used the Voronoi tessellation for the m-spacings estimator. Recently, Kybic and Vnučko [3] proposed to use an all nearest-neighbor (NN) Kozachenko-Leonenko entropy estimator. To solve the all-NN problem they evaluated several scatter space partitioning algorithms such as k-d trees, balanced box decomposition trees and locality sensitive hashing. Approaches based on entropic graphs [4,7,12] apply a minimal spanning tree (MST), which connects by a shortest overall path all the co-occurring image intensities that span the JDF. The length of the MST is a consistent estimator of the α-Rényi entropy [4]. Neemuchwala et al. [8] used a k-NN based entropic graph to estimate several different α-entropy measures. Each of the mentioned methods has at least one of the drawbacks: 1) lacks an efficient descent optimization method [14,5,8], 2) has high computational complexity, i.e. the all-NN problem [3], or 3) is sensitive to bad initialization [4,7,12].

In this paper, we propose a quad-tree (QT) based entropy estimator for image registration that is essentially an entropic graph entropy estimator [4,12], but can be adapted with minor modifications to work as a plug-in entropy estimator [14]. This duality was achieved by incorporating the Hilbert kernel density estimator [1,9]. A two 3-D rigid-body registration experiments were performed with multi-modal brain volumes to test the proposed QT-based registration methods and to compare them to the MST-based registration method [12]. The results indicate that the QT-based methods achieve similar registration accuracy as the MST-method, but have a higher success rate and a higher capture range, i.e. in the case of bad initialization the QT-based registration methods have a higher chance of convergence. Although the MST and the QT have similar computational complexities, the QT-based registration methods had about 50% shorter registration times.

2   Image Registration Methodology

Let $u_i = u(x_i)$ and $v_i = v(\mathcal{T}(x_i))$ be the intensities of the reference and the floating image, respectively, where $\mathcal{T}(x) : \mathbb{R}^n \to \mathbb{R}^n$ is a spatial transformation, n is the dimensionality of the images and $x_i \in \Omega$ are lexicographically ordered spatial coordinates for $i = 1, \ldots, N$ in the overlapping spatial domain Ω of the two images. Commonly, the spatial transformation $\mathcal{T}(x)$ is a function of some parameters θ, i.e. $\mathcal{T}(x) = f(x, \theta)$ and the floating image intensities are dependent on θ, noted as v_i^θ. Co-occurring intensity pairs in Ω can be compactly denoted as $z_i = [u_i, v_i^\theta]^{\mathrm{T}}$. The task now is to find the optimal parameters $\hat{\theta}$ that optimize a criterion $\mathcal{C}(\theta)$, which measures the degree of correspondence between the intensities u_i and v_i^θ. One such criteria that measures the statistical dependence between pixel pairs z_i is the joint entropy (or related mutual information [14]). The image registration problem can thus be formulated as:

$$\hat{\theta} = \operatorname{argmin}_\theta \hat{H}(z^\theta) , \tag{1}$$

where $\hat{\theta}$ are the optimal parameters with respect to (w.r.t.) the estimate of the joint entropy $\hat{H}(z^\theta)$. There are different ways to estimate the entropy, the most popular being the plug-in entropy estimate $\hat{H}(z) = - \sum_{i=1}^{N} \hat{p}(z_i) \log \hat{p}(z_i)$, which require an explicit model representing the JDF, i.e. $\hat{p}(z_i)$. Alternatively, an estimate of the entropy can be obtained by using entropic graphs.

2.1   Entropy Estimation Using Entropic Graphs

Entropic graphs refer to minimal graphs (e.g. MST, NN) on the i.i.d. samples z_i that define the JDF. Given a set $Z = \{z_i; i, \ldots, N\}$ in $\mathbb{R}^d$, let $G = (E, Z)$ be a graph with edge set E and vertex set Z. Edge $e = (z_i, z_j) \in E$ has length $\|e\| = \|z_i - z_j\|$, where $\| \cdot \|$ is the L_2 norm. For a graph G and $\gamma \in \mathbb{R}$, let $W_\gamma = \sum_{e \in E} \|e\|^\gamma$. For a fixed $G(Z)$, the minimal graph is defined as:

$$G^*(Z) = \operatorname{argmin}_{G \in G(Z)} W_\gamma(G) \tag{2}$$

and W_γ^* is the corresponding minimal graph weight. Ma et al.[4] have shown that the following quantity leads to an asymptotically unbiased estimate of the α-Rényi entropy:

$$\hat{H}_\alpha = \frac{1}{1 - \alpha} \log\left(\beta \frac{W_\gamma^*}{N^\alpha} \right) , \tag{3}$$

where $\alpha \in (0, 1)$ and β is a constant. Hence, by minimizing the minimal graph weight W_γ^*, the entropy estimate is effectively minimized, thereby solving the registration problem in (1).

The entropic graph is a special case of the plug-in entropy estimator. Let $A(G)$ represent the adjacency matrix of G, in which (ij)-th entry $A(G)(i,j)$ is the number of edges joining vertex i and j. For a family of minimal graphs, assume there exists a matrix L such that $L(G) + L(G)^{\mathrm{T}} = A(G)$ and each row of $L(G)$ has at most one non-zero entry equal to one. Then, the minimal graph weight is expressed as [12]:

$$W_\gamma^*(G) = \frac{1}{2} \sum_{i=1}^{N} \sum_{j=1}^{N} \|z_i - z_j\|^\gamma A(G^*)(i,j)$$

$$\sum_{i=1}^{N} \Big(\sum_{j=1}^{N} \|z_i - z_j\|^\beta L(G^*)(i,j) \Big)^{\gamma/\beta} . \tag{4}$$

Let $\gamma = d(1 - \alpha)$, then using (4) in the log-argument of (3) yields:

$$\beta \frac{W_\gamma^*(G)}{N^\alpha} = \sum_{i=1}^{N} \hat{p}(z_i; G^*)^{\alpha-1} , \tag{5}$$

where $\hat{p}(z_i; G^*)$ is a "graph-based" density estimate defined as:

$$\hat{p}(z_i; G^*) = \frac{\beta^{1/(\alpha-1)}}{N} \sum_{j=1}^{N} \|z_i - z_j\|^{-d} L(G^*)(i,j) . \tag{6}$$

By combining (5) and (3) one obtains the sample mean, plug-in approximation for the α-Rényi entropy, which becomes equal to the Shannon entropy estimate as $\alpha \to 1$; i.e. $\hat{H} = \mathbb{E}_i(\log \hat{p}(z_i))$ as proposed by Viola [14].

2.2 Plug-in Entropy Estimator Using Hilbert Kernel Density

For the plug-in entropy estimator we will employ the Hilbert kernel density proposed by Devroye and Krzyżak [1], defined as:

$$\hat{p}(z) = \frac{1}{V_d N \log N} \sum_{j=1}^{N} \|z - z_j\|^{-d} , \tag{7}$$

where V_d is the volume of the unit ball in $\mathbb{R}^d$. The Hilbert kernel density estimate in (7) is weakly consistent at almost all z, that is, $\hat{p}(z) \to p(z)$ in probability at almost all z [1]. Note that (7) is similar to (6) up to the choice of the neighboring samples defined by matrix L and the constant factors. By defining $L(G^*)(i,j)$ in (6) as the harmonic number we obtain exactly the Hilbert kernel density estimate, hence (7) is a harmonically weighted nearest-neighbor density estimate [1].

2.3 Quad-tree Based Entropy Estimator

The computational complexity of using (7) in (5) is of $\mathcal{O}(N^2)$. To break the $\mathcal{O}(N^2)$ complexity, we apply the quad-tree (QT) [3]. The idea is to group together increasingly large groups of z_j at increasingly large intensity differences from each z_i. In this way, interactions between z_i and the groups of z_j can be efficiently approximated in $\mathcal{O}(N \log N)$.

QT is constructed by iteratively subdividing the bounding box of all z_i into 2^d equal sub-cells up to depth level L. Let l_B be the length of cell B in QT and d_{iB} the difference between the cell's center-of-mass $\hat{z}_B$ to z_i. If $l_B/d_{iB}^\theta \leq \phi$, where ϕ is a fixed accuracy threshold, then we simplify $\sum_{j=1}^N \|z_i - z_j\| \sim N\|z_i - \hat{z}_B\|$. For $l_B/d_{iB} > \phi$, the current cell B is resolved into its 2^d subcells, which are then recursively examined one by one. Hence, sums in (7) can be computed fast, while the consistency of the QT-based entropy estimator relies on the consistency of the Hilbert kernel density estimate [1] and on the consistency of the sample mean, plug-in entropy estimator [14].

2.4   Gradient Descent Optimization

Registering images requires a minimization strategy for discussed entropy estimators. We will use a simple gradient descent optimization strategy, i.e. $\hat{\theta}^{k+1} = \hat{\theta}^k + \lambda \hat{g}(Z)$, where $\hat{g}(Z)$ represents the derivative of (5). According to Sabuncu and Ramadge [12], we can compute the derivative of the graph-theoretic entropy estimator as:

$$g(Z) = -C \sum_i \sum_{j \neq i} \hat{p}_i^{\alpha-2} \|z_i - z_j\|^{-d-2} (z_i - z_j) \nabla_\theta v_i^\theta , \qquad (8)$$

or the derivative of the plug-in entropy estimator as:

$$g(Z) = -C \sum_i \sum_{j \neq i} [\hat{p}_i^{\alpha-2} + \hat{p}_j^{\alpha-2}] \|z_i - z_j\|^{-d-2} (z_i - z_j) \nabla_\theta (v_i^\theta - v_j^\theta) , \qquad (9)$$

where $\hat{p}_i^\theta = \sum_{k \neq i} \|z_i - z_k\|^{-d}$. The QT is employed to obtain the estimates $\hat{g}(Z) \sim g(Z)$, i.e. the expressions for derivatives in (8) and (9).

3   Image Registration Experiments

Performance tests were carried out for the task of 3-D rigid-body registration of brain volumes using 1) simulated MR volumes from the BrainWeb project [2] and 2) the training set of the Retrospective Image Registration Evaluation (RIRE) project [15]. The simulated MR images (T1-, T2 and PD-weighted) from the BrainWeb project [2] had a volume of $181 \times 217 \times 181$ voxels and isotropic 1 mm spatial resolution, noise level of 3% relative to the brightest tissue and a 20% intensity non-uniformity. The RIRE training set consisted of a CT, PET and three PD-, T1- and T2-weighted MR brain volumes that were registered by a supplied gold standard registration, rescaled and zero padded to $80 \times 80 \times 32$ lattice so as to obtain without any upsampling the isotropic 4 mm spatial resolution of all volumes. To test the registration methods, each pair of volumes was initially displaced using randomly generated initial registration parameters relative to the gold standard position.

The initial displacements were generated in terms of mean target registration error (mTRE), computed as mTRE$= 1/|\Omega_B| \sum_{i \in \Omega_B} \|x_i - \mathcal{T}_{init}(x_i)\|$. Ω_B represents the set of voxels in the intracranium cavity that were used as targets. For the BrainWeb dataset $\mathcal{T}_{init}$ was generated by combining random translations (range [-70,70] pixels) and rotations (range [-35,35] degrees), such that initial mTRE was in the range of [0, 80] pixels, with 20 displacements per each 4 pixels subinterval. For the RIRE dataset the random translations (range [-20,20] pixels) and rotations (range [-10,10] degrees) were generated such that the initial mTRE was in the range of [0, 20] pixels, with 20 displacements per each 1 pixel subinterval. Hence, altogether 400 hundred initial displacements were generated for each image pair. The estimated final transformations $\mathcal{T}_{final}$ were then compared against the gold standard transformations to compute the final mTRE.

Registration was considered successful if the final mTRE was lower than 2 pixels. Three evaluation criteria were defined: 1) registration accuracy (ACC) as the average of mTRE of only the successful registrations, 2) success rate (SR) as the percentage of successful registrations and 3) capture range (CR) as the first mTRE subinterval, in which more than one of the 20 corresponding registrations failed. This setting corresponds to a 95% confidence level for the CR estimate.

The proposed QT-based entropy estimator was tested in two different settings. In the first setting, dubbed the QTG registration method, the gradient of the QT-based entropy estimator was computed as (8), which mimics the gradient of the MST-based [12] or other entropic graph entropy estimators [8]. In the second setting, dubbed the QTP registration method, the gradient was computed as (8), which mimics the plug-in entropy estimators of Viola [14].

Image pairs were registered in a multiresolution setting, running consecutively from lower to higher image resolution. For the BrainWeb image pairs, the resolutions scales were 1 : 8, 1 : 4, 1 : 2 and 1 : 1, while for the smaller RIRE volumes the resolution scales were 1 : 2 and 1 : 1. The QT-based methods were run by setting $L = 10$ and $\phi = 1$ and the MST-based method was initialized with $\gamma = 1.9$ and $\alpha = 0.5$. All the methods used a stochastic sampling scheme, in which only 1% of the co-occuring intensity samples at each resolution were used to estimate the entropy gradient. The entropy gradient was used in a fixed step gradient descent optimization with a maximum of 1000 iterations.

3.1   Results

For all registration trials on the BrainWeb dataset, the distribution of final mTRE w.r.t. the initial mTRE is shown on Fig. 1 for each of the image pairs and for each of the tested methods. For the RIRE dataset, the joint distributions for all image pairs are shown in Fig 2, i.e. only w.r.t. each of the tested methods due to space limitations. The three evaluation criteria, obtained by running 400 registration trials per each image pair are shown in Table 1 and Table 2 for the BrainWeb and the RIRE dataset, respectively. On the two tested image datasets, the MST- and QT-based methods achieved similar registration accuracy (ACC). Comparing the ACC between the BrainWeb and RIRE datasets, however, indicates that due to relatively low resolution the RIRE images might not be representative for studying the ACC. Nevertheless, the ACC of all tested methods could be improved by using a higher order (cubic instead of linear) interpolation method and by increasing the number of iterations. The latter might

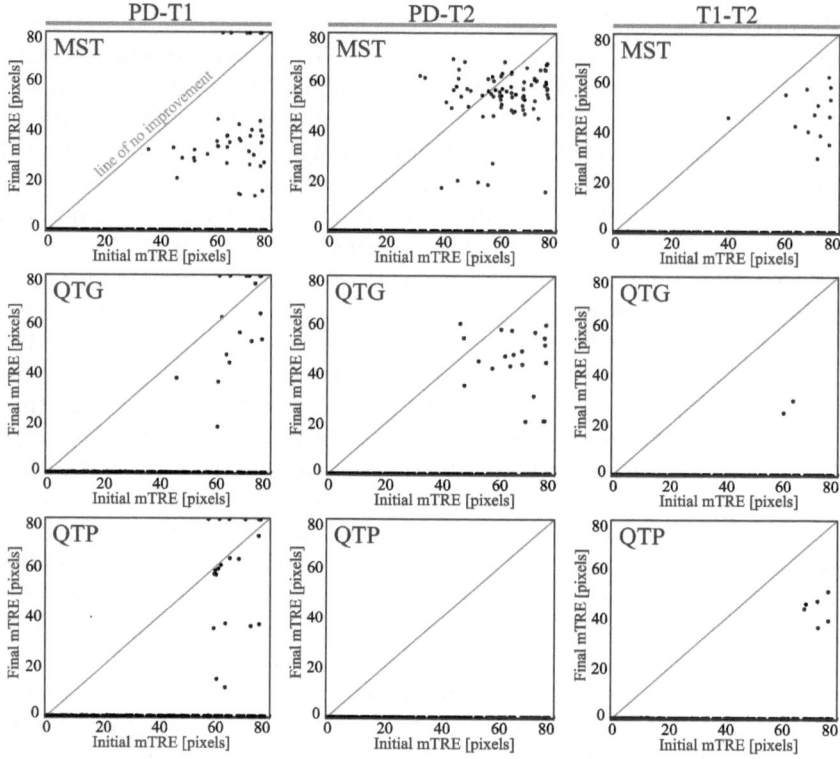

Fig. 1. Distributions of the final mTRE with respect to the initial mTRE shown for the BrainWeb image pairs and for the three tested methods

also require simultaneous regularization of the gradient step size to suppress the oscillatory effects of the stochastic sampling on the estimated entropy gradient.

The key advantage of the QT-based methods is observed in a much higher success rate (SR) and capture range (CR) compared to the MST-based registration method. For the MST, the overall SR (CR) were 89.0% (48.0 pixels) for the BrainWeb and 93.1% (14.8 pixels) for the RIRE datasets, respectively. For the QTG, that mimics the entropic graph entropy estimator, the respective values were 97.0% (62.7 pixels) for the BrainWeb and 95.6% (15.5 pixels) for the RIRE datasets. For the QTP, that mimics the plug-in entropy estimator, the respective values were the consistently the highest at 98.0% (69.3 pixels) for the BrainWeb and 96.6% (17.0 pixels) for the RIRE datasets. The advantageous convergence properties of the QTP method over both the QTG and the MST methods can also be clearly observed from the mTRE distributions in Figs. 1, 2, especially for the PD-T2 image pair in Fig. 1.

The proposed QT-based registration methods, i.e. the QTG and QTP methods, run significantly faster than the MST-based method. The box-whisker diagrams in Fig. 3 depicts the recorded registration times for each dataset and for

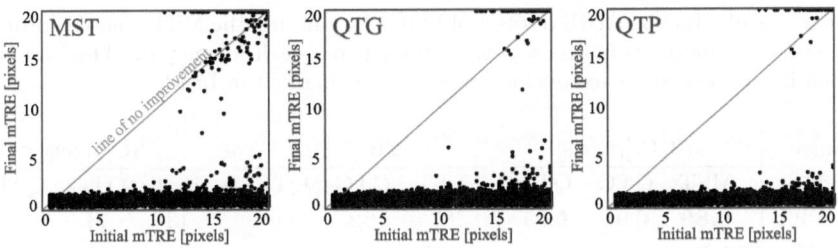

Fig. 2. Joint distributions of all 10 RIRE image pairs of the final mTRE with respect to the initial mTRE for the three tested methods

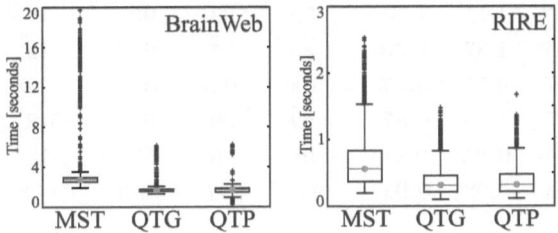

Fig. 3. Registration times for the BrainWeb dataset (*left*) and RIRE dataset (*right*) recorded for 1200 and for 4000 registration trials per each method, respectively

each tested registration method. Roughly, the QT-based methods require 50% less time to register a pair of 3-D volumes. The observed speedup can be attributed to the heuristic, and thus fast, subdivision scheme of the QT entropy estimator. For the BrainWeb dataset, the average registration times were 4.0, 1.7 and 1.8 seconds for the MST, QTG and QTP methods, respectively. For the RIRE dataset the respective average registration times were 0.7, 0.4 and 0.4 seconds. Due to smaller initial image resolution, the registration times were much shorter on the RIRE compared to the BrainWeb dataset.

Table 1. Results for the BrainWeb dataset obtained by running the MST, and the proposed QTG and QTP methods in 400 registration trials per each image pair. The best result for each image pair and each evaluation criteria is marked in **bold**.

Image	ACC [pixels]			SR [%]			CR [pixels]		
pair	MST	QTG	QTP	MST	QTG	QTP	MST	QTG	QTP
PD-T1	0.15	0.17	0.15	90	**96**	95	44	60	60
PD-T2	0.14	0.14	0.14	80	95	**100**	32	48	**80**
T1-T2	0.15	**0.13**	0.14	97	**100**	99	68	**80**	68
Mean	**0.14**	0.15	0.15	89.0	97.0	**98.0**	48.0	62.7	**69.3**

Table 2. Results for the RIRE dataset obtained by running the MST, and the proposed QTG and QTP methods in 400 registration trials per each image pair. The best result for each image pair and each evaluation criteria is marked in **bold**.

Image pair	ACC [pixels]			SR [%]			CR [pixels]		
	MST	QTG	QTP	MST	QTG	QTP	MST	QTG	QTP
CT-PET	**0.89**	0.94	0.95	87	**93**	89	13	14	14
CT-PD	0.73	0.67	0.67	100	100	100	20	20	20
CT-T1	**0.48**	0.49	0.52	97	99	99	11	**20**	17
CT-T2	**0.99**	1.46	1.09	100	98	100	20	10	20
PET-PD	**1.22**	1.31	1.33	82	91	91	12	12	**14**
PET-T1	**1.07**	1.11	1.10	79	89	**93**	10	**15**	13
PET-T2	1.55	1.37	**1.33**	89	94	**97**	12	14	**18**
PD-T1	0.57	0.55	**0.47**	100	100	100	20	20	20
PD-T2	1.07	1.16	**0.87**	99	99	99	12	16	16
T1-T2	0.95	**0.85**	0.86	98	96	98	18	14	18
Mean	0.94	0.98	**0.91**	93.1	95.6	**96.6**	14.8	15.5	**17.0**

4   Discussion

Performances of the information-theoretic multi-modality image registration methods crucially depend on the representation model of the JDF and on the implementation of the entropy estimator. We proposed an entropy estimator for image registration based on quad-tree (QT) that is essentially an entropic graph entropy estimator, but was also adapted to work as a plug-in entropy estimator by incorporating the Hilbert kernel density estimator. Results of 3-D rigid-body registration of multi-modal brain volumes indicate that the proposed QT-based methods achieve similar registration accuracies as the MST-based method, but have a consistently higher success rate (SR) and a higher capture range (CR).

Low capture range or the sensitivity to bad initialization is known to be one of the major drawbacks of the MST-based method [12]. This can be attributed to the fact that the MST takes into account only two edges connecting the vertex or sample z_i in the MST, while the QT-based methods consider all N samples (z_j) and approximate their contribution by grouping the distant samples. The grouping of z_j is controlled by the cell acceptance threshold ϕ and by the maximal tree depth L. Both of these parameters affect the level of approximation and the performance gains. In general, setting $\phi < 1.5$ and $L \geq 8$ should yield a good approximation of $\hat{g}(Z)$. For $\phi = 1$ and $L = 10$, the QT-based methods were more robust in terms of SR and CR, while they also required 50% less time than the MST-based method to register a pair of 3-D volumes. Although the MST and QT have similar computational complexities, the significant speedups achieved by the QT-based methods can be attributed to the heuristic, and thus fast, subdivision scheme of the QT entropy estimator.

In conclusion, to speedup and, especially, to robustify the MST-based method the QT-based methods present an attractive alternative approach. Furthermore, the QT-based methods provide a direct link between the entropic graph and plug-in entropy estimators, the only differences being 1) the weighting of the sample contributions to the joint entropy and 2) the inclusion (exclusion) of the mutual dependence of the density (graph) defining samples and the joint entropy defining samples on the parameters of the spatial transformation.

Acknowledgments. This research was supported by the Ministry of Higher Education, Science and Technology, Republic of Slovenia, under grants L2-2023, L2-4072, J2-2246 and an applied research grant ESRR-07-13-EU.

References

1. Devroye, L., Krzyżak, A.: On the Hilbert kernel density estimate. Stat. Probabil. Lett. 44(3), 299–308 (1999)
2. Kwan, R.K., Evans, A.C., Pike, G.B.: MRI simulation-based evaluation of image-processing and classification methods. IEEE T. Med. Imag. 18(11), 1085–1097 (1999)
3. Kybic, J., Vnučko, I.: Approximate all nearest neighbor search for high dimensional entropy estimation for image registration. Signal Process. 92(5), 1302–1316 (2012)
4. Ma, B., Hero, A., Gorman, J., Michel, O.: Image registration with minimum spanning tree algorithm. In: Dubois, E., Konrad, J. (eds.) Proc. IEEE ICIP, vol. 1, pp. 481–484. IEEE, Vancouver (2000)
5. Maes, F., Collignon, A., Vandermeulen, D., Marchal, G., Suetens, P.: Multimodality image registration by maximization of mutual information. IEEE T. Med. Imag. 16(2), 187–198 (1997)
6. Miller, E.G.: A new class of entropy estimators for multi-dimensional densities. In: Proc. IEEE ICASSP, vol. 3, pp. 297–300. IEEE, Hong Kong (2003)
7. Neemuchwala, H., Hero, A., Carson, P.: Image matching using alpha-entropy measures and entropic graphs. Signal Process. 85(2), 277–296 (2005)
8. Neemuchwala, H., Hero, A., Zabuawala, S., Carson, P.: Image registration methods in high-dimensional space. Int. J. Imag. Syst. Tech. 16(5), 130–145 (2006)
9. Špiclin, Ž., Likar, B., Pernuš, F.: Groupwise registration of multi-modal images by an efficient joint entropy minimization scheme. IEEE T. Image Process 21(5), 2546–2558 (2012)
10. Pluim, J.P.W., Maintz, J.B.A., Viergever, M.A.: Mutual-information-based registration of medical images: a survey. IEEE T. Med. Imag. 22(8), 986–1004 (2003)
11. Pluim, J.P.W., Maintz, J.B.A., Viergever, M.A.: f-information measures in medical image registration. IEEE T. Med. Imag. 23(12), 1508–1516 (2004)
12. Sabuncu, M.R., Ramadge, P.: Using spanning graphs for efficient image registration. IEEE T. Image Process. 17(5), 788–797 (2008)
13. Sheather, S.J.: Density estimation. Stat. Sci. 19(4), 588–597 (2004)
14. Viola, P.A.: Alignment by maximization of mutual information, Ph. D. thesis, Massachusetts Institute of Technology, Boston, MA, USA (1995)
15. West, J., et al.: Comparison and evaluation of retrospective intermodality brain image registration techniques. J. of Comput. Assist. Tomogr. 21(4), 554–566 (1997)

3D Tensor Normalization for Improved Accuracy in DTI Tensor Registration Methods

Aditya Gupta[1], Maria Escolar[1], Cheryl Dietrich[2], John Gilmore[2], Guido Gerig[3], and Martin Styner[2,4]

[1] Department of Pediatrics, University of Pittsburgh
[2] Department of Psychiatry, University of North Carolina at Chapel Hill
[3] Scientific Computing and Imaging Institute, University of Utah
[4] Department of Computer Science, University of North Carolina at Chapel Hill

Abstract. This paper presents a method for normalization of diffusion tensor images (DTI) to a fixed DTI template, a pre-processing step to improve the performance of full tensor based registration methods. The proposed method maps the individual tensors of the subject image in to the template space based on matching the cumulative distribution function and the fractional anisotrophy values. The method aims to determine a more accurate deformation field from any full tensor registration method by applying the registration algorithm on the normalized DTI rather than the original DTI. The deformation field applied to the original tensor images are compared to the deformed image without normalization for 11 different cases of mapping seven subjects (neonate through 2 years) to two different atlases. The method shows an improvement in DTI registration based on comparing the normalized fractional anisotropy values of major fiber tracts in the brain.

Keywords: Tensor Normalization, DTI Registration, DTITK.

1 Introduction

Diffusion tensor imaging (DTI) is a magnetic resonance imaging (MRI) technique that enables the measurement of restricted diffusion of water molecules in tissue to produce neural tract images. This technique has become increasingly important for studies of anatomical and functional connectivity of the brain regions. DTI is now extensively used to study the fiber architecture in the living human brain via DTI tractography. This technique has proven especially valuable in clinical studies of white matter (WM) integrity in the developing brain for diseases, such as metachromatic leukodystrophy (MLD), cerebral palsy and Krabbe. In this paper, the tensor normalization method is tested on a particular white matter demyelinating disease called Krabbe [1].

Krabbe disease (also called globoid cell leukodystrophy) is a rare, often fatal genetic disorder of the nervous system caused by a deficiency of an enzyme called galactocerebrosidase, which aids in the breakdown and removal of galactolipids found in myelin. Previous studies show that patients with infantile Krabbe disease have lower fractional anisotropy (FA) across the corpus callosum and along

B.M. Dawant et al. (Eds.): WBIR 2012, LNCS 7359, pp. 170–179, 2012.
© Springer-Verlag Berlin Heidelberg 2012

the DTI fiber bundle of internal capsules (IC) when compared with healthy age-matched controls [1]. Based on the above findings, atlas based fiber tract analysis is used for analyzing DTI of Krabbe subjects [2]. There are considerable anatomical variations between the Krabbe subjects and the atlas and hence for accurate analysis of white matter fiber tracts it is crucial to establish a registration based voxel-wise correspondence between a normal control neonate DTI atlas and the Krabbe subjects. To achieve this needed registration accuracy, the research presented in this paper provides a method to improve the state-of-the-art approach to individually register DTI images into the atlas space.

The registration of diffusion tensor images is particularly challenging when compared to registering scalar images as DTI data is multi-dimensional and the tensor orientations after image transformations must remain consistent with the anatomy. Prior to the development of full tensor based registration methods, DTI registration was performed with traditional image registration algorithms on scalar images derived from the DTI[3]. These methods discard the orientation component of the data and thus DTI registration algorithms that directly use higher order information of DTIs, such as the corresponding principal eigenvectors [4] and the full tensor information [5] are now preferred. In our recent publication [6], the performance of scalar and full tensor registration algorithms are compared for Krabbe neonates. In comparison to the commonly available regsitration packages, the full tensor based DTI-TK [5] method showed the most accurate registration performance. DTI-TK is a non-parametric, diffeomorphic deformable image registration that incrementally estimates its displacement field using a tensor-based registration formulation. It is designed to take advantage of similarity measures comparing whole tensors via explicit optimization of tensor reorientation. Hence, in this paper the method is tested with the DTI-TK registration tool.

Normalization of DTIs is challenging as the data is multidimensional and includes considering the shape of the tensors along with tensor properties such as FA. Methods to improve DTI registration have been proposed by determining the correspondence between tensors using Gabor filters [7]. For normalization, the full tensor registration methods like DTI-TK [5] uses the ADC profile information. The F-TIMER [4] method uses the local statistical information of underlying fiber orientations along with the edge strength of the FA and the ADC maps for normalization. In both methods, the normalization is specific to the methods developed and may not always result in good normalization if there are considerable differences in local tensor appearance between the case and the template, for example, in the mapping of a neonate to a 2 year template. In this paper, our aim is to develop a general tensor normalization step that can be incorporated in the analysis pipeline as a prior step to any full tensor based registration algorithms.

For DTI derived scalar image registration methods, a simple histogram normalization of the subject to the template improves the performance of registration considerably [8]. Motivated by these approaches, this paper presents a normalization method for full tensor registration methods that normalizes the 3 dimensional Eigenvalues of each tensor while maintaining similar FA values. The deformation fields are computed using the full tensor registration methods on the normalized DTI images, and the fields are applied on the original DTIs. The performance with and without normalization are compared based on normalized FA values of major fiber tracts of the brain.

2   Method

For scalar image registrations based on sum of squared differences, histogram based intensity normalization is commonly used prior to registration to improve the registration accuracy. Similarly for DTI derived scalar images such as FA images, histogram based intensity normalization is used to determine an improved deformation field. This normalization is achieved by computing the histograms of the subject I_{sub} and the template I_{temp} scalar image. From the histograms, the cumulative distribution functions (cdfs) of the two images C_{sub} and C_{temp} are determined. For each image intensity n_i, an intensity level n_o, for which $C_{sub}(n_i) = C_{temp}(n_o)$ is computed; this is the result of histogram matching function $M(n_i) = n_o$. The histogram matching function applied on each voxel of the subject image gives the normalized FA images. In this paper, we extend this idea of scalar intensity normalization 3D tensors in DTI.

Diffusion tensor MRI characterizes the diffusion of water molecules by measuring the apparent diffusion tensor in each voxel of an MRI volume. The method assumes that water molecules move according to a simple anisotropic diffusion process so that the displacement x of a water molecule over a fixed time t is modeled as a random variable that follows the multivariate normal distribution p with the mean at the origin and covariance $2tD$, where D is the diffusion tensor, a symmetric and positive-definite 3-by-3 matrix. The Eigenvalues $\lambda_1, \lambda_2, \lambda_3$ of D are used to determine the standard DTI properties like mean diffusivity (MD) and FA defined by:

$$MD = (\lambda_1 + \lambda_2 + \lambda_3)/3; FA = \sqrt{\frac{(\lambda_1 - \lambda_2)^2 + (\lambda_2 - \lambda_3)^2 + (\lambda_1 - \lambda_3)^2}{\lambda_1^2 + \lambda_2^2 + \lambda_3^2}} \quad (1)$$

Our proposed method, works in this three dimensional Eigenvalue space by first determining the cdf planes. The standard cdf equation for three values $\lambda_1, \lambda_2, \lambda_3$ is defined by the equation:

$$C_{in}(\lambda_{1a}, \lambda_{2a}, \lambda_{3a}) = p((0 \leq \lambda_1 \leq \lambda_{1a}), (0 \leq \lambda_2 \leq \lambda_{2a}), (0 \leq \lambda_3 \leq \lambda_{3a})) \quad (2)$$

In the 3D space, the summation cdf volume based on this equation is a rectangular box. Our aim in this paper is to nomalize two DTI volumes while maintaining a similar cumulative distribution function and also to maintain a similar distribution of mean diffusivity. To achieve this aim, we propose to modify this equation to have constant cdf planes rather than constant cdf rectangular volumes. The modified 3-D cdf equation is defined as:

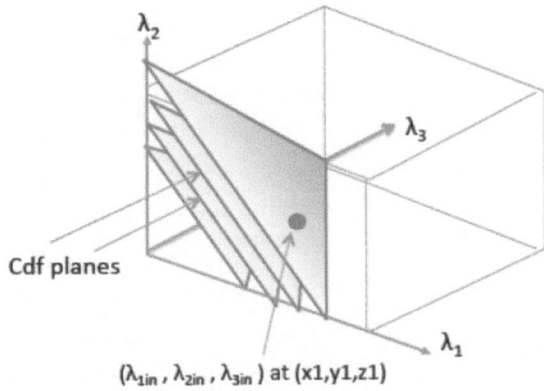

Fig. 1. Constant cdf planes - iso-MD planes defined in the subject and atlas eigen value space

$$C_{in}(\lambda_{1in}, \lambda_{2in}, \lambda_{3in}) = p((\lambda_1 + \lambda_2 + \lambda_3 \leq 3MD_i)) \tag{3}$$

where $MD_i = (\lambda_{1in} + \lambda_{2in} + \lambda_{3in})/3$. The summation volume is bound by a plane which has the same cdf values as shown in Fig. 2. The input cdf is a function of MD. Since these planes have constant MD values for all points $(\lambda_1, \lambda_2, \lambda_3)$ lying on the plane, in further discussion we refer to these constant cdf planes as iso-MD planes. Ji-Hee et. al. [9] presents a similar argument and result for color normalization in the r, g, b space.

The proposed method is discussed below step-by-step and is shown in Fig. 3. Based on the above proposed idea of constant cdf planes, the first step of the algorithm is to define iso-MD planes in the subject and the atlas eigen value space with fixed intervals $'\delta'$, a concept similar to defining histogram bins. The value of $'\delta'$ is selected based on the Eigenvalues of tensors of the subject and the atlas. The following steps are repeated for each tensor of the subject. Each subject tensor (for discussion consider tensor at particular location (x, y, z)) is mapped to the closest iso-MD plane. The atlas iso-MD plane with the closest cdf value to the selected subject iso-MD plane is determined based on the equation $C_{out}(MD_{out}) = C_{in}(\lambda_{1x1,y1,z1}, \lambda_{2x1,y1,z1}, \lambda_{3x1,y1,z1})$. This equation ensures a uniform cumulative distribution function between the normalized subject tensors and the atlas tensors. In fact, any selection of positive $\lambda_1, \lambda_2, \lambda_3$ value lying on this atlas iso-MD plane will lead to a uniform cdf. Let us refer to the set of points on the atlas iso-MD plane $'i'$ as $\lambda_{1i,MD}, \lambda_{2i,MD}, \lambda_{3i,MD}$, the subscript 'MD' indicating that all the points on this plane have constant MD. The next step is to find the particular $\lambda_1, \lambda_2, \lambda_3$ value on the iso-MD plane that best normalizes the subject case to the atlas space. For this, we need to determine the atlas normalized FA value for the tensor. This is achieved by applying a standard 2D histogram matching of the subject FA scalar image to the atlas FA scalar image as discussed below.

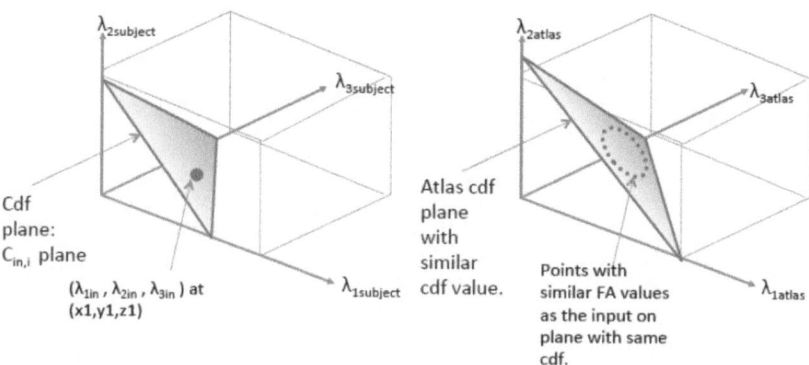

Fig. 2. Mapping from the subject eigen space to the template eigen space

The filter used to implement the standard 2D histogram matching normalizes the grayscale values of a source image (subject FA image in our case) based on the grayscale values of a reference image (atlas FA image in our case). This filter from Insight Toolkit[1] uses a histogram matching technique where the histograms of the two images are matched only at a specified number of quantile values. As a result of this histogram matching, each subject tensor has a corresponding atlas intensity normalized FA value. Let us denote the intensity normalized FA value for the location (x, y, z) as $FANormValue_{x,y,z}$. In our algorithm, after determining the matched iso-MD plane in the atlas space for each subject tensor, we determine the FA values of all the $(\lambda_1, \lambda_2, \lambda_3)$s on this plane based on the equation 1. The $(\lambda_1, \lambda_2, \lambda_3)$s with the most similar FA value to the tensor's intensity normalized FA value $FANormValue_{x,y,z}$ are selected.

$$argmin(FA_i - FANormValue_{x,y,z}) \qquad (4)$$

Substituting equation 1 in the above equation and computing the arg minimum leads to a set of points on the plane. These set of points represented as $(\lambda_{1i,MD,FA}, \lambda_{2i,MD,FA}, \lambda_{3i,MD,FA})$ ($'i'$ indicating the points on the selected iso-MD plane and $'MD'$ and $'FA'$ represent that these points satisfy the condition of closest MD and FA) form an ellipse on the iso-MD plane (Fig. 2). The final step in our method is to determine the point p_{min} from these set of points that satisfies the condition $(\lambda_1 > \lambda_2 > \lambda_3)$ and has the minimum Euclidean distance to the original tensor.

$$p_{min} = argmin((\lambda_{1x,y,z} - \lambda_{1i,MD,FA})^2 +$$
$$(\lambda_{2x,y,z} - \lambda_{2i,MD,FA})^2 + (\lambda_{3x,y,z} - \lambda_{3i,MD,FA})^2)^{0.5} \qquad (5)$$

This minimum Euclidean distance ensures that the normalized tensor has the most similar shape to the original tensor. Hence, this algorithm computes the

---

[1] www.itk.org

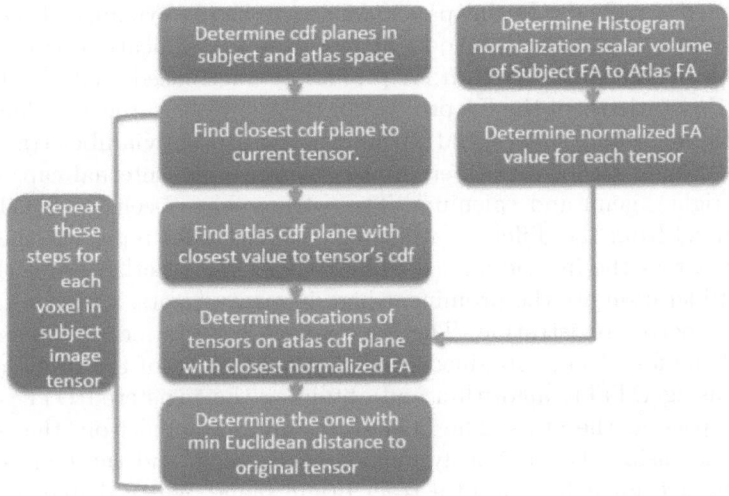

Fig. 3. Block diagram showing all the steps in the normalization algorithm

normalized tensor with the most similar tensor shape that satisfies the conditions of same cdf and closest normalized FA values. The normalized DTI volume is determined by computing the normalized tensor for each tensor of the subject based on the above steps. For clarity, the block diagram Fig. 3 illustrates all the steps.

3 Experiments

Subjects: The tensor normalization method is tested on Krabbe subjects in the age 10 days to 2 years. These subjects are registered to a neonate atlas (built from 377 age-matched neonate controls) and a 1-2 year atlas (from 283 controls age 1 to 2 year). Both atlases are built using a scalar, unbiased diffeomorphic atlas building method based on a nonlinear high-dimensional fluid deformation method [3]. Details of image acquisition of the controls and Krabbe can be found in [10].

Setup: Four Krabbe neonates are registered to a neonate atlas using the DTITK algorithm with and without the proposed normalization method. To test the robustness of the normalization wherein there are large anatomical variations between the subject and the atlas, we registered the same four neonates to a 1-2 year atlas (as there are considerable differences from a neonate to a 1-2 year brain). Three additional 1 to 2 year old Krabbe subjects are registered to the 1-2year atlas using the DTITK algorithm. An affine registration is implemented as a pre-processing step prior to DTITK registration. For all the Krabbe subjects, the DTI volumes are normalized using our proposed method and the DTITK deformation field for mapping the normalized subjects to the atlas is determined. The field is applied to the original (not normalized) DTI and the results are compared.

176   A. Gupta et al.

Tract-based Analysis: In this paper, we prove the performance of the method for atlas based registration methods. Since this is an application based methodology, we focus our evaluation on FA profiles of tract based analysis. The clinicians use the statistics of the FA profiles for their Krabbe subject evaluation. We evaluate the registration with and without normalization via fiber tractography based FA profiles [2] for four fiber tracts - corticospinal internal capsule tracts (left and right), genu and splenium. These tracts have been previously manually extracted from the different atlases. The FA profiles represent the average FA values across the individual streamlines along the tract[2]. Since the tracts under consideration are the prominent high intensity tracts, a higher FA profile indicates a better registration. The comparison is performed between the FA profiles of the four tracts obtained from: 1. Registration of the original DTI to the atlas using DTITK algorithm and obtaining the registered DTI volume in the same space as the atlas. The fiber tracts are extracted from the registered DTI volumes using the previously defined atlas tracts and the transformation field. Using a prior definition of a tract origin plane, which defines a curvilinear re-parameterization of the tracts, corresponding average tract property FA profiles are extracted from each individual fiber tract. 2. The original DTI is normalized using the proposed method. The normalized DTI is registered to the atlas and the deformation field is determined. This deformation field is applied to the original DTI to obtain the atlas registered DTI volume. The fiber tracts are extracted in the similar method as above. 3. A region of interest (ROI) in the tract that is under study is defined by a trained expert for the original DTI of each subject. The FA volume is used as a reference volume to trace the ROI. From the ROI, the fiber tracts are seeded using the tool Slicer3 [2]. The fiber tracts are cleaned to remove crossing fibers and the FA profiles are determined of these tracts using an in-house tool called FiberViewer [3].

Evaluation: The FA profiles from manual tractography ($MeanFA_{mt}$) are considered as the ground truth and compared to the FA profiles of the fiber tracts extracted from the registered original and normalized DTI ($MeanFA_{orig/norm}$). The mean absolute point-wise difference (MAD) normalized by the mean FA of the ground truth is used as the evaluation error metric:

$$E = \frac{MeanFA_{orig/norm} - MeanFA_{mt}}{MeanFA_{mt}} \qquad (6)$$

4   Results and Discussions

For the four fiber tracts, the tensor normalization resulted in FA profiles with higher values as compared to the profiles without normalization. In Table 1, we show the percentage error in registration of the major fiber tracts with and without normalization. Compared to the ground truth an average percentage decrease in error of 5 to 10% is observed. For example, for the Genu tract (Neonate3),

---

[2] `www.slicer.org`

[3] `www.na-mic.org`

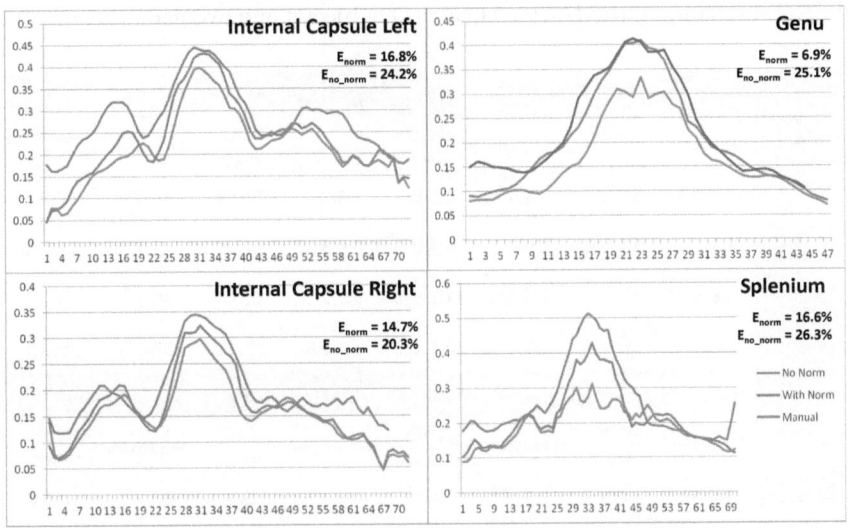

Fig. 4. Comparison of FA profiles for the four tracts. (x-axis:FA values; y-axis: points along the fiber tracts) For each tract - manual (highest FA), with normalization (middle) and without normalization (lowest FA).

normalization resulted in a 7% error as compared to 25% error without normalization i.e. an improvement in average FA values from 0.32 to 0.4 (18% improvement). The challenge of registration of Krabbe cases to a normal atlas has been discussed earlier, and a 2 to 18% improvement is substantial. Even in cases of poor registration (eg. left internal capsule Neonate1 mapped in 1-2 year atlas), the normalization improves the registration considerably (11%). The selected tracts are the tracts with the highest FA intensities and thus higher FA values indicate better mapping of the subject into the atlas template i.e. better registration. We observe a higher improvement in registration in the corpus collosum tracts compared to the cortico-spinal tracts. This is likely due to a higher reduction in registration errors that are normally seen in the central bends of the genu and splenium tracts without normalization (see splenium tract in Fig. 4. It is important to note that manual tractography, though performed to the best of our ability by a trained expert, is akin to manual segmentation and is subject to variability. Due to this factor, point-wise comparison and higher variability towards the ends of the tracts, the % error values in Table 1 appear high. Important to this evaluation is the percentage decrease in error rather than the absolute % error.

In most cases, the shape of the FA profile with normalization appears similar to the profile without normalization but with higher values. But in certain cases (splenium profile of Fig. 4), the shape of the FA profile from normalization appears more similar to the ground truth, again indicating an improvement in

Table 1. Table showing the $E\%$ for 11 cases (7 subjects) and average % error reduction

In Neonate Atlas	Neonate1		Neonate2		Neonate3		Neonate4	
	No Norm	With Norm	No Norm	With Norm	No Norm	With Norm	No Norm	With Norm
CSIC_left	22.0%	19.5%	25.7%	22.8%	24.1%	20.0%	24.2%	16.8%
CSIC_right	20.3%	14.7%	20.6%	19.0%	21.3%	17.0%	18.1%	11.2%
Genu	22.8%	15.7%	20.6%	15.6%	25.1%	6.9%	38.9%	23.2%
Splenium	26.3%	16.6%	22.6%	21.1%	30.2%	12.1%	38.1%	28.2%

In 1-2year Atlas	Neonate1		Neonate2		Neonate3		Neonate4	
	No Norm	With Norm	No Norm	With Norm	No Norm	With Norm	No Norm	With Norm
CSIC_left	43.6%	32.9%	51.4%	36.4%	25.1%	18.3%	26.2%	18.8%
CSIC_right	35.0%	25.7%	27.5%	18.1%	20.5%	10.9%	34.7%	30.4%
Genu	12.7%	0.6%	13.7%	4.8%	6.6%	2.7%	15.0%	9.7%
Splenium	22.8%	11.5%	27.1%	25.3%	13.3%	8.9%	22.8%	11.8%

In 1-2 year Atlas	1-2year1		1-2year2		1-2year3		Average % reduction in error for 11 cases
	No Norm	With Norm	No Norm	With Norm	No Norm	With Norm	
CSIC_left	24.9%	20.8%	34.0%	22.1%	36.8%	33.7%	5.99%
CSIC_right	28.7%	25.7%	37.4%	34.8%	34.5%	31.6%	5.42%
Genu	14.3%	9.2%	19.7%	14.5%	21.7%	11.0%	9.33%
Splenium	11.0%	6.1%	21.4%	9.1%	25.2%	16.8%	8.47%

registration along the entire tract. This method can be easily introduced as a pre-processing step in most analysis pipelines. On a typical workstation, the normalization takes less than 5 minutes. The code is open source and the binaries can be downloaded as a part of the "dtiprocess" package [4].

5   Conclusions

Based on the evaluation criteria, the proposed tensor normalization method considerably improves the registration of the subjects into the atlas template. Even for white matter demylinating diseases like Krabbe, where registration is a very crucial step for analysis, this method gives a significant improvement in

---

[4] www.nitrc.com

the registration accuracy. This method can be very easily introduced as a pre-processing step prior to registration in any analysis pipeline. The normalized DTI is only used for generating the registration diffeomorphic field, and this generated field is applied to the original DTI and hence no properties of the original DTI are altered in this pre-processing step. Our future work will be focused on testing this method on other tensor registration methods like MedINRIA and also on atlas building methods.

Acknowledgements. This work was supported by NIH U54 EB005149 (NAMIC), NINDS 5R01NS61965-2, DANA Foundation, NIH P30 HD03110 (NDRC), UNC-CH MH064065 (Conte Center) and UNC-CH NIH R01 HD055741 (Autism Center).

References

1. Escolar, M., Poe, M., Smith, J., Gilmore, J., Kurtzberg, J., Lin, W., Styner, M.: Diffusion tensor imaging detects abnormalities in the corticospinal tracts of neonates with infantile krabbe disease. American Journal of Neuroradiology 30(5), 1017–1021 (2009)
2. Goodlett, C.B., Fletcher, P.T., Gilmore, J.H., Gerig, G.: Group analysis of dti fiber tract statistics with application to neurodevelopment. NeuroImage 45(1, supplement 1), S133 – S142 (2009)
3. Joshi, S., Davis, B., Jomier, M., Gerig, G.: Unbiased diffeomorphic atlas construction for computational anatomy. NeuroImage 23(supplement 1(0)), S151–S160 (2004)
4. Yap, P.T., Wu, G., Zhu, H., Lin, W., Shen, D.: F-timer: Fast tensor image morphing for elastic registration. IEEE Transactions on Medical Imaging 29(5), 1192–1203 (2010)
5. Zhang, H., Yushkevich, P.A., Alexander, D.C., Gee, J.C.: Deformable registration of diffusion tensor mr images with explicit orientation optimization. Medical Image Analysis 10(5), 764–785 (2006)
6. Wang, Y., Gupta, A., Liu, Z., Zhang, H., Escolar, M.L., Gilmore, J.H., Gouttard, S., Fillard, P., Maltbie, E., Gerig, G., Styner, M.: Dti registration in atlas based fiber analysis of infantile krabbe disease. NeuroImage 55(4), 1577–1586 (2011)
7. Verma, R., Davatzikos, C.: Matching of diffusion tensor images using gabor features. In: IEEE International Symposium on Biomedical Imaging: Nano to Macro, vol. 1, pp. 396–399 (April 2004)
8. Salas-Gonzalez, D., Estrada, J., Gorriz, J.M., Ramirez, J., Segovia, F., Chaves, R., Lopez, M., Illan, I.A., Padilla, P.: Improving the convergence rate in affine registration of pet brain images using histogram matching. In: Nuclear Science Symposium Conference Record (NSS/MIC), 2010 IEEE, October 30-November 6, pp. 3599–3601 (2010)
9. Han, J.H., Yang, S., Lee, B.U.: A novel 3-d color histogram equalization method with uniform 1-d gray scale histogram. IEEE Transactions on Image Processing 20(2), 506–512 (2011)
10. Gilmore, J.H., Zhai, G., Wilber, K., Smith, J.K., Lin, W., Gerig, G.: 3 tesla magnetic resonance imaging of the brain in newborns. Psychiatry Research: Neuroimaging 132(1), 81–85 (2004)

A Method for Automated Cortical Surface Registration and Labeling

Anand A. Joshi[1], David W. Shattuck[2], and Richard M. Leahy[1],*

[1] Signal and Image Processing Institute, University of Southern California, Los Angeles, CA
[2] Laboratory of Neuro Imaging, University of California, Los Angeles, CA

Abstract. Registration and delineation of anatomical features in MRI of the human brain play an important role in the investigation of brain development and disease. Accurate, automatic and computationally efficient cortical surface registration and delineation of surface-based landmarks, including regions of interest (ROIs) and sulcal curves (sulci), remain challenging problems due to substantial variation in the shapes of these features across populations. We present a method that performs a fast and accurate registration, labeling and sulcal delineation of brain images. The new method presented in this paper uses a multiresolution, curvature based approach to perform a registration of a subject brain surface model to a delineated atlas surface model; the atlas ROIs and sulcal curves are then mapped to the subject brain surface. A geodesic curvature flow on the cortical surface is then used to refine the locations of the sulcal curves sulci and label boundaries further, such that they follow the true sulcal fundi more closely. The flow is formulated using a level set based method on the cortical surface, which represents the curves as zero level sets. We also incorporate a curvature based weighting that drives the curves to the bottoms of the sulcal valleys in the cortical folds. Finally, we validate our new approach by comparing sets of automatically delineated sulcal curves it produced to corresponding sets of manually delineated sulcal curves. Our results indicate that the proposed method is able to find these landmarks accurately.

1 Introduction

Human cerebral cortex is often modeled as a highly convoluted sheet of gray matter. Inter- and intra-subject comparison involving anatomical changes over time or differences between populations requires the spatial alignment of the cortical surfaces, such that they have a common coordinate system that is anatomically meaningful. Sulcal curves are fissures in the cortical surface and are commonly used as surrogates for the cytoarchitectural boundaries in the brain. Therefore, there is also great interest in direct analysis of the geometry of these curves for studies of disease propagation, symmetry, development and group differences (e.g. [10,8]). Labels of cortical regions of interest (ROIs) or sulcal curves that are often required for these studies and can be produced using manual [13] or automatic delineation [15,17]. Manual delineation is often performed using an interactive software tools [13]. This, however, can be a tedious and

* This work was supported by grants NIH-NIBIB P41 EB015922 / P41 RR 013642 and NIH-NINDS R01 NS074980.

B.M. Dawant et al. (Eds.): WBIR 2012, LNCS 7359, pp. 180–189, 2012.

subjective task that also requires substantial knowledge of neuroanatomy and is therefore confounded by intra- and inter-rater variability. This variability is reduced to some extent using rigorous definitions of a sulcal tracing protocol and extensive training as described in [9,13].

An alternative approach to this problem is to use automatic surface registration to align surface curvature or sulcal depth [2]. Sulcal curves can be delineated on a reference atlas brain surface, which is then aligned with the subject brain surface using automated registration. The sulci from the atlas are then transferred to the subject using the point correspondence defined by the surface mapping. While this approach can find the sulcal location approximately, there is often substantial residual error [9]. This is because automatic methods align the whole surface using curvature and do not focus specifically on the sulcal locations and label boundaries, which are sometimes biased by the reference atlas chosen. Also, the variability of the atlas and subject folds can be reflected in the misalignment of sulcal curves, thus the transferred sulcal curves may not lie at the valleys of the subject surfaces. A local refinement of the curves representing sulci and label boundaries can alleviate this problem. This paper describes a fast and accurate surface registration and curve refinement method based on 2D flat mapping and geodesic curvature flow on surfaces where the sulcal curves are represented as curvature weighted geodesics. The surface registration method presented here extends the surface registration method presented in [4] that required manually traced sulcal inputs. The cortical labels from the atlas cortex surface model are then transferred to the subject cortex surface model using the point correspondence. The local refinement of this registration is performed by using geodesic curvature flow of the label boundaries as described for parametric surfaces in [14]. Here, we use a level set based formulation similar to [19,6] and apply it to the label boundary refinement and sulcal detection problem. The curve evolution is defined in terms of evolution of a zero level set. The flow is discretized in the surface geometry using a finite element method.

2   Materials and Methods

We assume as input, an atlas brain surface mesh with manually delineated surface labels as well as sulcal landmarks and a subject brain surface mesh. The goal is to perform atlas to subject cortical surface registration and transfer cortical labels and delineated sulci from atlas surface to the subject surface. First, we briefly describe an automated curvature based registration approach that performs alignment of the atlas surface and the subject surface. The cortical labels and sulci from the atlas surface are then transferred to the subject surface.

2.1   Cortical Surface Registration

We developed a single subject anatomical atlas brain based on a T1-weighted MRI from which we generated inner cortical and pial surfaces using our BrainSuite software [12]. These surfaces were labeled with anatomical structures (35x2 ROIs) and sulcal curves (26x2) that were delineated manually by an expert neuroanatomist (Fig 1). We apply a surface-based registration method that establishes one-to-one correspondence between

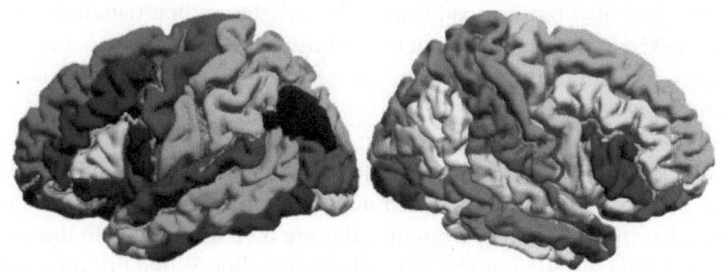

Fig. 1. Rendering of the brain atlas cortical surface used in this work. The gyri have been labeled manually and are coded with different colors on the surface. Manually traced sulcal curves are also shown.

the atlas surface $\mathscr{A}$ and the subject surface $\mathscr{S}$. The method for surface registration has three stages: (i) for subject and atlas, we generate a smoothed representation of the subject and atlas surfaces and then perform a L_2 energy based 3D matching, (ii) for each subject, we parameterize the surface of each cortical hemisphere to a unit square (iii) find a vector field with respect to this parameterization which aligns curvature of the surfaces and the 3D aligned coordinates from step (i).

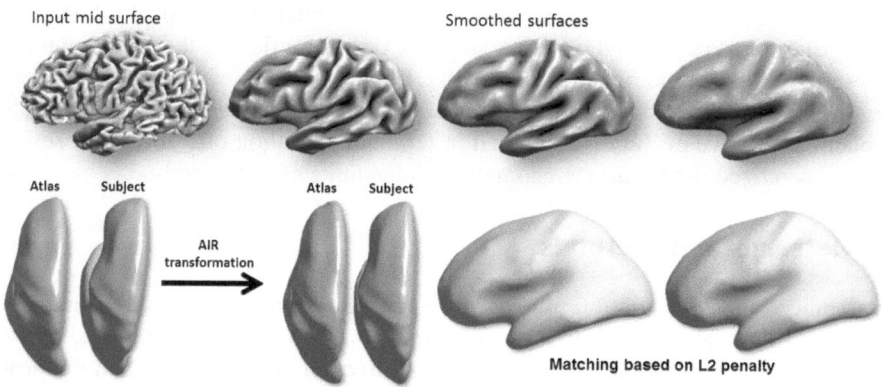

Fig. 2. (Top) Mid-cortical surface iteratively inflated by mean curvature flow to generate a multiresolution representation of the cortical surface. (Bottom) Initial 3D alignment of the cortex, first by using deformation field of AIR and later by L_2 energy minimization.

First, the multiresolution representation of curvature, as shown in Fig. 2, is generated using an iterative smoothing of the cortical surface and computation of the mean curvature at each iteration. The smoothing is performed by mean curvature flow [16]. Additionally, we also use the computed mean curvature as a feature for surface matching in the subsequent steps. The reason for using the mean curvature is that it represents the sulcal fundi with negative values and gyral crowns with positive values, therefore its alignment leads to accurate alignment of the cortex.

Next, we perform a coarse alignment of these smooth surfaces in 3D. For this purpose, we first apply a 5th order polynomial warping field to the subject and atlas surfaces; this field is computed using AIR [18] as part of BrainSuite's extraction sequence. This is followed by an L_2 surface registration procedure described in [5] as shown in Fig. 2. We chose initial alignment of the cortex based on the 5th degree polynomial initialization which is followed by L^2 surface registration. This rough alignment is fast because it is surface based and is performed in 3D rather than in the flat space. Additionally at this point our goal is compute an alignment of the major lobes and these are better defined by their 3D locations rather than local features such as curvature. Curvature registration in flat space then refines this alignment.

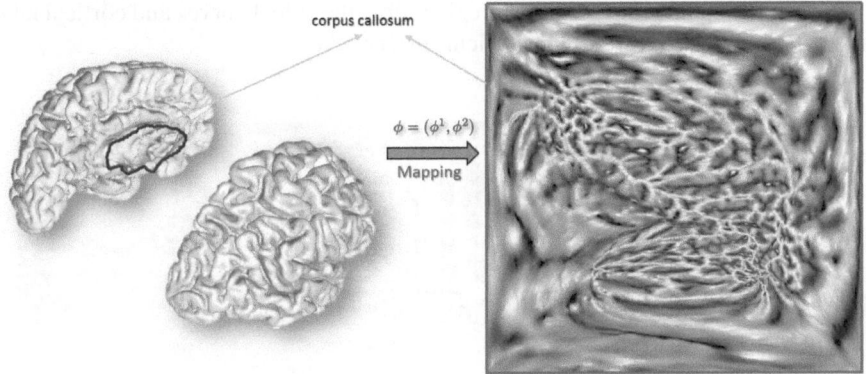

corpus callosum

$\phi = (\phi^1, \phi^2)$

Mapping

Flat-map color coded by curvature

Fig. 3. p-harmonic mapping of the cortex generated by p-harmonic energy minimization. The corpus callosum denoted by the blue boundary is mapped to the boundary of the square. After the energy minimization the cortical hemisphere maps to the inside of the square.

The subject and atlas surfaces are mapped to the unit square using p-harmonic mappings as described in [4]. The p-harmonic maps generate a one-to-one correspondence between a unit square and the cortical surfaces such that the inter-hemispherical fissure dividing the left and right hemisphere maps to the boundary of the unit square as a uniform speed curve. The cumulative curvature maps generated in the previous step are then transferred to the unit squares using the point correspondence established by the p-harmonic maps. To perform the curvature based alignment, we model the brain surface as an elastic sheet and solve the associated linear elastic equilibrium equation using the Finite Element Method (FEM) as described in [4]. The alignment of the curvature maps is then performed by minimizing a cost function with elastic energy as a regularizing penalty. This reparameterizes the cortical hemisphere surfaces and establishes a one-to-one point correspondence between subject and atlas surfaces. For every point s in the unit square space, let $C_{\mathscr{A}}(s)$ and $C_{\mathscr{S}}(s)$ denote the cumulative mean curvature values at s for atlas and subject, respectively. Also, $X(s) = [x(s), y(s), z(s)]^T$ denotes the 3D vertex coordinates of the surface at the mapped point s; $X_{\mathscr{A}}$ and $X_{\mathscr{S}}$ denotes aligned atlas and subject surfaces 3D coordinates described in the previous paragraph. Let E denotes elastic energy regularizer computed on the surface mesh. Then we find a deformation field ϕ that minimizes the cost function:

$$C(\phi) = E(\phi(s)) + \sigma_1 \|C_{\mathscr{A}}(\phi(s)) - C_{\mathscr{S}}(s)\|^2 + \sigma_2 \|X_{\mathscr{A}}(\phi(s)) - X_{\mathscr{S}}(s)\|^2. \quad (1)$$

The parameters $\sigma_1 = .5$, $\sigma_2 = .1$ were chosen empirically. The cost function minimizes the weighted sum of a curvature matching penalty and a 3D coordinate matching penalty, regularized by an elastic energy [4]. The optimization of the cost is performed by applying the L-BFGS optimization scheme [7]. The flat maps corresponding to the subject, atlas and warped subject are shown in Fig. 4.

After performing the atlas to subject registration, the sulcal curves and cortical labels from the atlas are transferred to the cortical surface (Fig. 5).

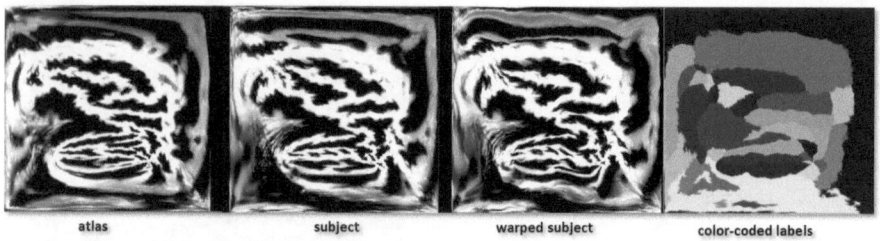

atlas   subject   warped subject   color-coded labels

Fig. 4. Flat maps produced by the automatic surface registration sequence. Shown are the atlas, subject, and warped subject flatmaps, shaded according to curvature (bright=positive; dark=negative); and the atlas-color flatmap colored according to anatomical ROI labels.

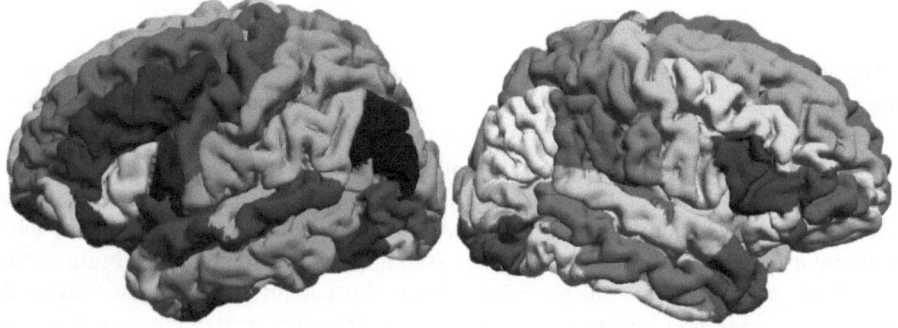

Fig. 5. Lateral views of the left and right hemispheres of an automatically labeled subject cortical surface. The labels from the atlas surface were transferred to the subject's surface by using the correspondence established by registration.

2.2   Geodesic Curvature Flow on Surfaces

The second major step in our method performs local refinement of the transferred sulcal curves and label boundaries using a geodesic curvature flow [6,19] so that these boundaries conform to sulcal fundi as represented by the curvature minima. In this section, we discuss the refinement of these sulcal curves, but note that the label boundaries are refined in a similar manner. The numerical implementation and FEM formulation of this method is described in detail in [3]; we describe it here briefly but omit the details. By using the point correspondence established by the registration, the sulcal curves on the atlas are transferred to the subject surface; we refer to these as the RT curves. The RT curves are typically in the correct sulcal valley, but are not precisely at their desired locations at the bottoms of these valleys. It has been noted that the sulci propagated by automatic registration generally lie withing 3cm of the true sulcal valleys [9]. Therefore, to reduce the computational burden, we calculate a surface patch around the sulcus of interest using front propagation for 3cm (Fig. 6).

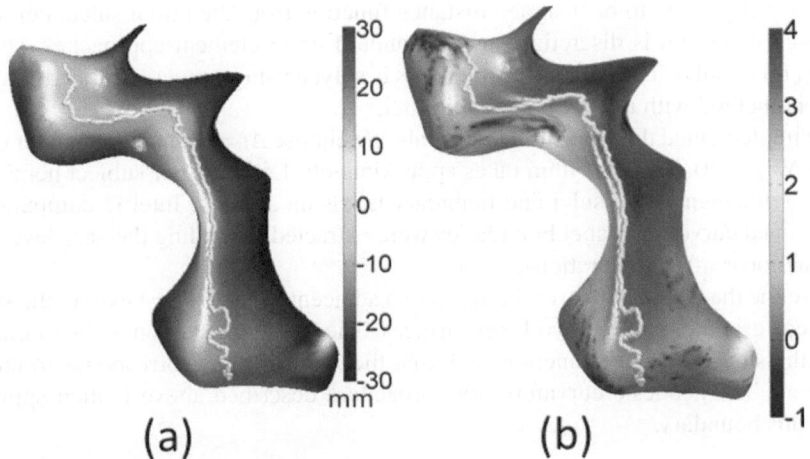

Fig. 6. (a) Initial sulcal curve and signed distance function; (b) curvature weighting function f shown as color-coded overlay on the surface patch around that sulcus

The geodesic curvature flow is performed over this surface patch around the sulcus of interest using a level set formulation. The approach presented here is based on [6], but in our case we add curvature weighting when computing minimizing geodesics. Assume $\mathcal{M}$ is a general 2D manifold representing the surface patch embedded in $\mathbb{R}^3$ and let Γ be the sulcal curve on the surface. Let the curve Γ be represented by the zero level set of a function $\phi : \mathcal{M} \to \mathbb{R}$, i.e., $\Gamma = \{s : \phi(s) = 0\}$. Suppose that $c : \mathcal{M} \to \mathbb{R}$ is the curvature of the surface $\mathcal{M}$. It has been noted that for sulcal tracing, a sigmoid function of the curvature works well as a weighting function on the paths for sulcal tracing [13]. Therefore, we define $f(s) = \frac{1}{1+e^{-2c(s)}}$ as the curvature based weights on the surfaces and seek to minimize the weighted length of Γ given by

$$E(\Gamma) = \int_{\Gamma:\phi=0} f\,dS \qquad (2)$$

where integration is computed over the surface at the curve points. Following [6,14,19], the Euler-Lagrange equations for the energy functional minimization of $E(\Gamma)$ yield

$$\begin{cases} -\mathrm{div}\left(f\frac{\nabla\phi}{|\nabla\phi|}\right) & = 0 \\ \frac{\partial\phi}{\partial n}\big|_{\partial\mathcal{M}} & = 0, \end{cases} \qquad (3)$$

where $\partial\mathcal{M}$ is the boundary of $\mathcal{M}$ and $\vec{n}$ is the intrinsic outward normal of $\partial\mathcal{M}$. A gradient descent flow of the equation [1] is given by:

$$\begin{cases} \frac{\partial\phi}{\partial t} = |\nabla\phi|\mathrm{div}\left(f\frac{\nabla\phi}{|\nabla\phi|}\right) \\ \frac{\partial\phi}{\partial n}\big|_{\partial\mathcal{M}} = 0 \\ \phi(0) = \phi_0 \end{cases} \qquad (4)$$

where we choose ϕ_0 to be a signed distance function from the initial sulcal curve. The boundary condition is discretized using standard finite element approaches (see [11] and [3] for details). This system of equations is solved using a preconditioned conjugate gradient method with a Jacobi preconditioner.

We implemented the algorithm in Matlab. We choose $\Delta t = .5$ and the number of iterations $N_{iter} = 20$. The algorithm takes approximately 1.5 hours per subject hemisphere for the refinement of all sulci and boundary labels on a 4 core Intel i7 computer. The final refined curves and label boundaries were extracted by finding the zero level set of the function ϕ after 20 iterations.

To refine the label boundaries between two adjacent ROIs, we first extract the surface patch corresponding to the two label surfaces. The level set function is then initialized using the signed distance function such that the zero level set corresponds to the ROI boundary. The geodesic curvature flow procedure described above is then applied to refine this boundary.

3   Results

To evaluate the performance of our method, we performed a validation study on a set of 6 subject brains. We used the ICBM Single Subject Template as our atlas (http://www.loni.ucla.edu/Atlases/Atlas_Detail.jsp?atlas_id=5). The BrainSuite software [12] was applied to extract cortical surface meshes from the subject and atlas MRI data. BrainSuite includes a multistage cortical modeling sequence. First, the brain is extracted from the surrounding skull and scalp tissues using a combination of edge detection and mathematical morphology. Next, the intensities of the MRI are corrected for shading artifacts. Each voxel in the corrected image is then labeled according to tissue type using a statistical classifier. A standard atlas with associated structure labels is aligned to the subject volume, providing a label for cerebellum, cerebrum, brainstem, and subcortical regions. These labels are combined with the tissue classification to identify the cerebral white matter automatically, to fill the ventricular spaces, and to remove the brainstem and cerebellum. This produces a volume whose boundary surface represents the outer white-matter surface of the cerebral cortex. Prior to tessellation, topological defects are identified and removed automatically from the binary volume using a graph based approach. An isosurface algorithm is then applied to the topologically corrected white matter volume, yielding a genus zero surface. This surface is then expanded to identify the pial surface, i.e., the boundary between grey matter and CSF. The inner cortical and pial surfaces are then split into left and right hemispheres based on the registered atlas labels.

We delineated sulcal curves using BrainSuite's interactive delineation tools [13] following a sulcal protocol with 26 sulcal curves [9]. These sulci are consistently seen in normal brains and are distributed throughout the entire cortical surface. A thorough description of the sulcal curves with instructions on how to trace them is available on the web site (http://neuroimage.usc.edu/CurveProtocol.html). The protocol specifies methods for identifying the 26 sulci by making consistent decisions in delineation in case of ambiguity in the brain anatomy. We traced the curves on the midcortical surface because it provides better access to the depth of the sulci than the pial surface, and the valleys of the sulci are more convex than they are on the white matter surface, thus allowing more stable tracing of the curves. The same procedure was repeated on the single subject atlas. Next, we performed the subject to atlas registration as described in Sec. 2.1 and transferred the curves of the atlas to the subject brains. The transferred curves were refined using the geodesic curvature flow as discussed in Sec 2.2. The evolution of one sulcal curve in shown in Fig. 7(online link:http://sipi.usc.edu/~ajoshi/GCF_Sulci.html).

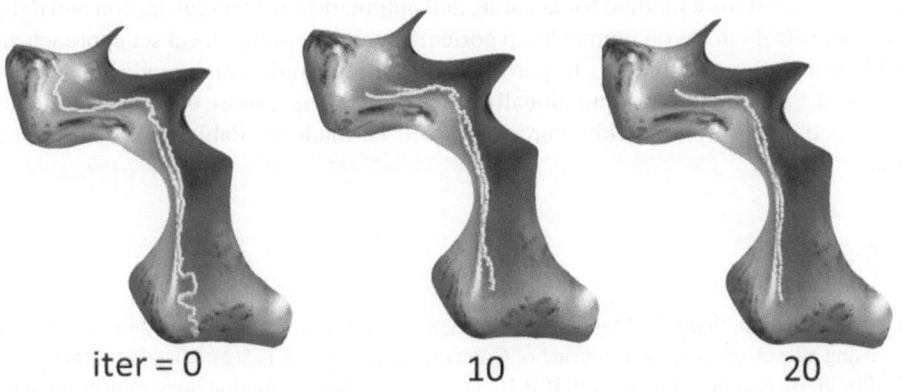

iter = 0   10   20

Fig. 7. Evolution of the sulcal curve by geodesic curvature flow for different iterations. The curvature weighting function f is shown as color-coded overlay

To compare the alignment of transferred curves, as well as the refined curves, we mapped the 26 protocol curves from all subjects to the target surface. We then quantified their accuracy using their variance on the subject surface, which is estimated as follows. We use a distance measure based on the Hausdorff distance metric:

$$d(D_i,D_j) = 0.5\frac{1}{N}\sum_{p\in D_i}\min_{p\in D_i}|p-q|^2 + 0.5\frac{1}{N}\sum_{p\in D_j}\min_{q\in D_j}|p-q|^2$$

where $d(D_i,D_j)$ is the distance between the curves D_i and D_j. This distance is computed between subject's manual curve and RT curve, as well as manual curve and GCF curve.

The results for some of the prominent sulci are presented in Table 1. It can be seen that the sulcal error is reduced substantially after geodesic curvature flow. This improvement is most pronounced in the sulci that are clearly defined by curvature extrema and shortest length paths on the cortex such as central sulcus and superior frontal sulcus.

Table 1. Sulcal errors measured by Hausdorff distance metric. The table shows mean error for N=6.

	manual vs transferred curves (*mm*)	manual vs refined curves (*mm*)
Cent. sulcus	1.9	1.4
Sup. Front. sulcus	2.9	1.9
Calc. sulcus	2.6	2.0
Sup. Temp. sulcus	3.9	3.4
Avg over all 26 sulci	3.6	2.9

4 Conclusion

This paper presents a method for accurate and automatic cortical registration and delineation of sulcal curves on human brain cortex. The 2D mapping, level set approach and FEM formulations enabled us to perform surface registration and geodesic curvature flow on the surface in a computationally efficient manner. A more extensive evaluation is planned. The software with source code will be made available online in the near future.

References

1. Cheng, L., Burchard, P., Merriman, B., Osher, S.: Motion of curves constrained on surfaces using a level-set approach. Journal of Computational Physics 175(2), 604–644 (2002)
2. Fischl, B., Sereno, M.I., Tootell, R.B.H., Dale, A.M.: High-resolution inter-subject averaging and a coordinate system for the cortical surface. Human Brain Mapping 8, 272–284 (1998)
3. Joshi, A., Shattuck, D., Damasio, H., Leahy, R.: Geodesic curvature flow on surfaces for automatic sulcal delineation. In: Proc. ISBI (2012)
4. Joshi, A.A., Shattuck, D.W., Thompson, P.M., Leahy, R.M.: Surface-constrained volumetric brain registration using harmonic mappings. IEEE Trans. Med. Imag. 26(12), 1657–1669 (2007)
5. Joshi, A., Chaudhari, A., Li, C., Dutta, J., Cherry, S., Shattuck, D., Toga, A., Leahy, R.: Digiwarp: a method for deformable mouse atlas warping to surface topographic data. Physics in Medicine and Biology 55, 6197 (2010)

6. Lai, R., Shi, Y., Sicotte, N., Toga, A.W.: Automated corpus callosum extraction via laplace-beltrami nodal parcellation and intrinsic geodesic curvature flows on surfaces. In: ICCV (2011)
7. Liu, D., Nocedal, J.: On the limited memory bfgs method for large scale optimization. Mathematical Programming 45(1), 503–528 (1989)
8. Narr, K., Thompson, P., Sharma, T., Moussai, J., Zoumalan, C., Rayman, J., Toga, A.: Three-dimensional mapping of gyral shape and cortical surface asymmetries in schizophrenia: gender effects. Am. J. Psychiatry 158(2), 244–255 (2001)
9. Pantazis, D., Joshi, A., Jiang, J., Shattuck, D., Bernstein, L., Damasio, H., Leahy, R.: Comparison of landmark-based and automatic methods for cortical surface registration. Neuroimage 49(3), 2479–2493 (2010)
10. Rettmann, M., Kraut, M., Prince, J., Resnick, S.: Cross-sectional and longitudinal analyses of anatomical sulcal changes associated with aging. Cerebral Cortex 16(11), 1584–1594 (2006)
11. Sadiku, M.N.O.: Numerical techniques in electromagnetics. CRC (2000)
12. Shattuck, D.W., Leahy, R.M.: Brainsuite: An automated cortical surface identification tool. Medical Image Analysis 8(2), 129–142 (2002)
13. Shattuck, D., Joshi, A., Pantazis, D., Kan, E., Dutton, R., Sowell, E., Thompson, P., Toga, A., Leahy, R.: Semi-automated method for delineation of landmarks on models of the cerebral cortex. J. Neuroscience Meth. 178(2), 385–392 (2009)
14. Spira, A., Kimmel, R.: Geodesic curvature flow on parametric surfaces. In: Curve and Surface Design, pp. 365–373 (2002)
15. Tao, X., Prince, J., Davatzikos, C.: Using a statistical shape model to extract sulcal curves on the outer cortex of the human brain. IEEE Transactions on Medical Imaging 21(5), 513–524 (2002)
16. Tosun, D., Prince, J.L.: Cortical Surface Alignment Using Geometry Driven Multispectral Optical Flow. In: Christensen, G.E., Sonka, M. (eds.) IPMI 2005. LNCS, vol. 3565, pp. 480–492. Springer, Heidelberg (2005)
17. Vaillant, M., Davatzikos, C.: Finding parametric representations of the cortical sulci using an active contour model. Medical Image Analysis 1(4), 295–315 (1997)
18. Woods, R., Grafton, S., Holmes, C., Cherry, S., Mazziotta, J.: Automated image registration: I. general methods and intrasubject, intramodality validation. Journal of Computer Assisted Tomography 22(1), 139 (1998)
19. Wu, C., Tai, X.: A level set formulation of geodesic curvature flow on simplicial surfaces. IEEE Transactions on Visualization and Computer Graphics 16(4), 647–662 (2010)

Registration of Dynamic Contrast Enhanced MRI with Local Rigidity Constraint

Lars Ruthotto[1], Erlend Hodneland[2,3], and Jan Modersitzki[1]

[1] Institute of Mathematics and Image Computing, University of Lübeck, Germany
[2] Department of Biomedicine, University of Bergen, Norway
[3] Department of Radiology, Haukeland University Hospital, Bergen, Norway
lars.ruthotto@mic.uni-luebeck.de
http://www.mic.uni-luebeck.de

Abstract. Dynamic Contrast Enhanced Magnetic Resonance Imaging (DCE-MRI) of the kidney provides important information for the diagnosis of renal dysfunction. To this end, a time series of image volumes is acquired after injection of a contrast agent. The interpretation and pharmacokinetic analysis of the time series data is highly sensitive to motion artifacts. Registration of these data is a challenging task as contrast uptake adds new image features and gives rise to intensity changes over time within the kidneys.

This paper presents a new registration pipeline for a time series of 3D DCE-MRI. The pipeline combines state-of-art modules such as a weighted and robust least squares type distance measure, a regularization that is based on hyperelasticity and thus ensures diffeomorphic transformations and enables the incorporation of local rigidity constraints on the kidneys. We provide results that indicate the necessity of these constraints and illustrate the superiority of the proposed pipeline as compared to other approaches.

Keywords: DCE-MRI, Motion Correction, Constrained Image Registration, Local Rigidity, Hyperelastic Registration.

1 Introduction

Dynamic Contrast Enhanced Magnetic Resonance Imaging (DCE-MRI) of the kidney provides in vivo information about the Glomerular Filtration Rate (GFR). The GFR is an important measure of renal function and useful in the diagnosis of chronic kidney diseases. To this end, a small dose of contrast agent, gadolinium, is administered and a time series of three dimensional images is acquired. Although the images are partly acquired during breath hold the time series can be affected by inconsistencies between the respiratory phases at the instance of recording. Even small displacements can affect the voxelwise pharmacokinetic analysis yielding incorrect estimates of the GFR [8] and thus limit the usability of DCE-MRI. In particular, when looking at the update rate in the cortex of the kidneys, this is an important issue.

B.M. Dawant et al. (Eds.): WBIR 2012, LNCS 7359, pp. 190–198, 2012.

Registration of DCE-MRI time series is a challenging task since intensity changes in the region of interest take place due to uptake of bolus, but also from geometrical changes due to inconsistent breath hold, free breathing after breath hold, patient movements and physiological pulsations. New features may appear during wash in and disappear during the wash out phase, which can mislead unimodal distance measures.

DCE-MRI registration is an important challenge and has thus drawn much attention. Melbourne et al. [7] proposed a nonlinear registration scheme based on repeated registrations of the data to a reference time series generated by a Principal Component Analysis (PCA). The reference volumes preserve long term contrast uptake but show less motion. Their approach is based on the assumption that the displacements between acquisitions is periodically or random. Alternatively the impact of intensity variations on nonlinear registration schemes can be suppressed by multi-modal distance measures such as mutual information [13,14] or normalized gradient fields [4,6]. Under the assumption that uptake of contrast agent is limited to the kidneys the registration problem is essentially uni-modal in large parts of the image. This assumption is also supported by our analysis of the results for kidney data from Haukeland University Hospital, Bergen, Norway. Another option to gain robustness against uptake-induced intensity modulations is to limit the flexibility of the transformation model. A direct comparison between nonlinear and rigid transformation models on the entire image and limited to rectangular regions around the kidneys was performed in [11]. The results suggest that rigidity is useful to describe the motion of the kidneys, however, improper to model the overall respiratory motion [11].

In this paper, we propose a novel nonlinear registration pipeline with local rigidity constraints on the kidneys [12,5]. Thereby we ensure that the relevant contrast variations related to blood clearance are preserved in the registered time series. Further the robustness of the registration against intensity changes related to contrast uptake is improved. Our comparison with an unconstrained approach demonstrates the improvement that can be gained by integrating the local rigidity constraints. In contrast to [11], a globally smooth and nonlinear transformation is estimated and the registration is driven by a very robust uni modal distance measure. Smooth transitions between the constrained and unconstrained regions are provided by a novel hyperelastic regularizer [2]. This remarkable regularizer prohibits tissue folding and thus it is guaranteed to compute a diffeomorphic transformation independent of the choice of regularization parameters.

First promising results on clinical data are presented and suggest that local rigidity is a useful option to reduce the degradation of DCE-MRI due to motion artifacts.

2   Locally Rigid Registration Scheme

Given a time series of three dimensional images $\mathcal{I}_1, ..., \mathcal{I}_T$ on a domain $\Omega \subset \mathbf{R}^3$ our goal is to eliminate the motion between the individual time points. To this end, we aim to register all image volumes to an assigned reference image – in the following

$\mathcal{R} := \mathcal{I}_1$. For ease of presentation, we limit the description to one subproblem, i.e. the registration of one arbitrary time frame $\mathcal{T} \in \{\mathcal{I}_2, ..., \mathcal{I}_T\}$ to $\mathcal{R}$.

Since displacements due to respiratory motion on the entire thorax are non-linear, we choose a non-parametric model for the mapping $y : \Omega \to \mathbf{R}^3$ [9].

In our application difficulties arise due to uptake related intensity variations within the kidneys. The goal is to preserve this essential piece of information, but nevertheless eliminate the displacement between the frames in the time series. As our analysis of the data indicates, the DCE-MRI registration problem is essentially unimodal outside the kidney regions. Therefore we choose a simple and robust weighted SSD distance measure

$$\mathcal{D}(\mathcal{T}, \mathcal{R}) := \frac{1}{2} \int_\Omega (\mathcal{T}(x) - \mathcal{R}(x))^2 \, v(x) \, dx. \tag{1}$$

The weighting function $v : \Omega \to \mathbf{R}^+$ is used to reduce the influence of regions with varying signal intensities, see Sec. 3 for details.

2.1   Locally Rigid Image Registration

To avoid misregistrations due to uptake induced contrast variations we aim to limit the flexibility of the transformation within the kidneys by adding rigidity constraints as motivated by [11].

Our notation and implementation follows [5]. Let $M_1, M_2 \subset \Omega$ denote the regions of the kidneys in the reference image $\mathcal{R}$. The idea is to restrict the nonlinear transformation y to be locally rigid on M_1 and M_2. This motivates the formulation of the constrained registration problem [5]

$$\min_{y, w} \frac{1}{2} \int_\Omega (\mathcal{T}(y(x)) - \mathcal{R})^2 \, |\det \nabla y(x)| \, v(x) \, dx \, + \, \mathcal{S}[y] \tag{2}$$

$$\text{subject to } y(x) = Q(x) f(w_i) \; \forall x \in M_i, \; i = 1, 2.$$

Note the appearance of $|\det \nabla y(x)|$ due to a change of the coordinate system and the transformation rule; see [5] for details. As for the constraints, $Q(x)$ describes a model for a linear transformation, w_1 and w_2 are the six parameters of the rigid transformations for the two kidney regions and f is the embedding of the rigid space into the space of affine linear transformations; see [5] for details. The regularization $\mathcal{S}$ is discussed in the next subsection.

2.2   Hyperelastic Regularization

To allow for large transformations and to enforce invertibility we choose a hyperelastic regularizer [2]

$$\mathcal{S}^{\text{hyper}}(y) = \alpha_l \mathcal{S}^{\text{length}}(y) + \alpha_a \mathcal{S}^{\text{area}}(y) + \alpha_v \mathcal{S}^{\text{volume}}(y). \tag{3}$$

This regularizer controls the changes in length, area and volume induced by the transformation y. Due to the growth behavior and since infinite energy is required to annihilate a volume element, $\mathcal{S}^{\text{hyper}}$ guarantees the invertibility of

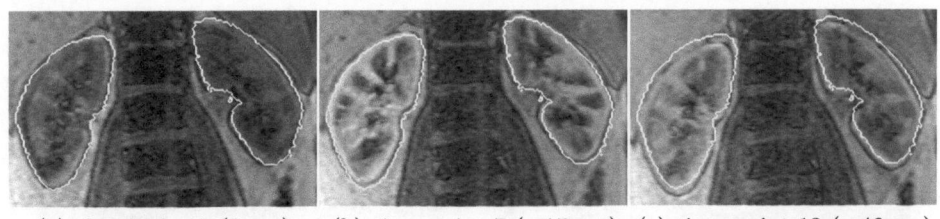

Fig. 1. Illustration of the motion problem in DCE-MRI. We exemplarily visualize three time points in coronal views. The semi automatic segmentation of the kidney obtained for the first image volume is represented by a white contour in (a) – (c). The appearance of new structures due to uptake of the contrast agent can for example be seen by comparing (a) to (b). The motion problem due to free breathing is observable for instance by comparing a) to (c).

the transformation even for large displacements and thus enforces diffeomorphic transformations. Moreover, the transformation field is very smooth and the hyperelastic regularizer is therefore especially attractive in combination with rigidity constraints to control volume changes in the neighborhood of the kidney cortices.

2.3   Numerical Implementation

The constrained registration algorithm is implemented using the publicly available toolbox FAIR in Matlab [9]. Important routines such as image interpolation, distance measures and hyperelastic regularizer are re-used. The problem is attacked in a multi-level strategy on a coarse-to-fine hierarchy of discretizations. Each discrete optimization problem is solved using a Newton-SQP optimizer [10]. The linear system is solved using a preconditioned minimum residual method [1] where the preconditioner is a slightly modified version of [3].

2.4   Test Data

A 1.5 Tesla MR-scanner (Avanto, Siemens) is used to acquire DCE-MRI data from a healthy volunteer. A breath-hold T1-weighted 3D single Gradient Recall Echo (GRE) pulse sequence was used to acquire signal-intensity time curves after administration of a small dose (2 ml) of gadolinium contrast media intravenously. The acquisition parameters for the examination was: Slice-thickness 3 mm, Repetition Time 3.3, Echo Time 1.79, Flip Angle 9, Acquisition Matrix 256×128, Parallel factor 2, Time resolution is 2.5 sec in the breath hold phase (first 11 time frames) and 30 sec in the free breathing phase. The voxel size is $1.48 \times 1.48 \times 3$ mm.

The kidney segmentation in the first image volume $\mathcal{R} = \mathcal{I}_1$ that was delivered with the data was obtained using a semi-automatic segmentation using temporal curve information [6]. A training mask for each desired phase was given initially by the user, representative for the tissue classes to be found. Thus, a large set of

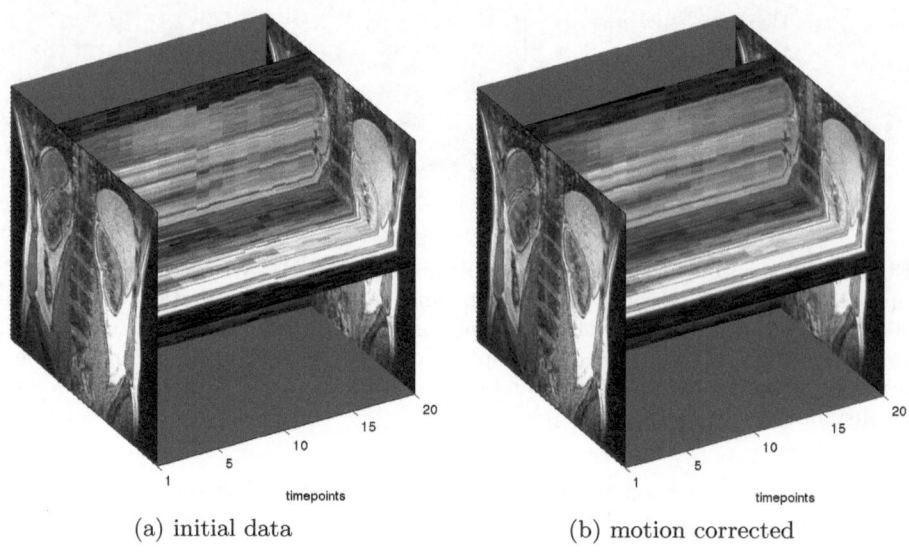

(a) initial data   (b) motion corrected

Fig. 2. 3D Motion correction results are visualized exemplarily for one coronal slice. The slice is shown at the first and last time point before (a) and after locally rigid registration (b). The time course is visualized by two planes. It is apparent, that the proposed scheme reduces motion artifacts as can be observed for example in the end of the breath hold at timepoint 11.

T-dimensional tissue vectors were obtained, where T is the number of time points. The algorithm uses the Mahalanobis distance between such temporal curve shapes to classify each voxel in space with KNN nearest-neighbor classification. Each voxel is assigned to the most abundant class within the K nearest neighbors in the training set. After classification, the voxel is assigned to the training set, and the algorithm runs iteratively until no voxels are changing class.

3   Results

We apply the proposed registration pipeline to the clinical data set consisting of 20 DCE-MRI image volumes. The template images $\mathcal{I}_2, .., \mathcal{I}_{20}$ are sequentially registered to the reference image $\mathcal{I}_1$ by solving the constrained registration problem (2). The distance measure (1) is weighted with arbitrarily chosen factors $v(x) = 0.05$ within the kidneys and $v(x) = 1$ elsewhere. For all 3D registration problems we use hand-picked regularization parameters, $\alpha_l = 300, \alpha_a = 30, \alpha_v = 300$, see (3).

The average reduction of the weighted distance measure $\mathcal{D}$ (1) over all 19 registration problems is 48%. For all transformations the Jacobian determinant $\det \nabla y$ is in the interval $[0.43, 1.49]$ and hence, as guaranteed by our regularization scheme, all mappings are diffeomorphic.

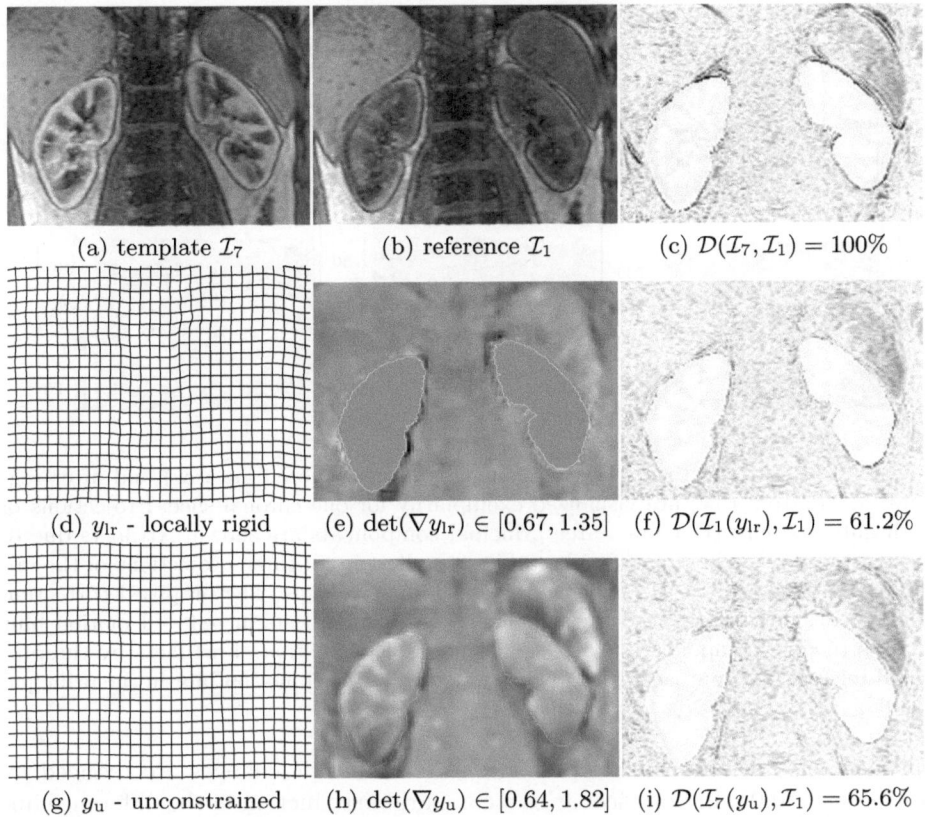

(a) template $\mathcal{I}_7$ (b) reference $\mathcal{I}_1$ (c) $\mathcal{D}(\mathcal{I}_7, \mathcal{I}_1) = 100\%$

(d) y_{lr} - locally rigid   (e) $\det(\nabla y_{\mathrm{lr}}) \in [0.67, 1.35]$ (f) $\mathcal{D}(\mathcal{I}_1(y_{\mathrm{lr}}), \mathcal{I}_1) = 61.2\%$

(g) y_{u} - unconstrained   (h) $\det(\nabla y_{\mathrm{u}}) \in [0.64, 1.82]$ (i) $\mathcal{D}(\mathcal{I}_7(y_{\mathrm{u}}), \mathcal{I}_1) = 65.6\%$

Fig. 3. Results of the 3D registration of the time points with most extreme variations in contrast uptake ($\mathcal{I}_1$ and $\mathcal{I}_7$) are visualized in one coronal slice. The template image $\mathcal{I}_7$ (a) is registered to the reference image $\mathcal{I}_1$ (b). The solutions of the registration with and without local rigidity constraints, y_{lr} and y_{u}, are visualized in (d) and (g). Both transformations are smooth and diffeomorphic indicated by the Jacobian determinants being positive and finite (e) and (h). However, (h) also shows volumetric changes in the kidney regions which can be avoided using the constrained approach (e). A comparable reduction of the distance is achieved by both transformations, compare the absolute weighted distance images with identical colormap (c),(f) and (i).

Fig. 2 illustrates the considerable reduction of motion artifacts due to inconsistencies between the respiratory phases and free breathing as well as the improvement that can be gained using the proposed pipeline. The impact of the registration pipeline is illustrated exemplarily for one coronal slice. The time courses before and after locally rigid registration are visualized by two orthogonal planes in time dimension.

We exemplarily show more detailed results of the 3D registration for the images with the most extreme variations in contrast uptake ($\mathcal{I}_1$ and $\mathcal{I}_7$) in Fig. 3. We also demonstrate the importance of local rigidity constrains for this application by comparing the constrained with an unconstrained approach. In the

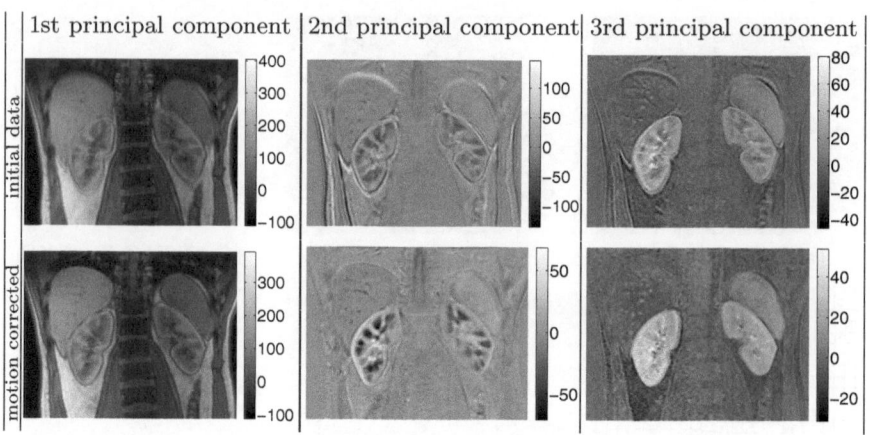

Fig. 4. 3D Results of Principal Component Analysis before (top row) and after registration (bottom row) are visualized exemplarily for one coronal slice. Projections of both datasets onto their first three principal components are shown. Artifacts due to inconsistent breath hold and free breathing manifest in all three projections of the initial data as shadows in the spleen, liver and kidney regions. The proposed correction scheme considerably reduced these artifacts, which manifests in reduced motion blur of the principal components. Note the considerable reduction of artifacts by the proposed registration approach as can be observed by reduced motion blur in the principal components.

unconstrained setting the regularization of volumetric changes are reduced by setting $\alpha_v = 0.01$. In both scenarios a comparable reduction in the difference images is achieved and essentially all structure outside the kidney regions vanishes, supporting our assumption that the registration problem is uni-modal outside the kidneys. Both transformations are very smooth and due to the hyperelastic regularizer also diffeomorphic. However, as to be expected the unconstrained registration introduces volumetric changes inside the kidneys to compensate the different uptake levels while the constrained scheme does not. Note that the underlying image differences relate to contrast uptake and not to tissue distortion. Hence the results of the constrained approach are superior.

As another indicator of the effectiveness of our method, we perform a Principal Component Analysis (PCA) of the time series before and after registration; see [7]. To this end, we remove the mean of each time point on the finest discretization level, compute the covariance matrices and their eigenvectors and eigenvalues. The projections onto the three principal components are shown in Fig. 4. The reduction of motion artifacts can be seen by comparing the respective projections. Before correction the first principal component is motion-blurred and contours of the spleen, liver and kidneys are shaded. Inconsistent respiratory phases and problems due to free breathing also manifest in the second and third principal component. After registration the first principal component is less blurred and the remaining projections describe the long term uptake behavior within the kidneys.

4   Discussion and Outlook

We present a novel image registration pipeline for Dynamic Contrast Enhanced MRI (DCE-MRI) of kidneys. The new pipeline combines a robust, weighted least squares based distance measure, a hyperelastic regularizer, and local rigidity constraints. The basic idea is to partition the domain into regions of primarily pharmacokinetic activities and remainder. In active regions tissue deformations are restricted to be locally rigid and thus uptake-induced intensity changes that are essential for pharmacokinetic analysis are preserved. The emphasis of the weighted distance measure is on the remainder, where the registration problem is approximately uni-modal. First promising results indicate that our pipeline considerably reduces motion artifacts related to inconsistencies between respiratory phases at the instance of recording and free breathing.

It is well known that unconstrained registration approaches may lead to incorrect changes of volume in kidneys. Synthetically generated reference images sharing the long term uptake behavior have been used to resolve this issue [7]. However, the synthesis is based on certain assumptions on the motion such as periodicity which can be questionable in acquisitions with breath hold and free breathing phases. We present experiments demonstrating that our new constrained approach is capable to register kidney DCE-MRI without making assumptions on the underlying motion.

Similar to [11] our findings suggest that local rigidity within the kidneys is a useful assumption to eliminate motion artifacts in DCE-MRI data related to respiration. Instead of computing separate rigid registrations of both kidneys as in [11], our scheme uses only one global transformation. Even though only the kidneys are of interest for the analysis of renal function, our experiments indicate that adjacent anatomical structures provide additional and useful information.

Our approach focuses on eliminating motion artifacts due to inconsistencies between respiratory phases at the instance of recording and free breathing. Further reasons for displacement between time frames such as physiological pulsations are not addressed. Obviously, our scheme is only indented for DCE-MRI of tissue where the local rigidity assumption holds. For DCE-MRI of tissue with severe non-rigid displacements our scheme may only serve as a rigid pre-registration step.

At present, the proposed scheme requires an initial segmentation of the kidneys in one reference image. In our case a semi automatic segmentation of the first time point was already provided with the data. In future work we will also investigate the integration of automatic kidney segmentations into our framework. We are positive that our scheme is robust against segmentation errors since the powerful hyperelastic regularization [2] gives a very smooth transition from the constrained to the unconstrained region.

Acknowledgements. We like to thank the *MR kidney function researchgroup* and Jarle Rørvik (MD, PhD) et al. from the Department of Surgical Sciences, University of Bergen and Department of Radiology, Haukeland University Hospital, Bergen, Norway for providing this interesting data. Furthermore we thank Åsmund Kjørstad for his segmentations of the kidneys.

References

1. Barrett, R.: Templates for the solution of linear systems. building blocks for iterative methods. Society for Industrial Mathematics (1994)
2. Burger, M., Modersitzki, J., Ruthotto, L.: A hyperelastic regularization energy for image registration. SIAM Journal on Scientific Computing (in revision) (2012)
3. Greif, C., Schötzau, D.: Preconditioners for saddle point linear systems with highly singular (1, 1) blocks. Electronic Transactions on Numerical Analysis 22, 114–121 (2006)
4. Haber, E., Modersitzki, J.: Intensity gradient based registration and fusion of multimodal images. Methods of Information in Medicine 46(3), 292–299 (2007)
5. Haber, E., Heldmann, S., Modersitzki, J.: A framework for image-based constrained registration with an application to local rigidity. Linear Algebra and its Applications 431, 459–470 (2009)
6. Hodneland, E., Kjorstad, A., Andersen, E., Monssen, J.A., Lundervold, A., Rørvik, J., Munthe-Kaas, A.: In vivo estimation of glomerular filtration in the kidney using DCE-MRI. In: Image and Signal Processing and Analysis (ISPA), pp. 755–761. IEEE (2011)
7. Melbourne, A., Atkinson, D., White, M.J., Collins, D., Leach, M., Hawkes, D.: Registration of dynamic contrast-enhanced MRI using a progressive principal component registration (PPCR). Physics in Medicine and Biology 52(17), 5147–5156 (2007)
8. Michoux, N., Vallee, J., Pechere-Bertschi, A., Montet, X., Buehler, L., Van Beers, B.: Analysis of contrast-enhanced MR images to assess renal function. Magnetic Resonance Materials in Physics, Biology and Medicine 19(4), 167–179 (2006)
9. Modersitzki, J.: FAIR: Flexible algorithms for image registration (2009)
10. Nocedal, J., Wright, S.J.: Numerical optimization. Springer (1999)
11. Rogelj, P., Zöllner, F.G., Kovačič, S., Lundervold, A.: Motion correction of contrast-enhanced MRI time series of kidney. In: Proceedings of the 16th International Electrotechnical and Computer Science Conference (ERK 2007), pp. 191–194 (2007)
12. Staring, M., Klein, S., Pluim, J.: A rigidity penalty term for nonrigid registration. Medical Physics 34, 4098 (2007)
13. Viola, P., Wells III, W.M.: Alignment by maximization of mutual information. International Journal of Computer Vision 24(2), 137–154 (1997)
14. Zöllner, F.G., Sance, R., Rogelj, P., Ledesma-Carbayo, M.J., Rørvik, J., Santos, A., Lundervold, A.: Assessment of 3D DCE-MRI of the kidneys using non-rigid image registration and segmentation of voxel time courses. Computerized Medical Imaging and Graphics 33(3), 171–181 (2009)

Diffeomorphic Cardiac Motion Estimation with Anisotropic Regularization along Myofiber Orientation

Zhijun Zhang[1], David J. Sahn[1,2], and Xubo Song[1]

[1] Department of Biomedical Engineering
[2] Department of Pediatric Cardiology
Oregon Health and Science University
20000 NW Walker Road, Beaverton, OR 97006, USA
{zhangzhi,songx,sahn}@ohsu.edu

Abstract. Quantitative motion analysis from cardiac imaging is an important yet challenging problem. Most of the existing cardiac motion estimation methods ignore the fact that the myocardium is a fibrous structure with elastic anisotropy. We propose a novel method in which an anisotropic regularization energy is used to favor the motion consistency with the myofiber orientation. The myofiber direction comes from a diffusion tensor image and it is mapped to the end-diastole frame by using nonrigid registration. We implement the method based on a diffeomorphic motion estimation framework in which a spatiotemporally smooth velocity field is estimated by optimization of a variational energy. We validate the proposed method by using cine magnetic resonance imaging (MRI) datasets and echocardiography of an open-chest pig with sonomicrometry. We compare the proposed method with a temporal diffeomorphic free form deformation method without consideration of myofiber orientation. Experiments results show that the proposed motion estimation method has higher accuracy.

Keywords: Diffeomorphic registration, nonrigid registration, motion estimation, myofiber orientation.

1 Introduction

Cardiovascular disease is the number one cause of casualties in the western world. Quantitative analysis of deformation and motion from cardiac image sequences has become an important research tool because of its invasiveness [1]. However cardiac motion estimation is still a challenging problem because the spatial and temporal resolution of the images are still less than desirable and the complexity of the cardiac motion makes the problem more difficult.

Standard motion estimation method using nonrigid registration pairwisely have been proposed in [2, 3]. Various constraints have been used to make the motion estimation to be more physically plausible. Deformation models with temporal smoothness constraints have been used in [4, 5]. Properties such as particle trajectory smoothness, transformation symmetry and temporal transitivity

B.M. Dawant et al. (Eds.): WBIR 2012, LNCS 7359, pp. 199–208, 2012.
© Springer-Verlag Berlin Heidelberg 2012

have also been used to constrain motion estimation [6–8]. Diffeomorphic registration has been proposed to estimate the transformation as end point of an
evolution process constrained by a transport equation so that it is inherently
smooth, invertible and one-to-one mapping [9, 10]. It has been extended to solve
motion estimation problem in [11, 12]. Myocardium incompressibility has been
used as a biological tissue constraint together with elastic models to improve the
motion estimation [12–14]. However, all of the above physical constraints are
added on the deformable solids which are isotropically elastic and it is inconsistent with the fact that the myocardium is anisotropically elastic.

In fact, the motion of heart such as twist and contraction is closely related to
the anisotropic structure of the myocardium. The myofiber is distributed in a he-
lix structure in the myocardium and the contraction and relaxation are primarily across and along the myofiber orientations. From apical view the apex rotates
counterclockwise and the base rotates clockwise during contraction, and reverses
in the relaxation phase [15]. Consideration of the myofiber orientation can help decrease the ambiguity of the myocardium deformation which is not clearly visible
in the image modalities such as MRI and echocardiography. Myofiber orientation
has been used to analyze the strain in cardiac mechanics studies [16, 17], and it has
been used to improve the biomechanical model performance [18]. However, few articles consider the myofiber orientation in motion estimation. Papademetris *et al.*
[19] used a finite element model (FEM) in which the myofiber orientation in each
element is predetermined by fitting the model with the myofiber angle measurements. The FEM nodes displacement between frames is estimated by minimizing
a weighted sum of a feature distance function and a strain energy function. The
strain tensor is defined by an anisotropic elastic model in which the stiffness factor
along the myofiber orientation is a multiple of those across myofiber. However, in
this method the feature points from the segmented myocardium are needed. We
propose a novel intensity-based motion estimation method with myofiber orientation considered. The myofiber orientation information comes from a diffusion tensor image (DTI). For tracking, the intensity image of DTI is first aligned with the
first frame of the sequence by using a nonrigid registration and the tensors are reori-
ented into the reference image. An anisotropic regularization is used in the motion
estimation which makes the motion to be smooth along and across the myofiber.
The method is implemented with a diffeomorphic motion estimation framework
which has the advantage of one-to-one, smooth and invertible.

2   Method

2.1   Diffeomorphic Motion Estimation

We start with the diffeomorphic registration problem between the reference
image I_0 and target image I_1. We define a flow $\phi(\mathbf{x}, t), t \in [0, 1], \mathbf{x} \in \Omega \subset R^3$
with its smooth velocity field $\boldsymbol{v}(\mathbf{x}, t)$ by using the differential equation of $\frac{d\phi}{dt} = \boldsymbol{v}(\phi(\mathbf{x}, t), t), \phi(\mathbf{x}, 0) = \mathbf{x}$. It has been proven in [20] that if $\boldsymbol{v}(\mathbf{x}, t)$ is smooth with
a differential operator L in a Sobolev space V, the transformation $\phi(\mathbf{x}, t)$ defines
a group of diffeomorphisms with t varying from 0 to 1. The diffeomorphic image

registration is stated as a variational problem to find an optimal velocity field $\hat{v}(\mathbf{x}, t)$ which minimizes an energy functional consisting of a weighted sum of a summed squared difference (SSD) between $I_0(\mathbf{x})$ and the unwarped target image $I_1(\phi(\mathbf{x}, 1))$ and a distance metric between transformations $\phi(\mathbf{x}, 0)$ and $\phi(\mathbf{x}, 1)$:

$$\hat{v} = arg \inf_{v \in V} \lambda \int_0^1 ||v(\mathbf{x}, t)||_V^2 dt + \int_\Omega (I_0(\mathbf{x}) - I_1(\phi_{0,1}(\mathbf{x})))^2 d\mathbf{x}, \tag{1}$$

with λ being the weighting to balance two metrics.

The Euler Lagrange equation of the variational functional in Eqn.(1) is derived in Beg *et al*'s work [9]. The optimal velocity field can be obtained by solving the partial differential equation (PDE). However, the approach is expensive. We here adopt a parameterized approach to find the optimal velocity field [21]. The velocity field is discretized with a series of 3D B-spline function at time $t_k(k = 0, 1, ...N_f, t_k = k\Delta t, \Delta t = 1/N_f)$. The B-spline function at time point t_k is defined as $v(\mathbf{x}, t_k) = \sum \mathbf{c}_{i;k}\beta(\mathbf{x} - \mathbf{x}_i)$, with $\mathbf{c}_{i;k}$ being the B-spline control vectors located on a uniform grid of $\mathbf{x}_i$ at t_k, $\beta(\mathbf{x} - \mathbf{x}_i)$ being the 3D B-spline kernel function which is the tensor product of the 1-D B-spline functions. The transformation $\phi(\mathbf{x}, t)$ can be expressed as the forward Euler integral of velocity field by assuming that the velocity is piecewise constant within a time step. The transformation ϕ_{0,t_k} is related with $\phi_{0,t_{k-1}}$ by:

$$\phi_{0,t_k} = \phi_{0,t_{k-1}} + v(\phi_{0,t_{k-1}}, t_{k-1})\Delta t = (\mathbf{Id} + v_{k-1}\Delta t) \circ \phi_{0,t_{k-1}}, \tag{2}$$

with $\mathbf{Id}$ the identity transformation and $v_{t_k} = v(\mathbf{x}, t_k)$ the velocity field at t_k. The transformation $\phi_{0,1}$ is represented by:

$$\phi_{0,1} = \phi_{0,t_{N_f}} = (\mathbf{Id} + v_{N_f-1}\Delta t) \circ ... \circ (\mathbf{Id} + v_0\Delta t) \circ (\mathbf{x}), \tag{3}$$

it is parameterized with a series of 3D B-spline parameters $\mathbf{c}_k(k = 0, 1, ..., N_f-1)$.

For the motion estimation problem, the spatiotemporal transformation is defined by a diffeomorphism flow $\phi(\mathbf{x}, t), t \in [0, N_s], \mathbf{x} \in \Omega$ with $N_s + 1$ being the number of frames. The flow is parameterized with a velocity field $v(\mathbf{x}, t)$ which minimizes a variational energy in form of:

$$\hat{v} = arg \inf_{v \in V} \lambda \int_0^{N_s} ||v(\mathbf{x}, t)||_V^2 dt + \sum_{n=1}^{N_s} E_{SSD}(I_{n-1}(\phi_{0,n-1}), I_n(\phi_{0,n})), \tag{4}$$

with $E_{SSD}(I_{n-1}(\phi_{0,n-1}), I_n(\phi_{0,n}))$ being the SSD metric of two consecutive frames unwarped to the reference frame I_0 respectively. The use of consecutive frames to evaluate similarity metric instead of the reference frame to following frame is because the consecutive frames usually have higher correlation than faraway frames [23]. Since $\phi_{0,n} = \phi_{n-1,n} \circ \phi_{0,n-1}$, the SSD metric between the unwarped image $I_{n-1}(\phi_{0,n-1})$ and $I_n(\phi_{0,n})$ is equal to that between images $I_{n-1}(\mathbf{x})$ and $I_n(\phi_{n-1,n})$, with $\phi_{n-1,n}$ being the transformation from $(n-1)$th frame to nth frame. Then the velocity field optimizes the variational energy which consists of a regularization term and the sum of SSD metrics between the consecutive frames:

$$\hat{v} = arg \inf_{v \in V} \lambda \int_0^{N_s} ||v(\mathbf{x}, t)||_V^2 dt + \sum_{n=1}^{n=N_s} E_{SSD}(I_{n-1}(\mathbf{x}), I_n(\phi_{n-1,n})). \tag{5}$$

By this definition, the SSD energy terms are only related to the velocity field within the consecutive frames instead of global velocity field evaluation, then the derivative of the SSD energy with respect to the velocity field can be evaluated as what is done in the two image registration. But the regularization term requires the velocity field at all time points to be optimized simultaneously.

We use an adaptive scheme to select the value of N_f, the number of time steps used between two consecutive frames. It is initialized as two. The B-spline parameters during optimization is checked at each iteration to make sure that the transformation between each two time points, that is $\mathbf{Id} + \boldsymbol{v}_k \Delta t$, is a diffeomorphism [22]. If the condition is broken due to large deformation between two frames, the number of N_f will be doubled to tolerate larger deformation while keeping the transformation between time points to be diffeomorphic.

2.2   Fiber Orientation and Diffusion Tensor Image

Diffusion tensor imaging is an MRI method which measures the water molecules diffusion process along any tissue directions. In each voxel, a diffusion tensor is a 3×3 symmetrical positive definite matrix is estimated. In cardiac DTI, assuming any tensor D is decomposed into the eigenvectors and eigenvalues of $\boldsymbol{q}_i$ and d_i (with $d_1 \geq d_2 \geq d_3$), then eigenvectors $\boldsymbol{q}_i, (i = 1, 2, 3)$ correspond with the direction of myofiber, the direction perpendicular to the myofiber in the laminar sheet and the direction perpendicular to the laminar sheet respectively.

In order to map the myofiber orientation of the DTI atlas to the subject in sequences, a diffeomorphic registration need to be done from the first frame of the sequence (usually the end-diastole) to the anatomical image of the DTI. Since the anatomical image and the myofiber orientations are aligned inherently, we can transform the eigenvectors to the first frame by using the estimated nonrigid transformation. The myofiber direction for each following frame is then estimated by reorientation it using the estimated transformation from the first frame to the following frame. Tensor reorientation method we used is the finite strain algorithm since it preserves the geometrical features [24].

2.3   Anisotropic Regularization

In order to assure the $\phi(\mathbf{x}, t)$ to be diffeomorphic, we need to define $\boldsymbol{v}(\mathbf{x}, t)$ to be spatiotemporally smooth under a differential operator L. The linear operator we choose is: $L(\boldsymbol{v}) = \sum\limits_{i=1}^{3} d_i \nabla^2 (\boldsymbol{v}\boldsymbol{q}_i) + w_t \frac{d\boldsymbol{v}}{dt}$, with $\nabla^2(\cdot)$ being a Laplacian operator and w_t a constant weight. With $\boldsymbol{q}_i$ and d_i are eigenvectors and eigenvalues which can be calculated from DTI images. The first term calculate the Laplacian of the velocity field projected along the myofiber direction and across fiber. It makes the velocity field spatially more smooth along the fiber orientation than cross the fiber since d_1 is the largest value and the diffusion effect along this direction is the most salient. This is consistent with the fact that the cross-fiber thickening strain is larger than the fiber strain. The second term keeps the particle velocity temporally smooth. When $d_i = 1$ and $\boldsymbol{q}_i$ are the unit vectors, this term becomes an isotropic regularization. The overall effect of this term is to keep the velocity field spatiotemporally smooth.

In the discrete time form of velocity field, the time integral of the norm in V space of Eqn.(6) will be approximated by:

$$E_{reg} = \sum_{k=0}^{N_t-1} \sum_{\mathbf{x}} \sum_{i=1}^{3} (d_i \nabla^2 \boldsymbol{v}_k \boldsymbol{q}_i)^2 + w_t \sum_{k=1}^{N_t} \sum_{\mathbf{x}} |\boldsymbol{v}_k(\mathbf{x} + \boldsymbol{v}_{k-1}\Delta t) - \boldsymbol{v}_{k-1}|^2, \quad (6)$$

with $N_t = N_s \times N_f$ being the number of time points used for the discrete velocity field. We denote the two terms with E_{sr} and E_{tr} respectively.

2.4   Optimization

We use a steepest descent method to optimize the parameterized function. The derivative of the total energy with respect to the B-spline parameters are calculated analytically. The derivative of the similarity metric with respect to the B-spline parameters $\mathbf{c}_{i;k'}$, $((k-1) * N_f \le k' < k * N_f)$ is:

$$\frac{\partial E_{SSD}}{\partial \mathbf{c}_{i;k'}} = (I_k(\phi_{k-1,k}) - I_{k-1})\nabla I_k(\phi_{k-1,k}) \frac{\partial \phi_{k-1,k}}{\partial \mathbf{c}_{i;k'}}, \quad (7)$$

and for other value of k' the gradient is zero.

For the derivative of the spatial and temporal regularization energies with respect to the mth component of $\mathbf{c}_{i;k}$, we have:

$$\frac{\partial E_{sr}}{\partial c_{i,m;k}} = \sum_{\mathbf{x}\in\Omega'} \beta''_m(\mathbf{x} - \mathbf{x}_i) \sum_{i=1}^{3} d_i^2 q_m \boldsymbol{v}_k \boldsymbol{q}_i, \quad (8)$$

with Ω' being the local support of the B-spline kernel function, and $\beta''_m(\cdot)$ being the second derivative of the B-spline function with respect to mth component. Considering that the displacement between two time step is small, we have:

$$\frac{\partial E_{tr}}{\partial c_{i,m;k}} \approx w_t \sum_{\mathbf{x}\in\Omega'} (2 * v_{i,m;k} - v_{i,m;k-1} - v_{i,m;k+1})\beta(\mathbf{x} - \mathbf{x}_i). \quad (9)$$

3   Dataset and Experiment

We use the cine MRI sequences to validate the proposed method. The datasets we used are from the cardiac atlas project [25]. In the first experiment, four normal subject image sequences are selected to validate the motion estimation method. Typical frame size is $256 \times 256 \times 10$ with voxel size of $1mm \times 1mm \times 8mm$ and the frame number is 20. The contours of the endocardium and epicardium in the end-diastole (ED) and end-systole (ES) phases are manually labeled by experts with the temporal consistency of the boundary enforced. The two ED contours are then transformed into the ES frame by using the estimated transformation. The mean and standard deviation (STD) of the contour distance errors are evaluated. It is defined as the average of shortest distance for the points in the first contour to those in the second contour.

In the second experiment, we evaluate the accuracy by using the landmarks extracted from the tagged MRI sequences. Four normal human subjects are used in this experiment. For each subjects, one mid short axis slice of grid tagged MRI are acquired. The crossing of grid tagging in myocardium in ED and ES frames are labeled by experts and they are used as landmarks to evaluate the motion estimation method. The landmarks in the ED phase are then transformed to the ES image space and the target registration error (TRE) with the ES landmarks are evaluated. The short axis slices of the ED and ES of one subject and the corresponding tagged MRI with labeled landmarks are shown in fig.(1).

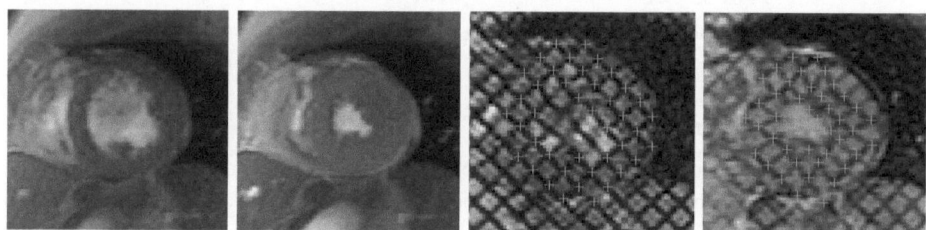

Fig. 1. Short axis slices of one subject and the tagged MRI slice with landmarks labeled with green crossing

In the third experiment, an open-chest pig heart sequence with normal condition is acquired with a Philips IE33 system. There are 26 frames and each frame is resampled into size of $137 \times 96 \times 124$ with voxel size $0.5mm^3$. For validation, we implanted six sonomicrometers in the myocardium. Sonomicrometry provides the ground truth distances between each pair of the crystals varying with time and they are compare with the algorithm-derived point pair distances. The sonomicrometers position are illustrated in fig.(2) together with the three orthogonal views of ED frame.

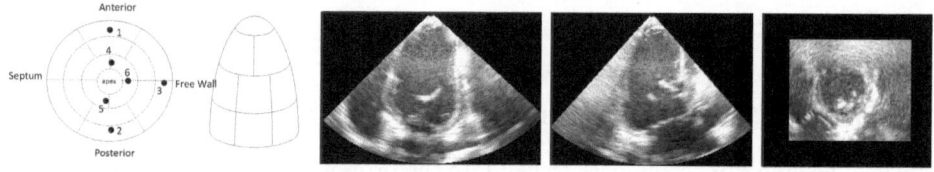

Fig. 2. The sonomicrometer location on the myocardium and the axial and sagittal views of the ED frame of the pig dataset

We compare the proposed method with a temporal diffeomorphic free-form deformation (TDFFD) method. In the TDFFD method no myofiber orientation is used while in the proposed method an anisotropic regularization term along and across myofiber is considered. The DTI is chosen as a public available statistical canine atlas [1]. The three orthogonal views of the anatomical MRI and the primary eigenvector direction are shown in Fig.(3). The similarity of the myofiber orientation between mammals makes the canine atlas a proper approximation of myofiber orientations for human and pig tests.

---

[1] http://www-sop.inria.fr/asclepios/data/heart/index.php

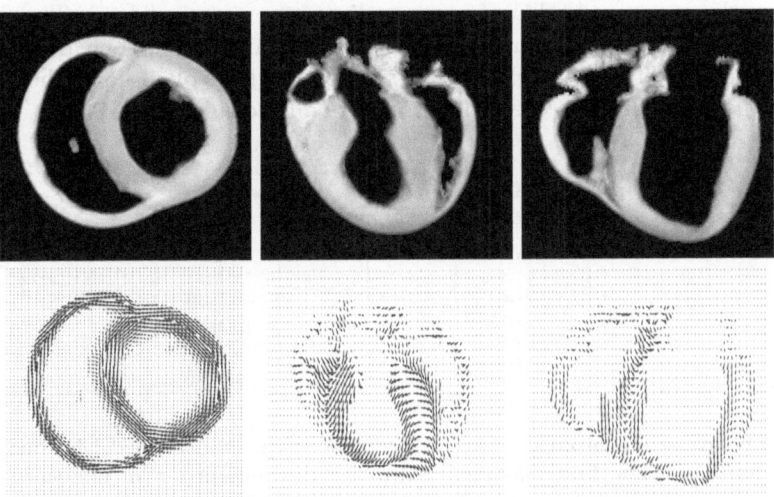

Fig. 3. The DTI canine atlas. The top row shows the three orthogonal view of the anatomical MRI. The bottom row shows the the primary eigenvector projected into the three central orthogonal planes.

4   Results

We use a series of 3D B-spline transformations with grid spacing of 10 in each spatial dimension for the velocity field. The values of λ and w_t are set to be 0.1 and 0.005. For a 3D sequence of 20 frames with frame size of $111 \times 91 \times 73$ the computing time is about 70 minutes.

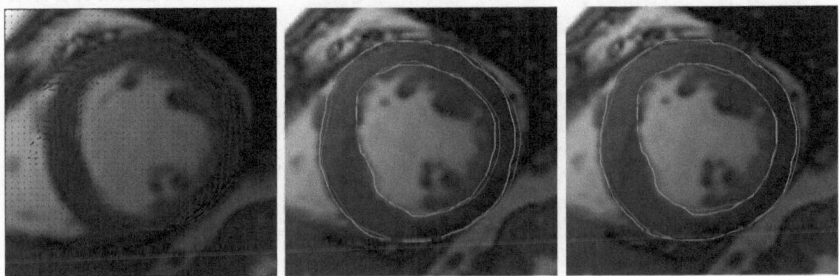

Fig. 4. From left to right, the first plot shows the nonrigid transformed myofiber direction. The second and third plots show the transformed epicardium and endocardium contours of ED (red) and those of ES(green).

We show the result of the first experiment in fig.(4). From left to right, the first image shows the nonrigid deformed myofiber orientation projected in the axial slice of the ED frame. The second and third plots show the transformed ED endocardium and epicardium contours (in red) together with ES contours (in green) by using the TDFFD method and the proposed method. We can see that both transformed ED contours are closer to the ES contours in the proposed method.

We show the mean and STD of contour distance errors in fig.(5). The first two plots show the contour distance errors of the endocardium and epicardium in apical, mid and basal slices of the first subject. The third plot shows the averaged contour distance errors in the endocardium of all the subjects.

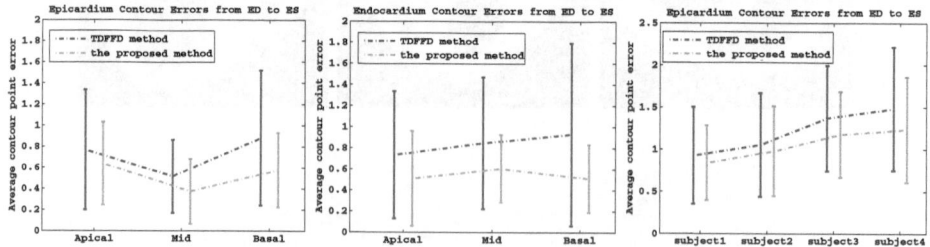

Fig. 5. The average contour distance error between the transformed ED contours and the ES contours. The first two plots show the distance errors of endocardium and epicardium in apical, mid and basal slices. The third plot shows the average errors of the endocardium of the four subjects.

The results of the tagged MRI experiment are shown in fig.(6). From left to right, the first two images shows the transformed ED landmarks (in red) with the ES landmarks (in green) in the TDFFD method and the proposed method. We can see the transformed ED landmarks are closer to ES landmark in the proposed method. The error bars show the average and STD of the TREs between the landmarks in all four subjects tests. We can see the proposed method has smaller mean and STD of TRE in all the four tests.

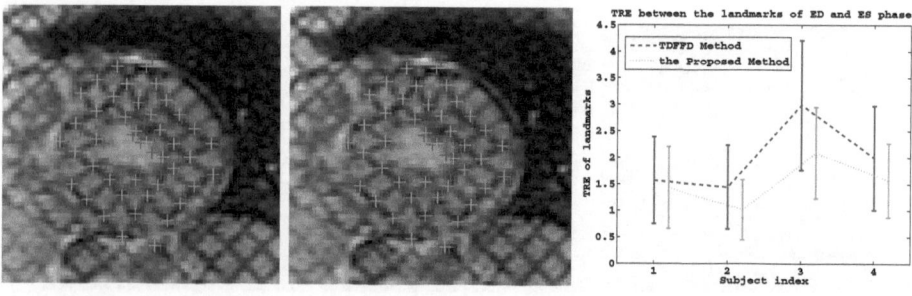

Fig. 6. Results of the tagged MRI tests. From left to right, the first two plots show the transformed ED landmarks (red) and the ES landmarks (green) in TDFFD and the proposed method. The error bar shows the mean and STD of the TRE between the landmarks in the two methods.

In the *in-vivo* open-chest pig test, we compare the performance of the two algorithms by computing the correlations between the time varying functions of algorithm-derived pair-wise distances and those of sonomicrometry, and the results are shown in table.1. We can clearly see the improvement of our proposed method.

Table 1. The correlations between the estimated pair-wise distances and those from the sonomicrometry, with TDFFD method (numbers to the left) and the proposed method (numbers to the right). Numbers 1-6 index the six sonomicrometry markers.

	1	2	3	4	5	6
1	1.0/1.0	0.875/0.910	0.784/0.836	0.861/0.888	0.912/0.941	0.915/0.943
2	0.875/0.910	1.0/1.0	0.766/0.794	0.965/0.983	0.789/0.807	0.879/0.902
3	0.784/0.836	0.766/0.794	1.0/1.0	0.952/0.975	0.867/0.899	0.947/0.975
4	0.861/0.883	0.965/0.983	0.952/0.975	1.0/1.0	0.895/0.899	0.897/0.919
5	0.912/0.941	0.789/0.807	0.867/0.899	0.895/0.899	1.0/1.0	0.784/0.828
6	0.915/0.943	0.879/0.902	0.947/0.975	0.897/0.919	0.784/0.828	1.0/1.0

5   Conclusion

We propose a diffeomorphic motion estimation method with anisotropic regularization of the velocity field. The anisotropic regularization is conducted primarily along the myofiber direction. We validate the proposed method with cine MRI and echocardiography with sonomicrometry. Experiments results show that the transformations estimated with the proposed method are more accurate and consistent with the ground truth. Currently, only canine DTI atlas is public available. In the future, we will use human DTI atlas image to improve the myofiber orientation accuracy and the motion estimation results.

Acknowledgement. This paper is supported by a NIH/NHLBI grant 1R01HL102407-01 awarded to Xubo Song and David Sahn.

References

1. Buckberg, G., Hoffman, J.I.E., Mahajan, A., Saleh, S., Coghlan, C.: Cardiac Mechanics Revisited The Relationship of Cardiac Architecture to Ventricular Function. Circulation 118, 2571–2587 (2008)
2. Elen, A., Choi, H.F., Loeckx, D., Gaom, H., Claus, P., Suetens, P., Maes, F., D'hooge, J.: Three-dimensional cardiac strain estimation using spatio-temporal elastic registration of ultrasound images: a feasibility study. IEEE Trans. Med. Imag. 27(11), 1580–1591 (2008)
3. Rougon, N., Petitjean, C., Preteux, F., Cluzel, P., Grenier, P.: A non-rigid registration approach for quantifying myocardial contraction in tagged MRI using generalized information measures. Med.l Imag. Anal. 9(4), 353–375 (2005)
4. Ledesma-Carbayo, M.J., Mah-Casado, P., Santos, A., Prez-David, E., GarMA, D.M.: Spatio-Temporal Nonrigid Registration for Ultrasound Cardiac Motion Estimation. IEEE Trans. Med. Imag. 24(9), 1113–1126 (2005)
5. Metz, C.T., Klein, S., Schaap, M., Walsum, T., Niessen, W.J.: Nonrigid registration of dynamic medical imaging data using nD+t B-splines and a groupwise optimization approach. Med. Imag. Anal. 15(2), 238–249 (2011)
6. Castillo, E., Castillo, R., Martinez, J., Shenoy, M., Guerrero, T.: Four-dimensional deformable image registration using trajectory modeling. Physics in Medicine and Biology 55(1), 305–327 (2010)
7. Sundar, H., Littb, H., Shen, D.G.: Estimating myocardial motion by 4D image warping. Pattern Recognition 42, 2514–2526 (2009)

8. Skrinjar, O., Bistoquet, A., Tagare, H.: Symmetric and Transitive Registration of Image Sequences. In: IJBI (2008)

9. Beg, M.F., Miller, M.I., Trouve, A., Younes, L.: Computing Large Deformation Metric Mappings via Geodesic Flows of Diffeomorphisms. IJCV 61(2), 139–157 (2005)

10. Vercauteren, T., Pennec, X., Perchant, A., Ayache, N.: Diffeomorphic Demons: Efficient Non-parametric Image Registration. NeuroImage 45(1,S1), 61–72 (2009)

11. Khan, A.R., Beg, M.F.: Representation of time-varying shapes in the large deformation diffeomorphic framework. In: ISBI 2008, pp. 1521–1524 (2008)

12. Craene, M.D., Piella, G., Camaraa, O., Duchateaua, N., Silvae, E., Doltrae, A., D'hooge, J., Brugadae, J., Sitgese, M., Frangi, A.F.: Temporal diffeomorphic free-form deformation: application to motion and strain estimation from 3D echocardiography. Med. Imag. Anal. 16(1), 427–450 (2012)

13. Bistoquet, A., Oshinski, J., Skrinjar, O.: Myocardial deformation recovery from cine MRI using a nearly incompressible biventricular model. Med. Imag. Anal. 12(1), 69–85 (2008)

14. Mansi, T., Pennec, X., Sermesant, M., Delingette, H., Ayache, N.: iLogDemons: A demons-based registration algorithm for tracking incompressible elastic biological tissues. International Journal of Computer Vision (IJCV) 92(1), 92–111 (2011)

15. Sengupta, P.P., Tajik, A.J., Chandrasekaran, K., Khandheria, B.K.: Twist Mechanics of the Left Ventricle. JACC 1(3), 366–376 (2008)

16. Rademakers, F.E., Rogers, W.J., Guier, W.H., Hutchins, G.M., Siu, C.O., Weisfeldt, M.L., Weiss, J.L., Shapiro, E.P.: Relation of regional cross-fiber shortening to wall thickening in the intact heart. Three-dimensional strain analysis by NMR tagging. Circulation 89(3), 1174–1182 (1994)

17. Ubbink, S.W.J., Bovendeerda, P.H.M., Delhaasb, T., Artsa, T., Vossea, F.N.: Towards model-based analysis of cardiac MR tagging data: Relation between left ventricular shear strain and myofiber orientation. Med. Imag. Anal. 10(4), 632–641 (2006)

18. Sermesant, M., Forest, C., Pennec, X., Delingette, H., Ayache, N.: Deformable biomechanical models: Application to 4D cardiac image analysis. Med. Imag. Anal. 7(4), 475–488 (2003)

19. Papademetris, X., Sinusas, A.J., Dione, D.P., Duncan, J.S.: Estimation of 3D left ventricular deformation from echocardiography. Med. Imag. Anal. 5(1), 17–28 (2001)

20. Dupuis, P., Grenander, U.: Variational problems on flows of diffeomorphisms for image matching. Quarterly Appl. Math. 56(3), 587–600 (1998)

21. Ashburner, J.: A fast diffeomorphic image registration algorithm. NeuroImage 38(1), 95–113 (2007)

22. Rueckert, D., Aljabar, P., Heckemann, R.A., Hajnal, J.V., Hammers, A.: Diffeomorphic Registration Using B-Splines. In: Larsen, R., Nielsen, M., Sporring, J. (eds.) MICCAI 2006, Part II. LNCS, vol. 4191, pp. 702–709. Springer, Heidelberg (2006)

23. Meunier, J.: Tissue motion assessment from 3D echographic speckle tracking. Phys. Med. Biol. 43, 1241–1254 (1998)

24. Peyrat, J.M., Sermesant, M., Pennec, X., Delingette, H., Xu, C.Y., McVeigh, E.R., Ayache, N.: A Computational Framework for the Statistical Analysis of Cardiac Diffusion Tensors: Application to a Small Database of Canine Hearts. IEEE Trans. Med. Imag. 26(11), 1500–1514 (2007)

25. Fonseca, C.G., Backhaus, M., Lima, J.A.C., Medrano-Gracia, P., Shivkumar, K., Suinesiaputra, A., Tao, W., Young, A.A.: The Cardiac Atlas Project C An imaging database for computational modeling and statistical atlases of the heart. Bioinformatics 27(16), 2288–2295 (2011)

Validation of DRAMMS among 12 Popular Methods in Cross-Subject Cardiac MRI Registration

Yangming Ou, Dong Hye Ye, Kilian M. Pohl, and Christos Davatzikos

Section of Biomedical Image Analysis (SBIA),
Department of Radiology, University of Pennsylvania

Abstract. Cross-subject image registration is the building block for many cardiac studies. In the literature, it is often handled by voxel-wise registration methods. However, studies are lacking to show which methods are more accurate and stable in this context. Aiming at answering this question, this paper evaluates 12 popular registration methods and validates a recently developed method DRAMMS [16] in the context of cross-subject cardiac registration. Our dataset consists of short-axis end-diastole cardiac MR images from 24 subjects, in which non-cardiac structures are removed. Each registration method was applied to all 552 image pairs. Registration accuracy is approximated by Jaccard overlap between deformed expert annotation of source image and the corresponding expert annotation of target image. This accuracy surrogate is further correlated with deformation aggressiveness, which is reflected by minimum, maximum and range of Jacobian determinants. Our study shows that DRAMMS [16] scores high in accuracy and well balances accuracy and aggressiveness in this dataset, followed by ANTs [13], MI-FFD [14], Demons [15], and ART [12]. Our findings in cross-subject cardiac registrations echo those findings in brain image registrations [7].

Keywords: Image Registration, Validation, Evaluation, Cardiac MRI.

1 Introduction

Cross-subject image registration rests in the core of many cardiac studies. Examples include atlas construction [3], atlas-based segmentation [4], and morphologic study to understand disease patterns [5].

In literature, cross-subject cardiac image registration is often handled by voxel-wise registration methods [6]. Voxel-wise registration methods rely on image information only, and do not require anatomic information or human intervention. Therefore, they can be applied to various organs including the heart [6]. Some basic question remains, however: 1) which voxel-wise registration methods are more accurate and more stable in cross-subject cardiac registration context; 2) whether those more accurate methods in cardiac registration coincide with those in brain image registrations (e.g., as found in [7]). The answers to these questions are not immediately clear, largely because the heart is usually imaged

B.M. Dawant et al. (Eds.): WBIR 2012, LNCS 7359, pp. 209–219, 2012.

with lower resolution, lower signal-to-noise ratio (SNR), more severe moving artifacts, and has a very different shape than the brain.

Towards answering these questions, this paper evaluates 12 commonly-used and publically-available registration methods and validates a recently developed method DRAMMS [16] in the context of cross-subject cardiac registrations. We have collected short-axis end-diastole magnetic resonance (MR) images of 24 subjects. By permuting source and target images, this dataset results in 552 possible pair-wise registrations for each of those 12 registration methods. The large number of experiments (perhaps largest to date in cardiac context) is **the first feature** of this study. **The second feature** of this study is the comprehensive evaluation criteria. Unlike other evaluation studies (e.g. [7]) that only measure accuracy, we measure both accuracy and aggressiveness of deformations, and visualize their relationship in a joint plot. A deformation is considered more "aggressive" if it leads to self-foldings at more locations, and if it takes greater expansions/shrinkages to capture cross-individual variations. Aggressiveness and accuracy are usually a pair of trade-off. Higher accuracy often comes from increased aggressiveness in deformation. On the other hand, too aggressive deformation will undesirably break topology. An ideal method should achieve high accuracy while accurately preserving topology. Measuring both accuracy and aggressiveness will help reveal which methods better balance the two. **The third feature** of this study is that, instead of using only one set of parameters, we have examined two parameter settings for the four more accurate methods – one more aggressive and one smoother version. This is important, because different cardiac studies will have different requirements on aggressiveness levels of deformation. It also helps reveal which methods achieve consistently high accuracy when aggressiveness levels change.

In the rest of the paper, we present evaluation protocol in Section 2 and evaluation results in Section 3. We discuss and conclude the paper in Section 4.

2   Evaluation Protocol

This section describes our evaluation protocol. It contains three parts: description of dataset (Section 2.1), brief review of registration methods included in this study (Section 2.2), and description of evaluation criteria (Section 2.3).

2.1   Dataset for Evaluation

We now describe the dataset and pre-processings. Three-dimensional short-axis cardiac MR images of 24 subjects are collected at end-diastole phase. The image dimension is $120 \times 120 \times 12$ and voxel size is $1.25 \times 1.25 \times 8.0 mm^3$. Common pre-processing steps include respiratory motion correction [19] and N3-based bias field correction [20]. Non-cardiac structures are removed by a semi-automatic process. In this process, the heart is first automatically outlined by a public software "Segment" [18]. Then, a cardiovascular expert refined the separation of cardiac and non-cardiac structures. Removal of non-cardiac structures is similar to skull-stripping in brain image registrations. The purpose is to remove

a) Images

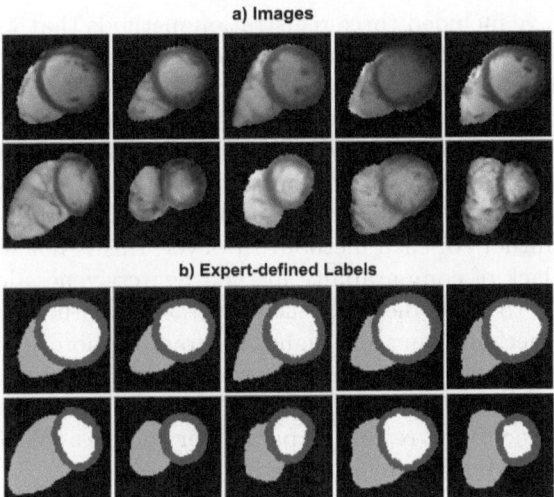

b) Expert-defined Labels

Fig. 1. Images (a) and expert-annotation of structures (b) for some 10 typical subjects from the dataset used in this study. Subjects in the first row in (a) are healthy controls and in the second row are with tetralogy-of-fallot (TOF) defect. In the expert annotation, white, orange and blue regions are LV, RV and myocardium, respectively.

unnecessary challenges, especially when different images may contain different non-cardiac structures due to different fields of view. Each cardiac image is further annotated by the same cardiologist into three structures – left ventricle (LV), right ventricle (RV) and myocardium. Some typical intensity images and expert-annotation images are shown in Fig. 1. We note that, except for removing non-cardiac structures, those expert annotations of LV/RV/myocardium are in no means used as any part of the registration process. They are only used to evaluate registration accuracy.

This dataset represents the common challenges in cardiac registrations – lower resolution, lower SNR, more severe moving artifacts and quite different shape from the brain. Besides, 11 out of 24 subjects have tetralogy-of-fallot (TOF) defect, hence having irregular ventricle shapes largely different from the remaining 13 normal subjects (Fig. 1).

2.2 Registration Methods to Be Evaluated

A total of 12 widely-used and publically-available methods are included in this study (Table 1). We note that they are only a small fraction of the vast number of registration methods developed in the community. The pool can be always expanded in the future to include other widely-acknowledged methods. In general, we chose those 12 methods because of the wide variety they represent. That is, they have different similarity measures, different deformation models and different optimization strategies, which are the most important components for registration algorithms (see Table 1). Out of those 12 registration methods, 9 methods were included in a recent brain registration evaluation study [7].

In addition, we have included three registration methods that were not included in that brain study [7]. Those three methods are: Demons [15] (a widely-used, ITK-based, public and fast software), DRAMMS [16] (our method that matches images by voxel-wise texture attributes instead of intensities), and DROP [17] (a novel discrete optimization strategy that is fast and accurate).

To encourage objectivity in evaluation, we need to take special care of parameters for different methods. In some previous evaluation studies [7,8], parameters are provided by authors of each method. However, this is not without problem. One issue is the lack of comparability in their aggressiveness levels, and hence possible unfairness to those methods that generate smoother deformations. Actually, almost all methods can score higher accuracy at more aggressive deformations. Ideally, we should require similar aggressiveness level for all methods, and then compare their accuracies. A second issue is the lack of information about sensitivity of accuracy with regard to parameter changes. With only one set of best parameters, it is hard to tell sensitivity.

To cope with those two issues and to promote objectivity, we set parameters by the following two rules. To settle the first issue, we tune parameters not just for best accuracy, but for best accuracy at similar aggressiveness level. Specifically, we start from parameters in a method's user manual or past papers. In each iteration, we keep other methods' parameters fixed, and slightly adjust one method's parameters until its deformations are at similar level with most other methods (few or no self-foldings, similar min, max and range of Jacobian determinants). We iterate on every method until they all converge to similar aggressiveness level. This provides common ground for more objectively evaluating their accuracies. To settle the second issue, we provide two sets of parameters, instead of only one most accurate set, for the four most accurate methods. One aggressive set for generally higher accuracy but increased risk of self-folding; and one smooth set for generally smoother deformation but lower

Table 1. Registration methods to be evaluated in this paper (diff.–diffeomorphism; MI – mutual information; NMI – normalized MI; SSD – sum of squared difference; SAD – sum of absolute difference; MSD – mean squared difference; CC – correlation coefficient; NCC – normalized CC)

Method	Deformation Model	Similarity	Regularization
flirt [9]	affine	SSD/(N)MI/CC	–
fnirt [10]	cubic B-spline	SSD	bending energy
AIR [11]	5th polynomial	MSD	by polynomial
ANTs [13]	symmetric diff.	CC	Gaussian smoothing
ART [12]	homeomorphism	NCC	Gaussian smoothing
CC-FFD [14]	cubic B-spline	CC	bending energy
MI-FFD [14]	cubic B-spline	MI	bending energy
SSD-FFD [14]	cubic B-spline	SSD	bending energy
DROP [17]	cubic B-spline	SAD	bending energy
Demons [15]	optical flow	SSD	Gaussian smoothing
Diff. Demons [15]	diff. optical flow	SSD	Gaussian smoothing
DRAMMS [16]	cubic B-spline	SSD of attributes	bending energy

accuracy. This reveals consistency of accuracy as parameters change. All parameters used in this paper can be found at http://www.seas.upenn.edu/ ouya/ documents/research/Ou12_WBIR_Supplementary.pdf.

To avoid bias in template selection, we have considered all possible images as source and target in registration. This results in a total of 552 (= 24 × 23) possible pair-wise registrations for each registration method.

2.3 Evaluation Criteria

This sub-section presents the criteria for evaluating both deformation accuracy and aggressiveness. Specifically, accuracy is implied by Jaccard Overlap between deformed expert-annotation of source image and the expert-annotation of target image. We measure overlaps in 3 regions: LV, RV, and myocardium. Larger overlap often indicates greater spatial alignment between subjects [7,21].

A deformation is considered more "aggressive" if it has self-foldings at more locations, and if it takes greater expansions/shrinkages to capture cross-individual variability. In measuring deformation aggressiveness, we have used Jacobian determinants. Jacobian determinant measures voxel-wise volumetric change ratio. It is > 1 for expansion, between 0 and 1 for shrinkage and < 0 if self-folding occurs. In particular, we measure 4 Jacobian-based metrics: 1) the number of deformations having negative Jacobian determinants; 2) the percentage of voxels having negative Jacobian determinants; 3) minimum and 4) maximum Jacobian determinants in a deformation. Finally, we use one metric, the range of Jacobian determinants (=maxJac-minJac), to quantify deformation aggressiveness.

For fairness, we used a standard ITK calculator to compute Jacobians of deformation. This requires converting deformation files from different software into a standard ITK-compatible MetaImage format. We carefully checked to assure the conversion reproduces the same exact warped images.

3   Results and Observations

We now present evaluation results (accuracy, aggressiveness, and their correlation) in this section. Observations follow each set of results. Average computational time of each method is listed in Appendix of this paper.

3.1   Deformation Accuracy Indicated by Jaccard Overlap is shown in Fig. 2 for myocardium, LV and RV. Several observations can be made:

a) in general, voxel-wise registration methods evaluated in this paper have obtained 0.6-0.9 Jaccard (roughly 0.75-0.95 Dice) overlap in left and right ventricles, and 0.4-0.7 Jaccard (roughly 0.55-0.85 Dice) overlap in myocardium.

b) DRAMMS scores highest Jaccard overlap in all three structures in this dataset – average 0.85 Jaccard (0.9 Dice) in LV and RV, 0.7 Jaccard (0.8 Dice) in myocardium. The margin is bigger in myocardium regions. A plausible explanation is that DRAMMS uses texture attributes other than solely intensity information to define similarity at each voxel.

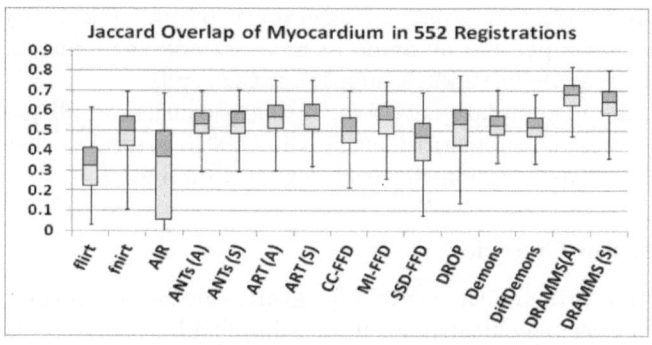

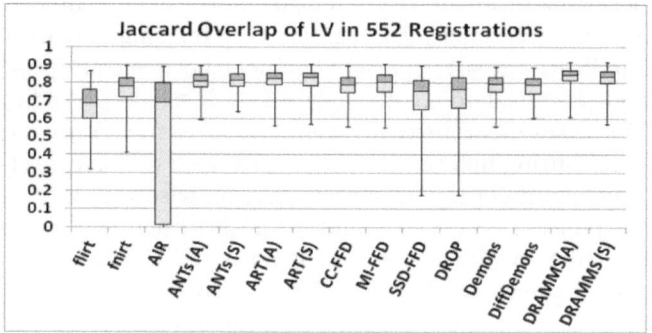

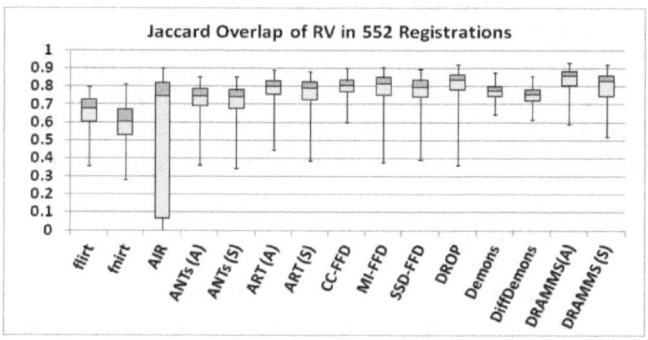

Fig. 2. Box-and-Whisker plots: accuracy indicated by Jaccard overlap in 3 expert-annotated structures. From top to bottom, results for myocardium, LV and RV regions. Letter "A" stands for aggressive version and "S" for smooth version of a method.

c) ANTs, MI-FFD, Demons, and ART also obtained high overlaps in this cardiac dataset. This echoes findings in brain registration evaluation study [7].

d) Methods using intensity differences (SSD) as similarity metric have reasonable Jaccard overlap on average. However, they have larger variations, and suffer in difficult cases. This shows that SSD metric is less likely to consistently capture large anatomical variations. One solution is to combine intensity difference with deformation mechanism of more degrees of freedom (like in ART and Demons).

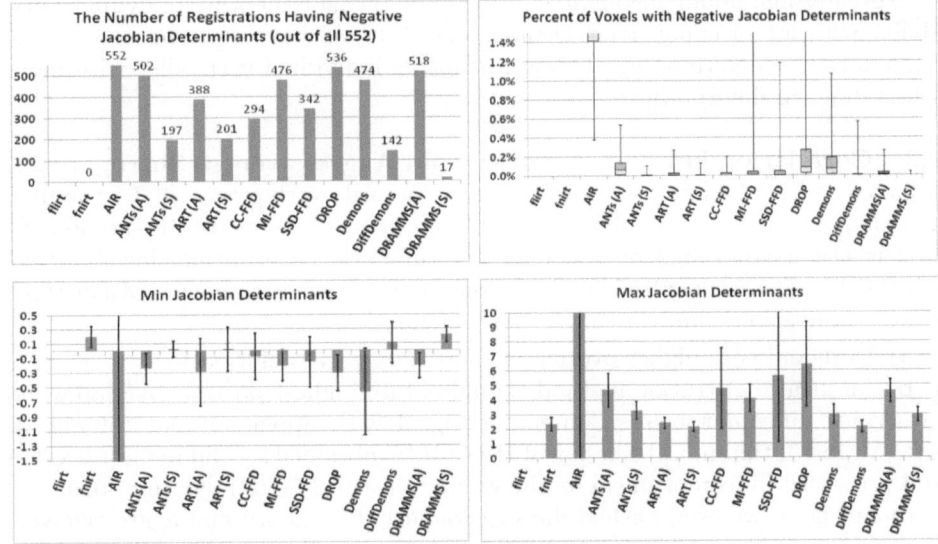

Fig. 3. Jacobian-based metrics to indicate deformation aggressiveness. Upper left: number of deformations (out of all 552) that have negative Jacobian determinants; Upper right: box-and-whisker plot of percentage of voxels having negative Jacobian determinants in a deformation; Lower row: min (left) and max (right) Jacobian determinants.

A perhaps better solution is to replace it with more robust similarity metric, such as correlation (like in ANTs), mutual information (like in MI-FFD), or attribute-based similarity (like in DRAMMS).

3.2   Deformation Aggressiveness is indicated by the four sets of results shown in Fig. 3. From left to right, top to bottom, they are: number of deformations with negative Jacobian determinants; percent of voxels having negative Jacobian determinants; minimum and maximum Jacobian determinants in deformations. We observe the following from those results:

a) From the top row in Fig. 3, fnirt is the only non-rigid registration method that guarantees diffeomorphism in this dataset. Diffeomorphism means no existence of negative Jacobian determinants (i.e. no self-folding) in deformations. It is a nice property that preserves topology and one-to-one forward and backward correspondences. fnirt guarantees diffeomorphism by directly checking and removing negativity in Jacobian map. However, this is at the cost of overlap-indicated registration accuracy, as reflected in Fig. 2. Actually, whether cross-subject deformation is a diffeomorphism is an unknown matter, especially when there are large anatomic variations.

b) DRAMMS(A), ANTs(A), MI-FFD, Demons and ART(A) scored higher overlap in Fig. 2. Interestingly, results in lower row of Fig. 3 show they have quite different deformation styles. In particular, DRAMMS(A), ANTs(A) and MI-FFD have greater maximum Jacobian determinants, trying to capture individual variability with larger expansions. Demons and ART(A) have more negative minimum Jacobian determinants, trying to capture individual variability with more self-foldings in deformations.

3.3   Correlation between Accuracy and Aggressiveness Surrogates is depicted in Fig. 4. Here y-axis is the mean Jaccard overlap over all 3 structures and all 552 registrations, indicating overall accuracy of a registration method. X-axis is the mean range of Jacobian determinants (=mean(maxJacobianDet-minJacobianDet)) over all 552 registrations, indicating aggressiveness of a method. Three observations can be made from this figure:

a) Methods score higher overlap at more aggressive deformations.

b) An ideal registration method should obtain highest possible overlap while preserving diffeomorphism. Combining Fig. 4 with upper left part of Fig. 3, DRAMMS(S), the smooth version of DRAMMS, obtained second highest overlap and preserved diffeomorphism in almost all but 3% (17/552) deformations.

c) In Fig. 4, we used dashed lines to connect the smooth and aggressive versions of four top-ranking methods. As a result, we observe that DRAMMS is general high in accuracy. More importantly, it has greater increase when going from smooth to aggressive version. It therefore offers wider range of choices for varying needs. That is, the aggressive version, DRAMMS(A), seems a good choice for single-/multi-atlas-based segmentation, where overlap is the focus. The smoother version, DRAMMS(S), is perhaps a better choice for finding common disease pattern in a population, where the key is to maximum possibly remove global difference and meanwhile preserve disease-induced individual variability.

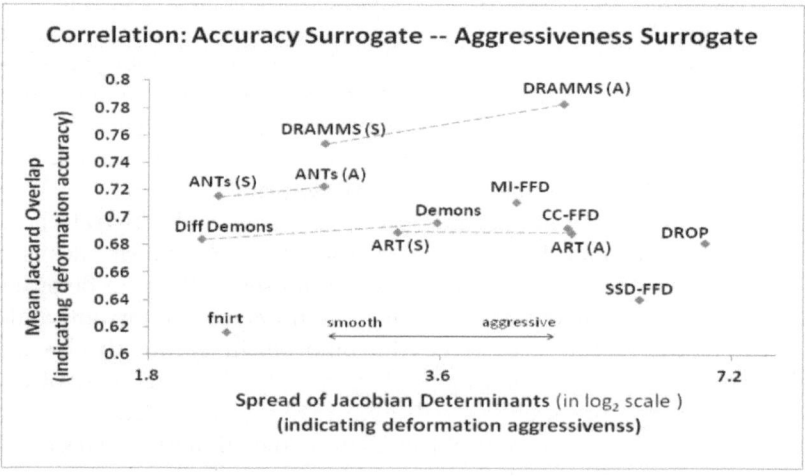

Fig. 4. Correlation between accuracy and aggressiveness surrogates. Letter "A" stands for aggressive and "S" for smooth versions for some methods.

4 Discussion

This paper evaluates 12 voxel-wise registration methods within the context of cross-subject cardiac registrations in a dataset of 24 subjects. Results show that those top-ranking registration methods – DRAMMS, ANTs, MI-FFD, Demons, ART – obtained average Jaccard overlap of 0.7-0.9 (i.e. Dice of 0.82-0.95) in left and right ventricles, and 0.5-0.7 (i.e., Dice of 0.66-0.82) in myocardium. In the following, we will discuss those important aspects of the paper.

Objectivity is a critical issue. In our study, it is encouraged by looking at accuracies when most methods are at similar aggressiveness levels. Deformation accuracy and aggressiveness are often a pair of trade-off. Reporting both and correlating them are a more comprehensive set of criteria than purely accuracy criterion. Their results (Figs. 2,3) and their correlation (Fig. 4) show that the smooth version of DRAMMS achieves best balance – high overlap and maximum preservation of diffeomorphism. ANTs, MI-FFD, Demons and ART also perform well in this cardiac dataset. This echoes findings in brain registration study [7].

On the note of similarity metrics, intensity difference is less stable than correlation (like in ANTs), mutual-information (like in MI-FFD) or attribute-based similarity (like in DRAMMS). On transformation models, different behaviors are observed. Transformation models behind DRAMMS, ANTs and MI-FFD tend to capture individual variability by larger deformation expansions and less severe self-foldings. Models behind Demons and ART tend to behave reversely.

One surprising observation is regarding diffeomorphism. fnirt is the only one that guarantees diffeomorphism in this dataset, as it directly checks and removes negative Jacobian determinants. Non-diffeomorphism occurs for many methods, although some were theoretically designed diffeomorphic. Numerical issues might be one reason. Or, perhaps the process of deforming subjects with large anatomical variability itself is not completely diffeomorphic in nature.

Future work includes additional validations that consist of additional registration methods, cardiac datasets, and accuracy surrogates like surface distance.

Acknowledgement. The project described was supported in part by Grant UL1RR024134 from the National Center for Research Resources, and in part by the Institute for Translational Medicine and Therapeutics (ITMAT) Transdisciplinary Awards Program at the University of Pennsylvania. We thank Dr. Litt Harold, from Cardiovascular Imaging Section of Hospital of the University of Pennsylvania, for annotating cardiac structures that serve as ground truth for our evaluation.

References

1. Chandrashekara, R., Rao, A., Sanchez-Ortiz, G.I., Mohiaddin, R.H., Rueckert, D.: Construction of a Statistical Model for Cardiac Motion Analysis Using Nonrigid Image Registration. In: Taylor, C.J., Noble, J.A. (eds.) IPMI 2003. LNCS, vol. 2732, pp. 599–610. Springer, Heidelberg (2003)

2. Isola, A., Grass, M., Niessen, W.J.: Fully automatic nonrigid registration-based local motion estimation for motion-corrected iterative cardiac CT reconstruction. Med. Phy., 1093–1109 (2010)
3. Perperidis, D., Mohiaddin, R., Rueckert, D.: Spatio-temporal free-form registration of cardiac MR image sequences. MedIA 9, 441–456 (2005)
4. Zhuang, X., Rhode, K.S., Razavi, R.S., Hawkes, D.J., Ourselin, S.: A Registration-Based Propagation Framework for Automatic Whole Heart Segmentation of Cardiac MRI. TMI, 1612–1625 (2010)
5. Ye, D.H., Litt, H., Davatzikos, C., Pohl, K.M.: Morphological Classification: Application to Cardiac MRI of Tetralogy of Fallot. In: Metaxas, D.N., Axel, L. (eds.) FIMH 2011. LNCS, vol. 6666, pp. 180–187. Springer, Heidelberg (2011)
6. Makela, T., Clarysse, P., Sipila, O., Pauna, N., Pham, Q., Katila, T., Magnin, I.E., Axis, L.L.: A review of cardiac image registration methods. TMI 21, 1011–1021 (2002)
7. Klein, A., et al.: Evaluation of 14 nonlinear deformation algorithms applied to human brain MRI registration. NeuroImage 46, 786–802 (2009)
8. Murphy, K., van Ginneken, B., Reinhardt, J.M., et al.: Evaluation of Registration Methods on Thoracic CT: The EMPIRE10 Challenge. TMI 30, 1901–1920 (2011)
9. Jenkinson, M., Smith, S.: A global optimisation method for robust affine registration of brain images. MedIA 5(2), 143–156 (2001)
10. Andersson, J., Smith, S., Jenkinson, M.: FNIRT–FMRIB's non-linear image registration tool. Human Brain Mapping (2008)
11. Woods, R., Grafton, S., Holmes, C., Cherry, S., Mazziotta, J.: Automated image registration: I. general methods and intrasubject intramodality validation. JCAT, 139–152 (1998)
12. Ardekani, B., Guckemus, S., Bachman, A., Hoptman, M.J., Wojtaszek, M., Nierenberg, J.: Quantitative comparison of algorithms for inter-subject registration of 3D volumetric brain MRI scans. J. Neu. Methods. 142, 67–76 (2005)
13. Avants, B., Epstein, C.L., Grossman, M., Gee, J.C.: Symmetric diffeomorphic image registration with cross-correlation: evaluating automated labeling of elderly and neurodegenerative brain. MedIA 12, 26–41 (2008)
14. Rueckert, D., Sonoda, L.I., Hayes, C., Hill, D.L.G., Leach, M.O., Hawkes, D.J.: Nonrigid registration using free-form deformations: application to breast MR images. TMI 18, 712–721 (1999)
15. Vercauteren, T., Pennec, X., Perchant, A., Ayache, N.: Diffeomorphic demons: Efficient nonparametric image registration. NeuroImage 45(1), 61–72 (2009)
16. Ou, Y., Sotiras, A., Paragios, N., Davatzikos, C.: DRAMMS: Deformable Registration via Attribute Matching and Mutual-Saliency Weighting. MedIA, 622–639 (2011)
17. Glocker, B., Komodakis, N., Tziritas, G., Navab, N., Paragios, N.: Dense image registration through MRFs and efficient linear programming. MedIA, 731–741 (2008)
18. Heiberg, E., Sjogren, J., Ugander, M., Carlsson, M., Engblom, H., Arheden, H.: Design and Validation of Segment - a Freely Available Software for Cardiovascular Image Analysis. BMC Medical Imaging 10, 1 (2010)
19. Zhang, H., Wahle, A., Johnson, R., Scholz, T., Sonka, M.: 4D Cardiac MR Image Analysis: Left and Right Ventricular Morphology and Function. TMI, 350–364 (2010)
20. Sled, J.G., Zijdenbos, A.P., Evans, A.C.: A nonparametric method for automatic correction of intensity nonuniformity in MRI data. TMI 17(1), 87–97 (1998)

21. Christensen, G.E., Geng, X., Kuhl, J.G., Bruss, J., Grabowski, T.J., Pirwani, I.A., Vannier, M.W., Allen, J.S., Damasio, H.: Introduction to the Non-rigid Image Registration Evaluation Project (NIREP). In: Pluim, J.P.W., Likar, B., Gerritsen, F.A. (eds.) WBIR 2006. LNCS, vol. 4057, pp. 128–135. Springer, Heidelberg (2006)

Appendix: Computational Time

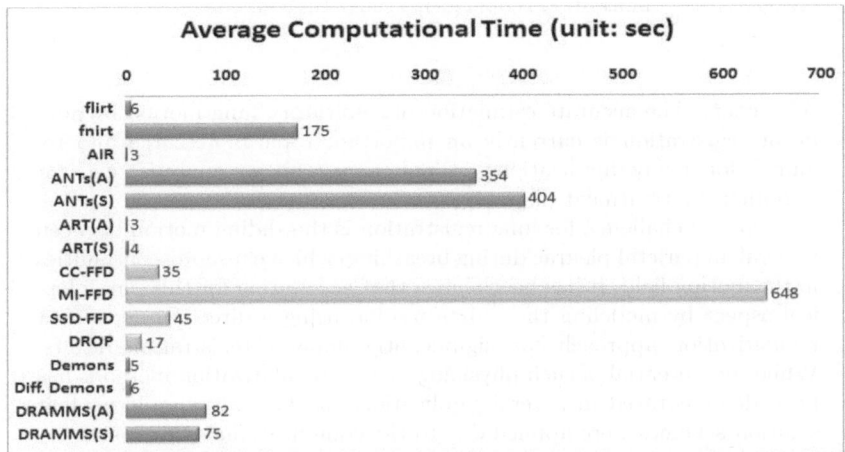

Fig. 5. Average computation time to register a pair of cardiac images in our dataset ($120 \times 120 \times 12 voxels$, $1.25 \times 1.25 \times 8.0 mm^3/voxel$). Blue bars are times in Linux centOS-5 Operating System, Xeon 2.80GHz CPU, 48GB memory. Green bars are times in Windows 7 Operating System, Intel i7 2.93GHz CPU, 4GB memory.

Fast Explicit Diffusion for Registration with Direction-Dependent Regularization

Alexander Schmidt-Richberg, Jan Ehrhardt, René Werner, and Heinz Handels

Institute of Medical Informatics, University of Lübeck, Lübeck, Germany
schmidt-richberg@imi.uni-luebeck.de

Abstract. The accurate estimation of respiratory lung motion by non-linear registration is currently an important topic of research and required for many applications in pulmonary image analysis, e.g. for radiotherapy treatment planning.

A special challenge for lung registration is the sliding motion between visceral an parietal pleurae during breathing, which causes discontinuities in the motion field. It has been shown that accounting for this physiological aspect by modeling the sliding motion using a direction-dependent regularization approach can significantly improve registration results. While the potential of such physiology-based regularization methods has been demonstrated in several publications, so far only simple explicit solution schemes were applied due to the computational complexity.

In this paper, a numerical solution of the direction-dependent regularization based on *Fast Explicit Diffusion* (FED) is presented. The approach is tested for motion estimation on 23 thoracic CT images and a significant improvement over the classic explicit solution is shown.

1 Introduction

Many clinical procedures and applications require a precise quantification of the anatomical motion of organs, for example to reduce motion-induced errors in treatment planning and intervention. Motion estimation is most commonly done by non-linear registration of two or more 3D images, each representing the anatomy at a different point of time. However, registration is challenging when two organs slide along each other causing discontinuous motion. Applied regularization schemes usually aim at avoiding such discontinuities, which entails incorrect registration results at the object boundaries. In particular, this problem arises for the estimation of lung motion where visceral and parietal pleurae slide along each other during the respiratory cycle.

Focusing on this application, many publications show that accounting for sliding motion can significantly improve registration accuracy and plausibility of the estimated motion fields [2,6,8,9,11]. In a straight-forward manner, this can be done by constraining the registration to the inside of the organ using binary lung masks [6,14]. Since this does neither model the exact physiological process nor allow a motion estimation on the whole image domain, many approaches for directly incorporating sliding motion in the regularization approach have

B.M. Dawant et al. (Eds.): WBIR 2012, LNCS 7359, pp. 220–228, 2012.

recently been presented. Nagel and Enkelmann [7] first proposed an image-driven regularizer for smoothing fields along strong edges but not across them. Based on a Helmholtz-Hodge decomposition of the motion field, Ruan et al. [10] propose to penalize only small shear values caused by noise. In Schmidt-Richberg et al. [11], a *direction-dependent regularization* (DDR) is formulated by splitting motion vectors at the object border (i.e. the area in which sliding motion potentially occurs) into normal- and tangential-directed motion and smoothing only the normal-directed part across the boundary. This idea was later adopted in other works, for example in Pace et al. [8] to formulate the problem as an anisotropic diffusion or in Delmon et al. [2] for a spline-based regularization. Risser et al. [9] applied a direction-dependent regularization within a diffeomorphic registration framework. While these approaches show very promising results, they usually suffer from the fact that simple explicit solution schemes with severe restrictions to the time step size are utilized. Advanced, for example semi-implicit schemes like *Additive Operator Splitting* (AOS) cannot be easily applied because they require solving large and non-trivial linear systems of equations. However, a *Fast Explicit Diffusion* (FED) scheme was recently presented by Grewenig et al. [4], in which cycles of explicit solution steps with varying step sizes lead to faster convergence and potentially better results.

In this work, we apply a FED solution scheme to registration with direction-dependent regularization and show its potential for improving both computation time and registration accuracy.

2 Methods

Let $R, T : \Omega \mapsto \mathbb{R}$ be two 3D images (i.e. time frames) of a 4D data set, called reference image $R(\boldsymbol{x})$ and template image $T(\boldsymbol{x})$ with the image domain $\Omega \subset \mathbb{R}^3$ and $\boldsymbol{x} = (x, y, z)^T \in \Omega$. Registration can be formulated as the task of finding a "plausible" displacement field $\boldsymbol{u} : \Omega \mapsto \mathbb{R}$ that transforms the template image to the domain of the reference image by minimizing the energy functional

$$\mathcal{J}[\boldsymbol{u}] := \mathcal{D}[R, T; \boldsymbol{u}] + \alpha \mathcal{S}[\boldsymbol{u}] . \tag{1}$$

Here, $\mathcal{D}$ is a distance measure quantifying the (dis-)similarity between reference and transformed template image. The plausibility of the motion field is controlled by the regularizer $\mathcal{S}$ with weighting parameter α, which smooths the field and thereby avoids discontinuities like gaps or foldings. A common choice is the diffusion regularization

$$\mathcal{S}^{Diff}[\boldsymbol{u}] := \frac{1}{2} \sum_{l=1}^{3} \int_{\Omega} \|\nabla u_l(\boldsymbol{x})\|^2 \, d\boldsymbol{x} , \tag{2}$$

where u_l is the l-th component of $\boldsymbol{u}$. This regularization can be expressed by the evolution equation

$$\partial_t \boldsymbol{u} = \Delta \boldsymbol{u} . \tag{3}$$

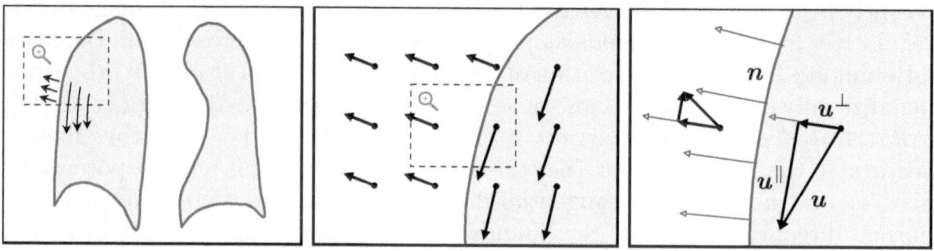

Fig. 1. In the center image the motion field along the border of the lung is visualized. This is not smooth according to a diffusion regularization. By decoupling $u^\perp$ and $u^\parallel$ we can demand the field to be smooth only in normal direction (right) [11].

However, a homogeneous smoothing contradicts physiology in the case of sliding objects and results in incorrect motion fields. This problem is addressed by direction-dependent regularization (DDR).

In the following section, DDR is briefly introduced. Its numerical stability in comparison to (anisotropic) diffusion its examined in section 2.2. Then, an overview of Fast Explicit Diffusion is given and it is applied to DDR in section 2.3.

2.1   Registration with Directional-Dependent Regularization

Registration with direction-dependent regularization was proposed in [11]. It is based on the common diffusion regularization and requires a segmentation of the object $\Gamma \subset \Omega$ that is supposed to slide along its surrounding tissue. The basic idea is to restrict regularization along the organ surface to the inside of the object (and simultaneously, the background) while maintaining smooth motion across the surface to avoid gaps or folding. This idea is illustrated in Fig. 1.

Let $n(x)$ be the normal vector on the segmentation at a point $x \in \Omega$. Without limiting the generality, we calculate it by $n = \nabla\phi/\|\nabla\phi\|$ with ϕ denoting the distance transformation of the segmentation. We proceed by splitting the motion field in two parts: the normal-directed part $u^\perp(x) = \langle u(x), n(x)\rangle n(x)$ on the one hand and the tangential-directed part $u^\parallel(x) = u(x) - \langle u(x), n(x)\rangle n(x)$ on the other hand. According to the assumptions, comprehensive (i.e. inter-object) smoothing is performed only in normal direction while object and background are smoothed separately in tangential direction. Assuming ∇n to be small, equation (2) can then be reformulated to

$$\mathcal{S}^{Diff}[u] := \frac{1}{2}\sum_{l=1}^{3}\left(\int_\Omega \|\nabla u_l^\perp\|^2 dx + \int_\Gamma \|\nabla u_l^\parallel\|^2\, dx + \int_{\Omega/\Gamma} \|\nabla u_l^\parallel\|^2\, dx\right)\ . \quad (4)$$

In this continuous formulation, equations (2) and (4) are equivalent but differences will occur in the discretization introducing Neumann boundary conditions.

In a second step, a weighting between the proposed regularization (4) and the common diffusive term (2) is included to restrict the calculation of the direction-dependent term to the region close to the object boundaries. This is mainly done because normals are only known in this region but it also entails a computational benefit. We use a continuous weighting function δ, which approximates the Dirac delta function and is 1 at the boundary of Γ and 0 elsewhere. This leads to the final energy term

$$\mathcal{S}^{DDR}[\boldsymbol{u}] := \frac{1}{2} \sum_{l=1}^{3} \left(\int_{\Omega} \delta \, \|\nabla u_l^{\perp}\|^2 + (1 - \delta) \, \|\nabla u_l\|^2 \, d\boldsymbol{x} \right.$$

$$\left. + \int_{\Gamma} \delta \, \|\nabla u_l^{\|}\|^2 \, d\boldsymbol{x} \ + \int_{\Omega/\Gamma} \delta \, \|\nabla u_l^{\|}\|^2 \, d\boldsymbol{x} \right) . \tag{5}$$

Minimizing this energy leads to the diffusion equation

$$\partial_t \boldsymbol{u} = \nabla \delta \nabla \boldsymbol{u}^{\perp} + \nabla (1 - \delta) \nabla \boldsymbol{u} + \overline{\nabla} \delta \overline{\nabla} \boldsymbol{u}^{\|} , \tag{6}$$

where $\overline{\nabla}$ implies that the gradient is calculated using Neumann boundary conditions at the borders of Γ.

2.2   Explicit Solution Schemes and Numerical Stability

To analyze the impact of using direction-dependent regularization on the numerical properties of the solution scheme, a stable step size τ_{max} is derived in the following.

For simplification, a discretized version of the one-dimensional the diffusion equation (3) is regarded:

$$U^{k+1} = (I + \tau A) U^k \tag{7}$$

This formulation can be adapted to the d-dimensional case by defining $A := \sum_{l=1}^{d} A_l$, where A_l corresponds to the derivatives along the lth coordinate axis and $U := (U_x^T, U_y^T, U_z^T)^T$ is a vector holding all entries of the displacement field component-wise.

The scheme (7) is stable if all Eigenvalues of the matrix $(I + \tau A)$ lie in the interval $[-1, 1]$. Therefore, the maximal eigenvalue λ_{max} of the matrix A is estimated in the following and a step size $\tau \leq \tau_{max}$ chosen such that this condition is satisfied.

Diffusion. First, the standard diffusion equation (3) is regarded. The matrix $A = A^{\triangle} = (a_{ij})$ is a discretization of the Laplace operator and writes

$$a_{ij} = \begin{cases} \frac{1}{h^2} & j \in \{i - 1, i + 1\}, \\ -\frac{2}{h^2} & j = i, \\ 0 & \text{else} \end{cases} .$$

Following the Gershgorin circle theorem, all eigenvalues λ_i of a square matrix $M = (m_{ij})$ lie in *discs* with the radius $r_i := \sum_{j \neq i} m_{ij}$ and the center $c_i := m_{ii}$ [4]. Therefore, we find for the matrix A that $\lambda_{max} \in [c_i - r_i, c_i + r_i] = [-\frac{4}{h^2}, 0]$. Accordingly, a step size $\tau_{max} = \frac{h^2}{2}$ has to be chosen to maintain numerical stability.

Anisotropic Diffusion. Before regarding the direction-dependent regularization, the anisotropic diffusion equation $\partial_t u = \nabla \delta \nabla u$ with a diffusivity map δ is considered [13]. The matrix $A = A^\delta = (a^\delta_{ij})$ then holds the entries

$$
a^\delta_{ij} = \begin{cases} \frac{\delta_i + \delta_j}{2h^2} & j \in \{i-1, i+1\}, \\ -\frac{\delta_{i-1} + 2\delta_i + \delta_{i+1}}{2h^2} & j = i, \\ 0 & \text{else} \end{cases} ,
$$

leading to $c_i = -r_i = -\frac{\delta_{i-1} + 2\delta_i + \delta_{i+1}}{2h^2}$. Since $\delta \in [0,1]$, the step size $\tau_{max} = \frac{h^2}{2}$ is still applicable to maintain numerical stability.

Direction-Dependent Regularization. For the direction-dependent regularization (6) the matrix $A = A^\rightleftharpoons$ can be written as

$$
\begin{aligned}
A^\rightleftharpoons U &= A^\delta U^\perp + A^{1-\delta} U + \bar{A}^\delta U^\| \\
&= A^\delta N U + A^{1-\delta} U + \bar{A}^\delta (I - N) U \\
&= \left(A^\delta N + A^{1-\delta} + \bar{A}^\delta (I - N) \right) U
\end{aligned}
\tag{8}
$$

with

$$
N := \begin{pmatrix} N_{xx} & N_{xy} & N_{xz} \\ N_{xy} & N_{yy} & N_{yz} \\ N_{xz} & N_{yz} & N_{zz} \end{pmatrix} ,
$$

and N_{xy} being diagonal matrices holding the product $n_x n_y$ in the main diagonal. The matrix $\bar{A}^\delta$ resembles A^δ but features Neumann boundary conditions at the object borders. If these matrices were equal (i.e. if there is no sliding object in the image domain), the first and third term in (8) would sum up to the anisotropic diffusion matrix A^δ and together with the second term, $A^\rightleftharpoons$ would be equal to $A^\triangle$.

After some calculations, we find in agreement with the previous observations that for rows without voxels corresponding to an object boundary $\lambda_i \in [-\frac{4}{h^2}, 0]$ still holds. However, for rows featuring Neumann boundary conditions and again assuming ∇n to be small, we get $c_i = -\frac{2}{h^2} - (1 - n^2_{x_d})(a^\delta_{i,i-1} - a^\delta_{i,i+1})$ and $r_i = \frac{2}{h^2} + (1 - n^2_{x_d})(a^\delta_{i,i-1} - a^\delta_{i,i+1})$ with $x_d \in \{x, y, z\}$. We know that $(1 - n^2_{x_d}) \in [0,1]$ and it will be small in most places because the normal is orthogonal to the object boundary. While also $(a^\delta_{i,i-1} - a^\delta_{i,i+1}) \in [-1,1]$ is evident, the value can be computed exactly depending on the image spacing and the parameters of the function δ. A worst-case estimation leads to a stable step size $\tau_{max} = \frac{h^2}{2+h^2}$.

2.3   Fast Explicit Diffusion

Solving the registration problem with direction-dependent regularization using an explicit scheme allows a simple implementation but requires a small step size, which entails slow convergence and the risk of getting stuck in a local minimum. However, advanced semi-implicit schemes like AOS demand for an inversion of the matrix $A^\rightleftharpoons$, which is not trivial [13].

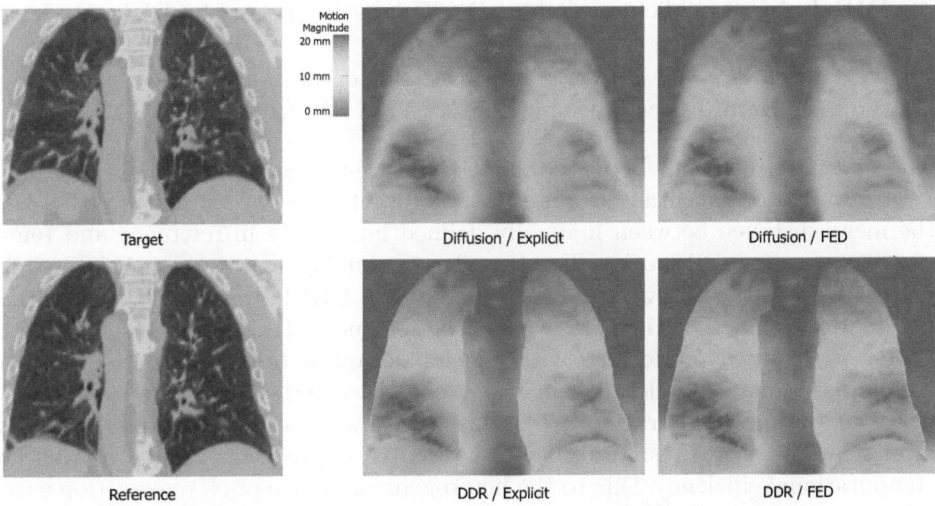

Fig. 2. Visualization of the motion magnitudes of the registration results for the different approaches. Sliding motion with DDR regularization is visible along the lung boundaries. Explicit and FED schemes are very similar but FED features larger displacements in some regions – presumably because local minima are bypassed during iterations with large step sizes.

Grewenig et al. recently proposed *Fast Explicit Diffusion* (FED) schemes for solving diffusion problems [4]. The main idea is to perform cycles of n explicit 1-D diffusion steps with varying step sizes

$$\tau_i = \frac{\tau_{max}}{2 \cos^2 \left(\pi \frac{2i+1}{4n+2} \right)}$$

to approximate a box filtering. Since box filtering is always stable, FED cycles are also stable even though individual steps violate the stability conditions.

Instead of approximating a box filter by simple diffusion steps, the approach can be adapted for arbitrary diffusion problems taking the maximal step size τ_{max} as derived in section 2.2 into account.

3   Results

Evaluation aims at comparing on the one hand diffusion (2) and direction-dependent regularization (5) and on the other hand explicit and FED schemes. The algorithms are tested on images of multiple data sets of which some are publicly accessible. The following thoracic CT images are considered for the estimation of respiratory lung motion:

– **WashU:** 12 thoracic 4D CT data sets, acquired by Low et al. [5] and reconstructed as described in [3].

- **DIR-Lab:** 10 publicly available 4D CT data sets hosted by DIR-Lab, University of Texas, US [1].
- **POPI:** The *Point-validated Pixel-based Breathing Thorax Model*, hosted by the Léon Bérard Cancer Center & CREATIS lab, Lyon, France [12].

The spatial resolution is between $0.97 \times 0.97 \times 1.5$ mm and $1.16 \times 1.16 \times 2.5$ mm.

For evaluation, accuracy is quantified as target registration error (TRE), i.e. the mean distance between manually defined landmarks in reference and template image after registration. Further, the maximal error was regarded for each patient to quantify the worst alignment. For the DIR-Lab and POPI data, the landmarks provided by the hosts were used (300 and 80 landmarks, respectively).

Registration was performed with end inhalation as reference and exhalation as template image. As detailed in [11], Normalized SSD (NSSD) forces are applied for optimal registration of regions with low contrast. Moreover, a multi level strategy with 4 resolution levels is used to improve the results as well as computational efficiency. Due to the heterogeneous image pool, registration with a fixed number of iterations is not applicable. Instead, computation is automatically stopped if the MSD between reference and transformed template image is not improved in the course of 10 iterations. Additionally, to avoid long run time on the finest level, a straight line is fitted on the MSD values of the 20 most recent iterations and registration is halted if its slope is below a certain threshold ($t = 0.001$). The number n of iterations per FED cycle is set to 5, but the method is very robust to this value.

For the explicit scheme step size and regularization weight were optimized empirically ($\tau = 0.01$, $\alpha = 0.25$). Although this step size is slightly larger than τ_{max} and therefore bears the risk of numerical instability, it provides the best results in practice and is therefore considered for comparison. For FED, τ_i are computed based on τ_{max} as derived in section 2.2.

The results are visualized in Fig. 2 and quantified in Table 1. For all image sets, registration with direction-dependent regularization yields better results than the common diffusion approach. This improvement is statistically significant in 17 of 23 cases (paired t-test on the landmark distances of each patient, significance level $p \leq 0.05$). These numbers show that it is of eminent importance for lung registration to take motion physiology into account.

Comparing the solution schemes, FED yields considerably better results than the simple explicit scheme with fixed step sizes. All together, the combination DDR with FED results in the most accurate registration.

Contrary to the expectations, registration with FED takes longer than with the explicit scheme (explicit: between approx. 2 and 25 minutes; FED: between 3 and 90 minutes). This is due to the automatic stop criterion: using the explicit scheme, registration stops after considerably less iterations than with FED because the MSD no longer decreases – presumably because a registration gets stuck in a local minimum. Using FED, however, minima can be bypassed during iterations with large step sizes. The increased number of iterations also explains the vast improvement of the DDR/FED approach over DDR with explicit solution.

Table 1. Results for the comparison of diffusion and direction-dependent regularizer as well as explicit, FED and AOS solution schemes. The best results are shown in bold font. For the WashU and DIR-Lab data, the average over 12 and 10 data sets is given.

Dataset	Regul.	Before Reg. Mean	Max	Explicit Mean	Max	FED Mean	Max
EXECUTION OF ALL ITERATIONS UNTIL CONVERGENCE							
WashU	Diffusion	6.59 ± 4.49	19.63	1.80 ± 1.84	9.63	1.74 ± 1.86	10.10
	DDR			1.48 ± 1.28	7.12	$\mathbf{1.31 \pm 0.95}$	**5.51**
DIR-Lab	Diffusion	8.46 ± 5.48	22.25	3.02 ± 2.79	15.53	2.91 ± 2.88	15.70
	DDR			2.22 ± 1.89	10.90	$\mathbf{1.55 \pm 1.11}$	**8.29**
POPI	Diffusion	7.15 ± 13.0	20.00	1.27 ± 1.02	5.64	1.21 ± 0.98	6.15
	DDR			1.14 ± 0.55	4.62	$\mathbf{1.02 \pm 0.29}$	**3.45**
EXECUTION FOR 10 (DIR-LAB, POPI) OR 15 (WASHU) MINUTES							
WashU	Diffusion	6.59 ± 4.49	19.63	1.84 ± 1.86	9.60	1.79 ± 1.87	9.86
	DDR			1.60 ± 1.33	7.03	$\mathbf{1.53 \pm 1.15}$	**6.45**
DIR-Lab	Diffusion	8.46 ± 5.48	22.25	3.08 ± 2.75	15.40	2.98 ± 2.75	15.48
	DDR			2.49 ± 1.99	11.43	$\mathbf{2.28 \pm 1.73}$	**10.61**
POPI	Diffusion	7.15 ± 13.0	20.00	1.27 ± 1.02	5.64	1.22 ± 0.99	6.24
	DDR			1.14 ± 0.55	4.62	$\mathbf{1.02 \pm 0.29}$	**3.32**

To avoid this bias, a second run is performed for each registration in which the computation is stopped after a maximal run time, such that a similar number of iterations is performed with the explicit as with the FED scheme (complete FED cycles are maintained). To cope with the different sizes, time was set to 10 (DIR-Lab, POPI) and 15 (WashU) minutes on an Intel Xeon machine with 2.67 GHz. However, it should be mentioned that one iteration with DDR takes approximately 35% longer than with diffusion regularization, resulting in considerably less iterations. The results are shown on the bottom of Table 1. Due to its faster convergence, FED is still superior to the explicit scheme. The DDR/FED approach still performs best but the improvement is less prominent than with all iterations since computation is stopped before full convergence.

4   Discussion and Conclusion

The goal of this work was to examine the potential of Fast Explicit Diffusion schemes for solving registration with direction-dependent regularization for the estimation of sliding organ motion. Registration was tested on 23 inhale/exhale CT scan pairs, of which 11 are publicly accessible. The results show that FED provides faster convergence per iteration than the explicit solution scheme. Moreover, it features considerably better accuracy since local minima are bypassed in iterations with a large step size. Using an automatic stop criterion, this can result in an effectively longer computation time.

In summary, the experiments demonstrate the capability of improving medical registration algorithms using Fast Explicit Diffusion.

References

1. Castillo, R., Castillo, E., Guerra, R., Johnson, V.E., McPhail, T., Garg, A.K., Guerrero, T.: A framework for evaluation of deformable image registration spatial accuracy using large landmark point sets. Phys. Med. Biol. 54, 1849–1870 (2009)
2. Delmon, V., Rit, S., Pinho, R., Sarrut, D.: Direction dependent B-splines decomposition for the registration of sliding objects. In: Fourth International Workshop on Pulmonary Image Analysis, MICCAI 2011, pp. 45–55 (2011)
3. Ehrhardt, J., Werner, R., Saering, D., Lu, W., Low, D.A., Handels, H.: An optical flow based method for improved reconstruction of 4D CT data sets acquired during free breathing. Med. Phys. 34(2), 711–721 (2007)
4. Grewenig, S., Weickert, J., Bruhn, A.: From Box Filtering to Fast Explicit Diffusion. In: Goesele, M., Roth, S., Kuijper, A., Schiele, B., Schindler, K. (eds.) DAGM 2010. LNCS, vol. 6376, pp. 533–542. Springer, Heidelberg (2010)
5. Low, D.A., Nystrom, M., Kalinin, E., Parikh, P., Dempsey, J.F., et al.: A method for the reconstruction of four-dimensional synchronized CT scans acquired during free breathing. Med. Phys. 30(6), 1254–1263 (2003)
6. Murphy, K., van Ginneken, B., Reinhardt, J.M., Kabus, S., Ding, K., et al.: Evaluation of Registration Methods on Thoracic CT: The EMPIRE10 Challenge. IEEE Trans. Med. Imag. 30(11), 1901–1920 (2011)
7. Nagel, H.H., Enkelmann, W.: An Investigation of Smoothness Constraints for the Estimation of Displacement Vector Fields from Image Sequences. IEEE Trans. Pattern Anal. Mach. Intell. (5), 565–593 (1986)
8. Pace, D.F., Enquobahrie, A., Yang, H., Aylward, S.R., Niethammer, M.: Deformable Image Registration of Sliding Organs Using Anisotropic Diffusive Regularization. In: Proc IEEE Int. Symp. Biomed. Imaging, pp. 407–413 (2011)
9. Risser, L., Baluwala, H., Schnabel, J.A.: Diffeomorphic registration with sliding conditions: Application to the registration of lungs CT images. In: Fourth International Workshop on Pulmonary Image Analysis, MICCAI 2011, pp. 79–90 (2011)
10. Ruan, D., Esedoglu, S., Fessler, J.: Discriminative sliding preserving regularization in medical image registration. In: Proc. IEEE Int. Symp. Biomed. Imaging, pp. 430–433 (2009)
11. Schmidt-Richberg, A., Werner, R., Handels, H., Ehrhardt, J.: Estimation of Slipping Organ Motion by Registration with Direction-Dependent Regularization. Med. Image Anal. 16(1), 150–159 (2012)
12. Vandemeulebroucke, J., Sarrut, D., Clarysse, P.: The POPI-model, a point-validated pixel-based breathing thorax model. In: International Conference on the Use of Computers in Radiation Therapy, ICCR (2007)
13. Weickert, J., Romeny, B.M.T.H., Viergever, M.A.: Efficient and Reliable Schemes for Nonlinear Diffusion Filtering. IEEE Trans. Image Process 7(3), 398–410 (1998)
14. Werner, R., Ehrhardt, J., Schmidt-Richberg, A., Handels, H.: Validation and comparison of a biophysical modeling approach and non-linear registration for estimation of lung motion fields in thoracic 4D CT data. In: Proc. SPIE, p. 72590U (2009)

Early DCE-MRI Changes after Longitudinal Registration May Predict Breast Cancer Response to Neoadjuvant Chemotherapy

Xia Li, Lori R. Arlinghaus, A. Bapsi Chakravarthy, Jaime Farley, Ingrid A. Mayer, Vandana G. Abramson, Mark C. Kelley, Ingrid M. Meszoely, Julie Means-Powell, and Thomas E. Yankeelov

Institute of Imaging Science, Vanderbilt University, Nashville, Tennessee, USA
{xia.li.1,lori.Arlinghaus,Bapsi.chak,Jaime.farley,ingrid.mayer,
vandana.abramson,mark.kelley,ingrid.meszoely,Julie.means,
tom.yankeelov}@vanderbilt.edu

Abstract. To monitor tumor response to neoadjuvant chemotherapy, investigators have begun to employ quantitative physiological parameters available from dynamic contrast enhanced MRI (DCE-MRI). However, most studies track the changes in these parameters obtained from the tumor region of interest (ROI) or histograms, thereby discarding all spatial information on tumor heterogeneity. In this study, we applied a nonrigid registration to longitudinal DCE-MRI data and performed a voxel-by-voxel analysis to examine the ability of early changes in parameters at the voxel level to separate pathologic complete responders (pCR) from non-responders (NR). Twenty-two patients were examined using DCE-MRI pre-, post one cycle, and at the conclusion of all neoadjuvant chemotherapy. The fast exchange regime model (FXR) was applied to both the original and registered DCE-MRI data to estimate tumor-related parameters. The results indicate that compared with the ROI analysis, the voxel-based analysis after longitudinal registration may improve the ability of DCE-MRI to separate complete responders from non-responders after one cycle of therapy when using the FXR model (p = 0.02).

Keywords: Longitudinal registration, DCE-MRI, breast cancer.

1   Introduction

Early investigations in monitoring tumor response to neoadjuvant chemotherapy focused on semi-quantitative analyses based on changes in morphology and/or anatomical measures [1-7]. More recently, investigators have begun to employ the quantitative physiological parameters available from dynamic contrast enhanced MRI (DCE-MRI). For example, Ah-See *et al* [8] acquired DCE-MRI data on thirty-seven patients with primary breast cancer. Through calculating the changes in seven kinetic parameters, they reported the that change in the volume transfer constant (K^{trans}) was the best predictor of pathologic nonresponse. In performing their analysis, the

B.M. Dawant et al. (Eds.): WBIR 2012, LNCS 7359, pp. 229–235, 2012.
© Springer-Verlag Berlin Heidelberg 2012

investigators tracked the changes in parameters obtained from tumor ROI or histogram data. While this approach is the current standard, it does discard all spatial information on tumor heterogeneity. Li *et al* presented [9] and validated [10] a method for the registration of breast MR images obtained at different time points throughout the course of neoadjuvant chemotherapy. In this study, we applied the approach to longitudinal pharmacokinetic parameters estimated by the fast exchange regime model (FXR) and performed a voxel-by-voxel analysis to examine the ability of early changes in parameters at the voxel level to separate pathologic complete responders (pCR) from non-responders (NR). The FXR model assumes that tissue is not homogeneous and water exchange between the vascular, extravascular intracellular space, and the extravascular extracellular spaces are not sufficiently fast. To the best of our knowledge, it is the first work to report the ability of the FXR model to predict breast cancer response and demonstrate the influence of tumor heterogeneity on the analysis of treatment response.

2   Patients and Methods

2.1   MRI Data Acquisition

Twenty-two patients with Stage II/III breast cancer were enrolled in an IRB-approved clinical trial where serial breast MRI scans were acquired pre-therapy (t_1) and after one cycle (t_2), and at the completion of neoadjuvant chemotherapy (t_3). Imaging was performed on a 3.0 T Achieva MR scanner (Philips Healthcare, Best, The Netherlands). The DCE-MRI acquisition employed a 3D spoiled gradient echo sequence with TR\TE\α =7.9ms\1.3ms\20°. The acquisition matrix was 192×192×20 over a sagittal $(22 \text{ cm})^2$ field of view with a slice thickness of 5 mm. Each 20-slice set was collected in 16.5 seconds at 25 time points and 0.1 mmol/kg of Magnevist was injected at 2 mL s^{-1} after the third dynamic scan. Responders (n=11) were defined as those patients who had a pathologic complete response at time of surgery. Non responders (n=11) were defined as patients with residual invasive cancer at the primary tumor site.

2.2   Data Registration

The purpose of the registration in this study is to align DCE-MRI data acquired at three time points: pre-, post-one cycle, post-all cycles of neoadjuvant chemotherapy. Since the DCE-MRI data at each imaging session consists of 25 dynamic scans, we apply the registration to the average of the post-contrast DCE-MRI data (i.e., the average of the 4th – 25th scans; this is done to increase the SNR of the data to yield a more accurate registration). First, the average DCE data pre- and post-one cycle of therapy are aligned to the data at the conclusion of all therapy by a rigid body registration algorithm [11], which searches the optimal rotation and translation parameters through maximizing the normalized mutual information (NMI). A nonrigid registration method [9] is then applied to refine the registration. This method extends the adaptive bases algorithm (ABA) [12] through incorporating an additional term designed to preserve the tumor volume during the registration process. The reason the tumor volume must be preserved is that compressing or expanding the tumor during the registration process could provide results that are misleading in regard to assessing biological changes in the tumor (e.g., disease progression or response) that occur between imaging sessions.

Both the ABA and the extended ABA algorithm with a tumor volume conserving constraint employ NMI as the similarity measure, and the deformation field is modeled by a linear combination of radial basis functions. To constrain the tumor volume, we compute the Jacobian determinant over the tumor regions in the MR images:

$$f_{con} = \alpha \int_T \left| log \left(J_T \left(x \right) \right) \right| dx, \tag{1}$$

where $J_T \left(x \right)$ is the Jacobian determinant on the tumor area and α is the parameter to control the weight of this constraint term, which is set to $0.15 - 0.3$ based on empirical evidence. Hence the cost function is composed of the negative NMI term and the tumor volume constraint term:

$$f_{cost} = -NMI + \alpha \int_T \left| log \left(J_T \left(x \right) \right) \right| dx, \tag{2}$$

Through minimizing Eq. (2), the algorithm can optimally register the normal tissues while simultaneously minimizing tumor distortion. The generated transformation is applied to each dynamic scan to obtain the registered DCE-MRI data.

2.3   Data Analysis

The fast exchange regime model (FXR) is applied to both the original and serially registered DCE-MRI data to estimate the volume transfer constant (K^{trans}, related to tumor perfusion and permeability), efflux rate constant (k_{ep}), extravascular extracellular volume fraction (v_e), and the average intracellular water lifetime of a water molecule (τ_i).

In order to perform quantitative DCE-MRI, the arterial input function (AIF) must be measured. Individual AIFs are detected by a semi-automatic AIF tracking algorithm, the details of which can be found in reference [13]. Here we use a population-averaged AIF which is calculated through averaging fifty individual AIFs.

For each patient at each time point, a conservative ROI is manually drawn around the contrast enhanced tumor region; that is, the ROI encompasses the entire tumor as well as surrounding healthy appearing tissue. Given this set of voxels, eleven subsets of enhancing tumor voxels are constructed on the basis of their averaged post-contrast signal intensity increase over the average of the three pre-contrast time points. Each subset is defined for different percent enhancement thresholds ranging from 10% to 110% in 10% increments. This allows us to establish an optimal "cut-off" point for selecting enhancing voxels to include in the analysis.

To evaluate the effectiveness of the longitudinal registration algorithm, both ROI and voxel-based analyses are performed. The ROI analysis is based on the unregistered DCE-MRI data and three parameters are computed: the change of mean, median, and mean of the top 15% parameters. The voxel analysis is performed on the registered data and the same parameters are calculated on voxels showing an increase in the parameter from t_1 to t_2. A Wilcoxon rank sum test is then used to determine if there is a significant difference between the pCR and NR groups.

3   Results

Figure 1 shows the registered DCE-MRI data at three time points with the corresponding K^{trans} maps superimposed; the top row shows a representative patient achieving a pCR, while the bottom row is a NR.

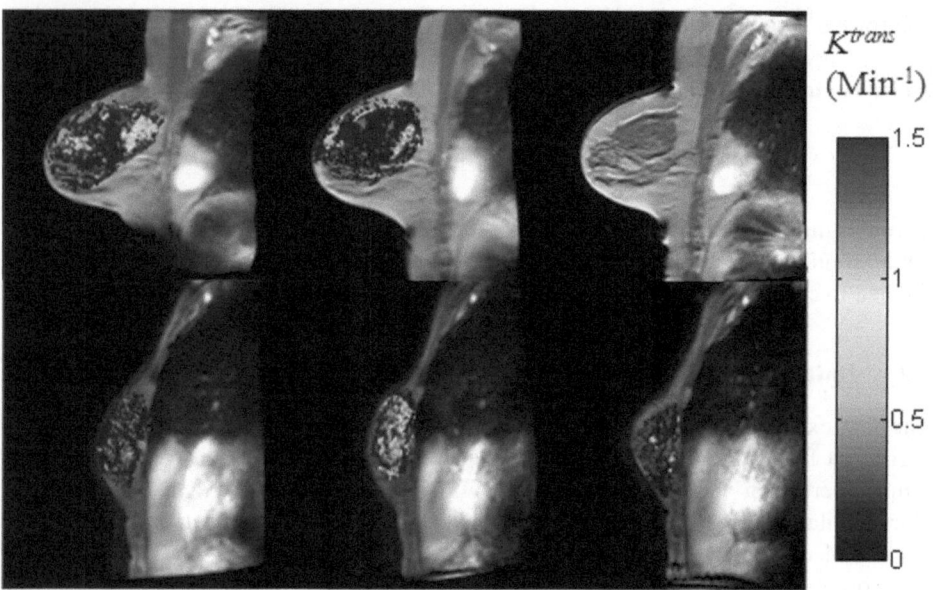

Fig. 1. The registered DCE-MRI data at three time points (columns) with the corresponding K^{trans} superimposed; the top row shows a patient with pCR, while the bottom row is a NR.

Figure 2 shows the p values obtained by both the ROI and voxel-based analyses at different enhancement thresholds. Before registration, only two ROI analyses are significant (the median K^{trans} when the 20% and 30% enhancement rates used as the cut-off) at the $p < 0.05$ level (indicated by the solid black line in the figure). However, after the longitudinal registration, p values are significant when the enhancement rates ranging from the 20% to 70% are used, indicating the parameters estimated by the FXR model with registration can distinguish the differences between two groups.

Table 1 lists the p values of three ways of summarizing different pharmacokinetic parameters by the ROI and voxel-based analyses. The results indicate that the registration makes the change in mean K^{trans} move from a not significant (p = 0.12 in the ROI analysis) to a significant difference (p = 0.02 in the voxel analysis). Similar conclusions can be made for the change in mean of the top 15% of K^{trans} and k_{ep}. The other parameters studied in this effort, v_e and τ_i, do not yield significant results in either analysis.

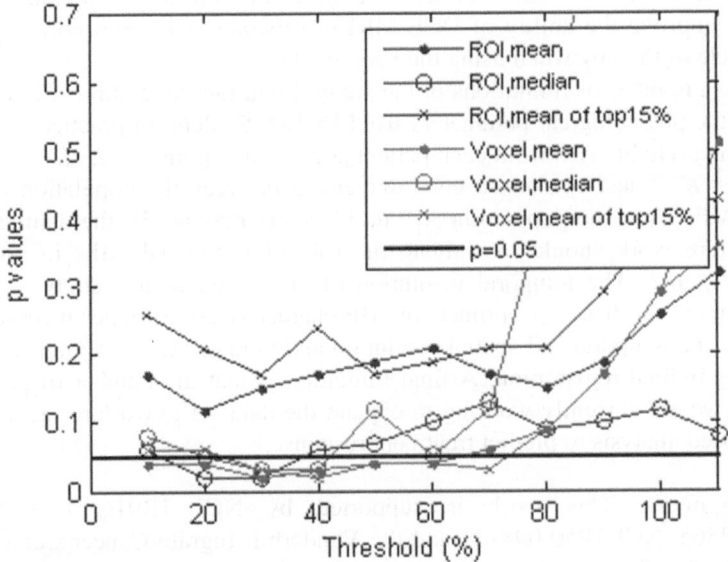

Fig. 2. The p values of k^{trans} obtained by both the ROI and voxel-based analyses at different enhancement thresholds. Most p values in the voxel-based analysis are significant (< 0.05) when the enhancement rates ranging from the 20% to 70% are used, compared with two significant p values in the ROI analysis, indicating the longitudinal registration may improve the ability of DCE-MRI data to predict treatment response.

Table 1. The table lists the p values of three ways of summarizing different pharmacokinetic parameters by the ROI and voxel-based analyses. The results after the voxel-based analysis, in general, lead to smaller p values, indicating the longitudinal registration may improve the ability of DCE-MRI data to separate pCR from NR patients.

Analysis	K^{trans} ROI	K^{trans} Voxel	k_{ep} ROI	k_{ep} Voxel	v_e ROI	v_e Voxel	τ_i ROI	τ_i Voxel
Δmean	0.12	**0.02**	**0.04**	**0.04**	0.12	0.39	0.69	0.26
Δmedian	**0.02**	**0.03**	0.08	0.06	0.17	0.15	0.51	0.13
Δmean of top15%	0.15	**0.02**	0.07	**0.04**	0.74	0.13	0.51	0.13

4   Conclusions

A nonrigid registration algorithm has been employed to retain the spatial information in DCE-MRI parameter maps obtained before and after neoadjuvant chemotherapy, thereby enabling a voxel-based analysis to be performed to predict response. The quantitative analysis demonstrates that K^{trans} and k_{ep} can separate pCR from non-responding patients after the parameters are aligned by this algorithm. Although v_e and τ_i cannot lead to any significant results, the p values trend to smaller values after registration. The results indicate that the voxel-based analysis after longitudinal registration may improve the ability of DCE-MRI to separate pCR from non-responders after one cycle of therapy when using the FXR model.

There are a number of limitations in the study. First, the population AIF was used to estimate the physiological parameters from DCE-MRI data. In practice, it is difficult to obtain a reliable AIF from each patient at each time point. Li *et al.*'s study [13] indicates that K^{trans} and v_p show a good agreement between the population AIF and individual AIF. Thus, the population AIF in this study may not be the main concern, although future work should investigate the role of individual AIFs in predicting treatment response. The temporal resolution of 16 s used in this study is also an important limitation. It is not optimal for AIF characterization; rather it represents a balance between temporal and spatial resolution and field of view coverage so we can perform longitudinal registration. A final limitation is that the number of patients is modest and we are currently working to expand the data set to explore the ability of the voxel-based analysis to predict treatment response.

Acknowledgments. This work is supported by NCI 1R01CA129961, NCI 1U01CA142565, NCI 1P50 098131 and the Vanderbilt-Ingram Cancer Center Grant (NIH P30 CA68485).

References

1. Cheung, Y.C., Chen, S.C., Su, M.Y., See, L.C., Hsueh, S., Chang, H.K., et al.: Monitoring the size and response of locally advanced breast cancers to neoadjuvant chemotherapy (weekly paclitaxel and epirubicin) with serial enhanced MRI. Breast Cancer Res. Treat. 78, 51–58 (2003)
2. Chou, C.P., Wu, M.T., Chang, H.T., Lo, Y.S., Pan, H.B., Degani, H., Furman-Haran, E.: Monitoring breast cancer response to neoadjuvant systemic chemotherapy using parametric contrast-enhanced MRI: a pilot study. Acad. Radiol. 14, 561–573 (2007)
3. Martincich, L., Montemurro, F., De Rosa, G., Marra, V., Ponzone, R., Cirillo, S., Gatti, M., Biglia, N., Sarotto, I., Sismondi, P., Regge, D., Aglietta, M.: Monitoring response to primary chemotherapy in breast cancer using dynamic contrast-enhanced magnetic resonance imaging. Breast Cancer Res. Treat. 83, 67–76 (2004)
4. Wasser, K., Klein, S.K., Fink, C., Junkermann, H., Sinn, H.P., Zuna, I., Knopp, M.V., Delorme, S.: Evaluation of neoadjuvant chemotherapeutic response of breast cancer using dynamic MRI with high temporal resolution. Eur. Radiol. 13, 80–87 (2003)

5. Drew, P.J., Kerin, M.J., Mahapatra, T., Malone, C., Monson, J.R., Turnbull, L.W., Fox, J.N.: Evaluation of response to neoadjuvant chemoradiotherapy for locally advanced breast cancer with dynamic contrast-enhanced MRI of the breast. Eur. J. Surg. Oncol. 27, 617–620 (2001)
6. Abraham, D.C., Jones, R.C., Jones, S.E., Cheek, J.H., Peters, G.N., Knox, S.M., Grant, M.D., Hampe, D.W., Savino, D.A., Harms, S.E.: Evaluation of neoadjuvant chemothera-peutic response of locally advanced breast cancer by magnetic resonance imaging. Cancer 78, 91–100 (1996)
7. Gilles, R., Guinebretiere, J.M., Toussaint, C., Spielman, M., Rietjens, M., Petit, J.Y., Con-tesso, G., Masselot, J., Vanel, D.: Locally advanced breast cancer: contrast-enhanced sub-traction MR imaging of response to preoperative chemotherapy. Radiology 191, 633–638 (1994)
8. Ah-See, M.L., Makris, A., Taylor, N.J., Harrison, M., Richman, P.I., Burcombe, R.J., Stirl-ing, J.J., d'Arcy, J.A., Pittam, M.R., Ravichandran, D., Padhani, A.R.: Early changes in functional dynamic magnetic resonance imaging predict for pathologic response to neoad-juvant chemotherapy in primary breast cancer. Clin. Cancer Res. 14, 6580–6589 (2008)
9. Li, X., Dawant, B.M., Welch, E.B., Chakravarthy, A.B., Freehardt, D., Mayer, I., Kelley, M., Meszoely, I., Gore, J.C., Yankeelov, T.E.: A nonrigid registration algorithm for longi-tudinal breast MR images and the analysis of breast tumor response. Magn. Reson. Imag-ing 27, 1258–1270 (2009)
10. Li, X., Dawant, B.M., Welch, E.B., Chakravarthy, A.B., Xu, L., Mayer, I., Keley, M., Meszoely, I., Means-Powell, J., Gore, J.C., Yankeelov, T.E.: Validation of an algorithm for the nonrigid registration of longitudinal breast MR images using realistic phantoms. Med. Phys. 37, 2541–2552 (2010)
11. Maes, F., Collignon, A., Vandermeulen, D., Marchal, G., Suetens, P.: Multimodality image registration by maximization of mutual information. IEEE Trans. Med. Imaging 16, 187–198 (1997)
12. Rohde, G.K., Aldroubi, A., Dawant, B.M.: The adaptive bases algorithm for intensity-based nonrigid image registration. IEEE Trans. Med. Imaging 22, 1470–1479 (2003)
13. Li, X., Welch, E.B., Chakravarthy, A.B., Lei, X., Arlinghaus, L.R., Farley, J., Loveless, M.E., Mayer, I., Kelley, M., Meszoely, I., Means-Powell, J., Abramson, V., Grau, A., Gore, J.C., Yankeelov, T.E.: A Novel AIF Detection Method and a Comparison of DCE-MRI Parameters Using Individual and Population Based AIFs in Human Breast Cancer. Phys. Med. Biol. 56, 5753–5769 (2011)

SUPIR: Surface Uncertainty-Penalized, Non-rigid Image Registration for Pelvic CT Imaging

Cheng Zhang[1], Gary E. Christensen[1], Sebastian Kurtek[2], Anuj Srivastava[2], Martin J. Murphy[3], Elisabeth Weiss[3], Erwei Bai[1], and Jeffrey F. Williamson[3]

[1] Department of Electrical and Computer Engineering,
University of Iowa, Iowa City, IA, USA
cheng-zhang@uiowa.edu
[2] Department of Statistics,
Florida State University, Tallahassee, FL, USA
[3] Department of Radiation Oncology,
Virginia Commonwealth University, Richmond, VA, USA

Abstract. Intensity-driven image registration does not always produce satisfactory pointwise correspondences in regions of low soft-tissue contrast characteristic of pelvic computed tomography (CT) imaging. Additional information such as manually segmented organ surfaces can be combined with intensity information to improve registration. However, this approach is sensitive to non-negligible surface segmentation errors (delineation errors) due to the relative poor soft-tissue contrast supported by CT. This paper presents an image registration algorithm that mitigates the impact of delineation errors by weighting each surface element by its segmentation uncertainty. This weighting ensures that portions of the surface that are specified accurately are used to guide the registration while portions of the surface that are uncertain are ignored. In our proof-of-principle validation, Monte Carlo simulations based on simple 3D phantoms demonstrate the strengths and weaknesses of the proposed method. These experiments show that registration performance can be improved using surface uncertainty in certain circumstances but not in others. Results are presented for situations when intensity only registration performs best, when intensity plus equally weighted surface registration performs best, and when intensity plus uncertainty weighted surface registration performs best. The algorithm has been applied to register CBCT and FBCT prostate images where the uncertainty of the prostate surface segmentation was estimated using contours drawn by five experts.

1   Introduction

Deformable image registration is needed for mapping organ segmentations from the planning fan-beam CT (FBCT) onto daily cone-beam CT (CBCT) images for adaptive replanning and for cumulative dose reconstruction in which individual fraction dose distributions are deformably mapped onto a single reference imaging study. Ideally, this problem would be solved by an intensity-driven registration algorithm that takes CBCT and FBCT images as input and returns the correspondence function. However due to the low contrast of soft tissue in CT imaging, the boundaries of the prostate and other organs are often difficult to distinguish from neighboring organs and tissue.

B.M. Dawant et al. (Eds.): WBIR 2012, LNCS 7359, pp. 236–245, 2012.

Therefore pure intensity-based volumetric registration often cannot obtain sufficiently accurate results especially in the pelvis. One approach to improving registration accuracy is to manually segment organ boundaries on both source and target image sets and utilize them, in the form of binary masks, as landmarks to guide the otherwise ill-conditioned intensity-based registration process [1, 3]. Another approach [4, 5, 8] is to register the source and target surfaces first and then using the obtained transformation as the initial condition or extra constraint in volume registration. To date, these methods ignore the uncertainty of manual segmentations due to contouring variability among different observers, known formally as interobserver delineation error [13]. For the prostate gland boundary, previous studies have shown that such errors vary dramatically (from 1-4 mm) with location on the prostate surface and adjacent organs at risk (OARs) [9]. Although the landmark uncertainty in the context of landmark-only registration have been studied [10, 14], the combination of surface and volume registration in the presence of boundary uncertainty has not been actively studied. As such this work proposes a registration algorithm that combines intensity and surface information using a probabilistic model to account for the surface segmentation error.

2   Method

We call our method Surface Uncertainty Penalized Image Registration (SUPIR). As illustrated in Fig. 1, SUPIR consists of two components: modeling the 3D positional boundary uncertainty from training dataset (Box 1, purple) and registering images with this surface uncertainty penalty (Box 2, green).

Box 1 shows how the a priori boundary position uncertainty is modeled. We start by collecting training FBCT and CBCT pelvic images. For each image, multiple experts segment the structure of interest (the prostate in this paper) individually and save them as 3D triangulated meshes. These meshes are then mapped into a spherical coordinate system and aligned with each other so that the interoperator discrepancies between any pair of experts can be quantified as a function of location in the spherical coordinate system. The segmentation error or boundary location uncertainty as a function of location on prostate surface in a FBCT image is modeled via the principal component analysis (PCA). PCA segmentation uncertainty model is constructed for CBCT image set as well.

In addition to the boundary-location PCA models, SUPIR requires both template and target images along with the corresponding segmented organ surfaces. Box 2 shows how the surface-uncertainty information is used to constrain volume registration solution space. It is assumed that the images to be registered each have a surface segmentation provided to help guide the registration. It is also assumed that the surface segmentation is an instance of a random process described by the underlying boundary location uncertainty model. That is, we assume that deviations of the supplied expert surface segmentation from the true surface are consistent with the boundary uncertainty model constructed from the training data. After the template and target surfaces are aligned with the training surfaces in the spherical coordinate system, the boundary uncertainty information is mapped to them. Finally, the images are registered by jointly minimizing the intensity and surface differences while taking into account the boundary uncertainty penalty.

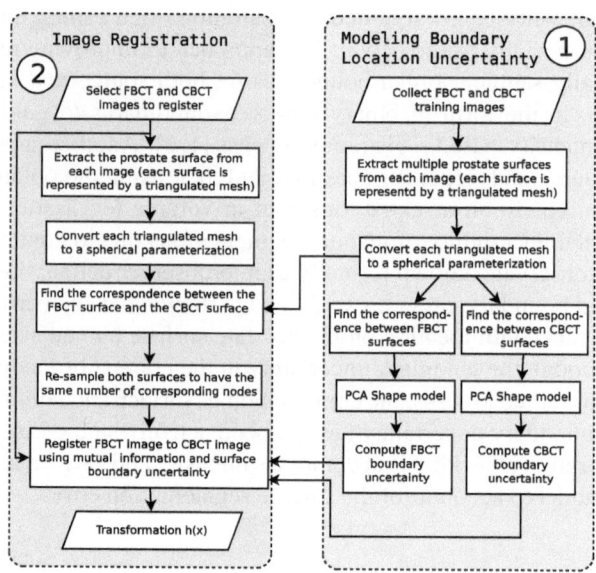

Fig. 1. Algorithm flowchart of SUPIR. Box 1 summarizes the steps to model the a priori boundary uncertainty. Box 2 summarizes the steps to use the surface uncertainty information to assist volume registration.

2.1   Volume and Surface Registration with Boundary Location Uncertainty

Denote the FBCT and CBCT images by $I_f : \Omega \mapsto \mathbb{R}$ and $I_c : \Omega \mapsto \mathbb{R}$, respectively, where $\Omega = [0,1]^3$ is the image domain. Let $X : S^2 \mapsto \Omega$ and $Y : S^2 \mapsto \Omega$ denote the parameterized embeddings of the prostate surfaces in the FBCT and CBCT, respectively, where S^2 is the unit sphere. The image registration problem can be cast as a search for the transformation $h : \Omega \mapsto \Omega$ that minimizes the cost function

$$C_{\text{Total}}(h) = \alpha C_{\text{Image}}(h) + \rho C_{\text{Surface}}(h) + \lambda \, C_{\text{Smooth}}(h) \tag{1}$$

where C_{Image} is the similarity cost between the FBCT and CBCT images, C_{Surface} is the similarity cost between the prostate surfaces, and C_{Smooth} is regularization cost that penalizes transformations that are not smooth. The weighting constants α, ρ and λ control the relative influence or priority of each of the individual cost functions.

For computational purposes, the transformation h is parameterized using a B-spline basis [11]. Let $c_i = [c_x(\mathbf{x}_i), c_y(\mathbf{x}_i), c_z(\mathbf{x}_i)]^T$ be the coefficients of the i-th control point $\mathbf{x}_i$ on the spline lattice G along each direction. $\mathbf{h}(\mathbf{x}) = \mathbf{x} + \sum_{i \in G} c_i B^{(3)}(\mathbf{x} - \mathbf{x}_i)$, where $B^{(3)}(\mathbf{x}) = B^{(3)}(x) B^{(3)}(y) B^{(3)}(z)$ is a separable convolution kernel. $B^{(3)}(x)$ is the uniform cubic B-spline basis function.

Since FBCT and CBCT are two different imaging modalities, C_{image} in Eq. 1 is given by the negative mutual information (MI) [12] between two images. MI indicates the amount of information that two image share. It is assumed that good correspondence is achieved when MI is maximized. In this paper C_{image} is defined as

$$C_{\text{MI}} = -\sum_i \sum_j p(i,j) \log \frac{p(i,j)}{p_{I_1 \circ h}(i) p_{I_2}(j)} \tag{2}$$

where $p(i,j)$ is the joint intensity distribution of transformed template image $I_1 \circ h$ and target image I_2; $p_{I_1 \circ h}(i)$ and $p_{I_2}(j)$ are their marginal distributions, respectively. The histogram bins of $I_1 \circ h$ and I_2 are indexed by i and j.

A commonly used Laplacian smoothness constraint is used to regularize the space of possible transforms:

$$C_{\text{Smooth}} = \frac{1}{2} \int \sum_{i=1}^{3} (\frac{\partial u_i(x)}{\partial x_i})^2 \, dx \tag{3}$$

where $u(x)$ is the displacement vector field (DVF) and is related to the transformation h by $h(x) = x + u(x)$.

The surface similarity metric used in Eq. 1 is defined as

$$C_{\text{Surface}} = \int_0^{2\pi} \int_0^{\pi} \frac{1}{\omega(u,v)} \|h(Y(u,v)) - X(\phi(u,v))\| \sin v \, du dv \tag{4}$$

where $\phi(u,v)$ defines the pointwise correspondence between surfaces $Y(u,v)$ and $X(u,v)$ and $\omega(u,v)$ is the uncertainty metric that is proportional to the segmentation error at (u,v). Details of how the uncertainty function $\omega(u,v)$ is estimated are discussed in Sec. 2.3.

2.2 Surface Registration

The correspondence between two surfaces needs to be established before the computation of $\omega(u,v)$ or C_{Surface}. In case of two closed surfaces, $X(u,v)$ and $Y(u,v)$, a common method is to conformally map each surface to a unit sphere and resample this spherical parametric domain to the necessary resolution. Then the two surfaces are aligned in this spherical space via the re-parameterization $\phi(u,v)$ which optimizes the correspondence between $X(u,v)$ and $Y(u,v)$ to give $X(u,v) \sim Y(\phi(u,v))$, where $\sim$ means "corresponds to" [2]. This work follows the same idea but uses a recently proposed parameterization-invariant approach which guarantees $\|Q(Y(u,v)) - Q(X(u,v))\| = \|Q(Y(\gamma(u,v))) - Q(X(\gamma(u,v)))\|$ when aligning surfaces where γ is a diffeomorphic transformation and Q is a novel representation of the given surfaces. We refer readers to [6] for more details.

2.3 Surface Uncertainty Model

The uncertainty of the boundary location is modeled using a principal component analysis (PCA) [7] of segmentations drawn of the same object by multiple experts. Let $X_i(u,v)$ and $Y_i(u,v)$, $i = 1$ to n, denote the manually segmented prostate surfaces traced on FBCT and CBCT images, respectively, by the i-th expert. Each randomly sampled FBCT prostate surface, $X(u,v)$, can be represented as

$$X(u,v) = \bar{X}(u,v) + \sum_{i=1}^{n} B_i \beta_i(u,v) \tag{5}$$

where $\bar{X}(u,v)$ is the mean prostate surface, B_i is a random variable with normal distribution $B_i \sim N(0, \sigma_i^2)$, σ_i^2 is the i-th eigenvalue of the covariance matrix, and $\beta_i(u,v)$ is the corresponding vector-valued eigenfunction, representing the i-th variation mode. Similarly, $Y(u,v)$ can be represented as

$$Y(u,v) = \bar{Y}(u,v) + \sum_{i=1}^{n} C_i \psi_i(u,v) \tag{6}$$

where $\bar{Y}(u,v)$ is the mean shape of CBCT prostate, $C_i \sim \mathcal{N}(0, \epsilon_i^2)$, and $\psi_i(u,v)$ is the corresponding variation mode.

$\omega(u,v)$ is required to have the following property. In regions where the experts closely agree and therefore are confident about the boundary location, the uncertainty is low and $\frac{1}{\omega(u,v)}$ is large suggesting that more surface matching weight should be given to these regions to guide registration. Whereas, at regions of large interoperator discrepancies, indicating lack of expert consensus on boundary location, the uncertainty is high and $\frac{1}{\omega(u,v)}$ is small indicating less surface matching weight should be given. To simplify the computation we define

$$\omega(u,v) = \mathrm{tr}(\mathrm{Cov}\,(X(u,v))) + \mathrm{tr}(\mathrm{Cov}\,(Y(u,v))) \tag{7}$$

At each point (u_0, v_0), the trace of the covariance $\mathrm{Cov}\,(X(u_0,v_0))$ is derived as

$$\begin{aligned}
\mathrm{tr}(\mathrm{Cov}\,(X(u_0,v_0))) &= \mathrm{tr}(\mathrm{E}\,\{[X(u_0,v_0) - \bar{X}(u_0,v_0)][X(u_0,v_0) - \bar{X}(u_0,v_0)]^{\mathsf{T}}\}) \\
&= \mathrm{tr}(\mathrm{E}\,\{[\sum_{i=1}^{n} B_i \beta_i(u_0,v_0)][\sum_{i=1}^{n} B_i \beta_i(u_0,v_0)]^{\mathsf{T}}\}) \\
&= \sum_{k=1}^{3} \sum_{i=1}^{n} \sum_{j=1}^{n} \mathrm{E}\,\{B_i B_j\} \beta_{ik}(u_0,v_0) \beta_{jk}(u_0,v_0) \\
&= \sum_{k=1}^{3} \sum_{i=1}^{n} \sigma_i^2 \beta_{ik}^2(u_0,v_0)
\end{aligned}$$

where i has the same meaning in Eq. 5 and k represents the k-th direction among x, y and z axises. Similarly, $\mathrm{tr}(\mathrm{Cov}\,(Y(u_0,v_0))) = \sum_{k=1}^{3} \sum_{i=1}^{n} \epsilon_i^2 \psi_{ik}^2(u_0,v_0)$.

3 Experiment and Result

3.1 Phantom Experiment

Monte Carlo simulation and simple 3D phantoms were used to investigate how the intensity and surface similarity costs affect the registration result. To this end, the following five registration algorithms derived from Eq. 1 were studied.

1. Intensity-only registration (SSD): $\alpha = 1$, $\rho = 0$ and $\lambda = 0.05$.
2. Equally-weighted surface-driven only registration (EWS): $\alpha = 0$, $\rho = 5$, $\lambda = 0.05$ and $\omega(u, v) = 1$.
3. Uncertainty-weighted surface-driven only registration (UWS): $\alpha = 0$, $\rho = 20$, $\lambda = 0.05$ and $\omega(u, v)$ defined by Eq. 7.
4. Equally-weighted surface-penalized intensity-driven image registration (ESPIR): $\alpha = 1$, $\rho = 5$, $\lambda = 0.05$ and $\omega(u, v) = 1$.
5. Surface uncertainty-penalized image registration (SUPIR): $\alpha = 1$, $\rho = 20$, $\lambda = 0.05$ and $\omega(u, v)$ defined by Eq. 7.

Note that ρ was set to 20 in the UWS and SUPIR methods while it was set to 5 in the EWS and ESPIR methods so that the total weight along the surface was similar.

As shown in Fig. 2, each phantom data set consists of a constant intensity 3D general ellipsoid shape centered in the image domain. It is assumed that there is an object of interest in the center of the ellipsoid to be registered that cannot be seen in the intensity image. Since the object of interest cannot be seen, we assume that we are given a surface segmentation of the object via some other means to aid in the registration. The figure of merit for a good registration is that the true object of interest in the template and target images are aligned. It is further assumed that surfaces that were provided have segmentation errors associated with them. The surface segmentation error is modeled probabilistically by a mean shape plus a spatially varying error term. To simplify the analysis, we will assume that one of the surfaces has no segmentation error and the other surface is a random sample from our uncertainty model. The registration experiments are repeated using 50 random surfaces to find the average performance of each algorithm.

The surface of interest is defined by $Y_p(u, v) = (a \cos u \sin v, a \sin u \sin v, b \cos v)$ where $u \in [0, 2\pi]$ and $v \in [0, \pi]$. Initially we set $a = b = 24$ mm to create a prostate-size sphere $Y_{p_m}(u, v)$ as the mean surface. Then a Gaussian random variable $\mathcal{N}(0, \sigma^2)$, $\sigma = 4$ mm is added to a and 50 random surfaces $Y_{p_i}(u, v)$ are sampled, where $\sigma = 4$ mm simulates the real case in Sec. 3.2. In this simplified experiment, there is only one variation mode in the phantom surfaces where the largest variance happens along the equator and the least at the poles. Also note that these parametric surfaces require no alignment between each other so their boundary uncertainty can be directly computed as Sec. 2.3.

All phantom surfaces are positioned at the center of a $128 \times 128 \times 128$ mm^3 co-ordinate system (see Fig. 2, where the blue contours are the sampled surfaces, the red ones are the true surfaces). Two phantom intensity images are created as one horizontal rasterized ellipsoid $S(x)$ with $a = 56$, $b = 40$ mm centered at $(64, 64, 64)$, and one vertical rasterized ellipsoid $T(x)$ with $a = 40$, $b = 56$ mm centered at $(64, 64, 64)$. These two images serve as the context intensity profile around the phantom surfaces.

Three phantom experiments were performed to study how the intensity and uncertainty weighted surface cost functions interact. In the first experiment, the true template and target surfaces of the object of interest were aligned before any registration but the shapes of the ellipsoids differed. This experiment was designed to study how matching the image intensity with imperfect knowledge of the surface position would affect the pre-aligned objects of interest. The second and third experiments are similar to the first except the shapes of the objects of interest in the template and target images differed.

Three 3D template surfaces $X_1(u, v)$, $X_2(u, v)$, $X_3(u, v)$ (red contours in the top row of Fig. 2 were chosen to simulate three different template surface configurations. We jointly registered $T(x)$ to $S(x)$ and each $Y_{p_i}(u, v)$ to $X_1(u, v)$, $X_2(u, v)$, $X_3(u, v)$ using the five aforementioned methods, giving rise to a family of DVFs, one for each randomly sampled observer contour.

The registration performance of the five algorithms was measured using the relative overlap (RO) and surface dissimilarity (SD) between the deformed *true* target surface and the template surface. Here, the RO was quantified as the Dice coefficient and the SD is defined as Eq. 4 with $\omega(u, v) = 1$. The statistical results are reported in Table. 1 and displayed graphically in the bottom of Fig. 2.

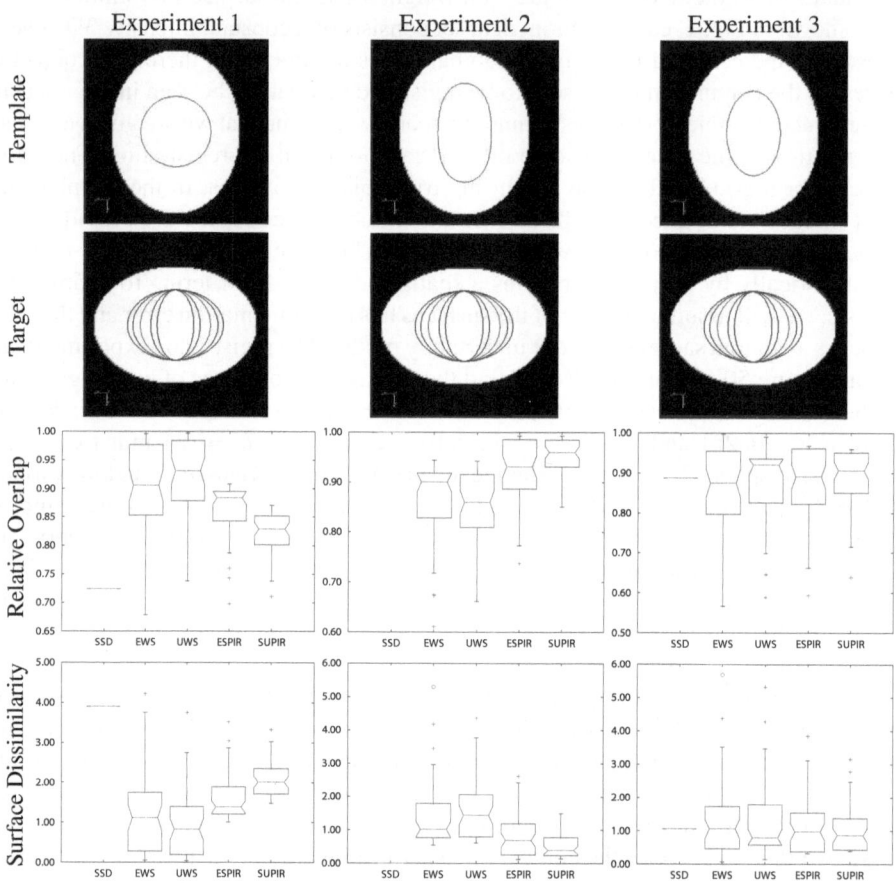

Fig. 2. Digital phantom geometry and registration evaluation results. The top two rows show cross-sections of the 3D phantoms constructed by revolving ellipses about the vertical axis of symmetry. The red contours denote the true boundaries while the blue contours illustrate for individual observer contours sampled from the normal ellipsoid diameter probability density distribution (only 4 of 50 are shown).

Table 1. Results of Monte Carlo stimulation with five algorithms on phantoms

	*Experiment*1				*Experiment*2				*Experiment*3			
	ROM	ROS	SDM	SDS	ROM	ROS	SDM	SDS	ROM	ROS	SDM	SDS
NOREG	0.874	0.118	1.476	1.304	0.704	0.079	4.120	1.204	0.738	0.103	3.771	1.423
SSD	0.724	0.000	3.899	0.000	**1.000**	0.000	**0.000**	0.000	**0.888**	0.000	1.065	0.000
EWS	0.900	0.083	1.208	1.039	0.859	0.081	1.471	1.001	0.862	0.112	1.339	1.188
UWS	**0.923**	0.066	**0.935**	0.820	0.856	0.067	1.561	0.850	0.868	0.098	1.326	1.097
ESPIR	0.864	0.047	1.592	0.586	0.923	0.065	0.815	0.642	0.878	0.091	1.125	0.838
SUPIR	0.823	0.037	2.081	0.432	0.951	0.039	0.550	0.384	**0.888**	0.075	**1.013**	0.672

ROM: Relative overlap mean, ROS: Relative overlap std.dev. SDM: Surface dissimilarity mean, SDS: Surface dissimilarity std.dev., the bold font indicates the best result under the corresponding metric

3.2 Prostate Cancer Case Study

We investigated how incorporating surface uncertainty into the registration process affects the FBCT-to-CBCT registration of a typical prostate patient. The prostate surface was segmented in the FBCT and CBCT by 5 experienced radiation oncology staff using a commercially available treatment planning system (Pinnacle version 8.1, Philips Medical Systems, Milpitas, CA). Contouring of FBCT and CBCT images was performed independently on each modality according to a detailed contouring protocol that provided instructions on the choice of window level and anatomical guidance on defining the surface. The 3D prostate surfaces were smoothed to remove high frequency noise resulting from surface reconstruction. The FBCT and CBCT images were aligned via a global affine transformation that minimized a mutual information dissimilarity cost. This transformation was applied to the associated surfaces which serve as the FBCT and CBCT training surfaces $X_i(u, v)$ and $Y_i(u, v)$, $i = 1$ to 5.

The correspondences among the training surfaces were established using the method described in [7]. The boundary variances of the training surfaces were computed as described in Sec. 2.3 and illustrated in Fig. 3. In this case, the largest uncertainty regions are near the prostate apex and at the interface between the prostate base and the bladder base.

The protrusion of the surface at the base of the prostate derived from the CBCT is not representative of the "true" surface because it is missing in the FBCT surface and it is a region where the experts did not agree. Therefore we chose the surface cost defined in Eq. 4 to evaluate the registration results. Additionally, we assume that the local contraction and expansion of prostate is small which implies the Jacobian should be approximately one in the prostate.

The FBCT and CBCT images were registered with the corresponding average surfaces using intensity-only registration (SSD), ESPIR and SUPIR. Before the registration the surface cost was 0.172, and after the registration the surface costs were 0.134, 0.043 and 0.044 for the three algorithms, respectively. It was observed that Jacobian of the SUPIR transformation was closer to unity than that of the ESPIR.

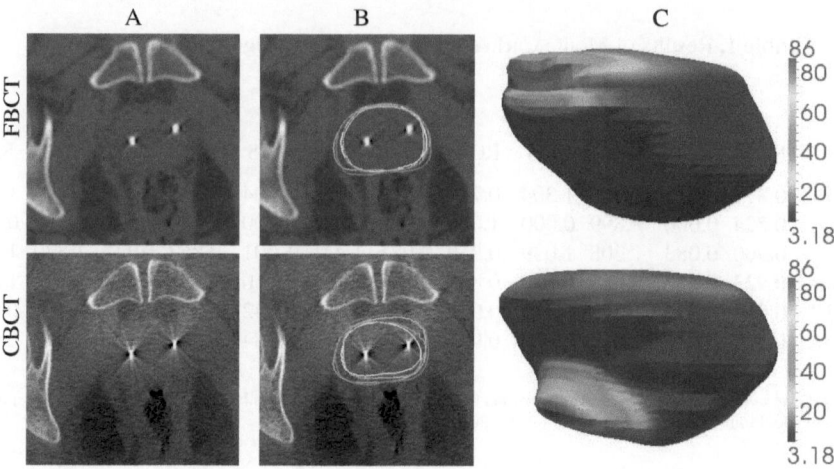

Fig. 3. The top and bottom rows illustrate the patient's FBCT and CBCT images respectively: A. The original gray-scale image, B. The same image overlaid by five prostate contours delineated by five experts marked as different colors, C. the interobserver variances about the mean surface (top: [2.02, 57.97] mm^2, bottom: [3.18, 86.00] mm^2)

4   Discussion and Conclusion

In contrast to traditional registration methods in which the template and target surfaces (or other features) are assumed as ground truth, our method takes segmentation error into account. In the case of bladder/prostate CT imaging, slice-by-slice 2D manual contouring is highly time-consuming and has limited accuracy. Any single observer's delineation may have large deviations over part of the pelvic organ surface. Therefore registration with a statistical model that accounts for surface segmentation errors may provide improved registration performance in clinical treatment.

Aiming to reduce the impact of delineation error on non-rigid registration of multi-modality pelvic image sets, this paper presented a non-rigid image registration framework that incorporates the intensity and surface segmentation error. Proof-of-principle experiments were presented for 3D idealized digital phantoms and one real patient case. By comparing the results with registration algorithms without considering the surface segmentation error, our method has shown the potentials under specific scope of applicability.

Acknowledgments. This work was supported by the National Cancer Institute Grant No P01CA116602.

References

1. Christensen, G., Carlson, B., Chao, K., Yin, P., Grigsby, P., Nguyen, K., Dempsey, J., Lerma, F., Bae, K., Vannier, M., et al.: Image-based dose planning of intracavitary brachytherapy: registration of serial-imaging studies using deformable anatomic templates. International Journal of Radiation Oncology Biology Physics 51(1), 227–243 (2001)

2. Davies, R., Twining, C., Cootes, T., Waterton, J., Taylor, C.: A minimum description length approach to statistical shape modeling. IEEE Transactions on Medical Imaging 21(5), 525–537 (2002)
3. Greene, W.H., Chelikani, S., Purushothaman, K., Knisely, J.P.S., Chen, Z., Papademetris, X., Staib, L.H., Duncan, J.S.: Constrained non-rigid registration for use in image-guided adaptive radiotherapy. Medical Image Analysis 13(5), 809 (2009)
4. Hartkens, T., Hill, D.L.G., Castellano-Smith, A.D., Hawkes, D.J., Maurer Jr., C.R., Martin, A.J., Hall, W.A., Liu, H., Truwit, C.L.: Using Points and Surfaces to Improve Voxel-Based Non-rigid Registration. In: Dohi, T., Kikinis, R. (eds.) MICCAI 2002, Part II. LNCS, vol. 2489, pp. 565–572. Springer, Heidelberg (2002)
5. Joshi, A.A., Shattuck, D.W., Thompson, P.M., Leahy, R.M.: Surface-constrained volumetric brain registration using harmonic mappings. IEEE Transactions on Medical Imaging 26(12), 1657–1669 (2007)
6. Kurtek, S., Klassen, E., Ding, Z., Jacobson, S., Jacobson, J., Avison, M., Srivastava, A.: Parameterization-invariant shape comparisons of anatomical surfaces. IEEE Transactions on Medical Imaging 30(3), 849 (2011)
7. Kurtek, S., Klassen, E., Ding, Z., Avison, M.J., Srivastava, A.: Parameterization-Invariant Shape Statistics and Probabilistic Classification of Anatomical Surfaces. In: Székely, G., Hahn, H.K. (eds.) IPMI 2011. LNCS, vol. 6801, pp. 147–158. Springer, Heidelberg (2011)
8. Postelnicu, G., Zollei, L., Fischl, B.: Combined volumetric and surface registration. IEEE Transactions on Medical Imaging 28(4), 508 (2009)
9. Remeijer, P., Rasch, C., Lebesque, J.V., van Herk, M.: A general methodology for three-dimensional analysis of variation in target volume delineation. Medical Physics 26(6), 931–940 (1999)
10. Rohr, K., Stiehl, H., Sprengel, R., Buzug, T., Weese, J., Kuhn, M.: Landmark-based elastic registration using approximating thin-plate splines. IEEE Transactions on Medical Imaging 20(6), 526–534 (2001)
11. Rueckert, D., Sonoda, L.I., Hayes, C., Hill, D.L.G., Leach, M.O., Hawkes, D.J.: Nonrigid registration using free-form deformations: application to breast mr images. IEEE Transactions on Medical Imaging 18(8), 712 (1999)
12. Wells, W.M., Viola, P., Atsumi, H., Nakajima, S., Kikinis, R.: Multi-modal volume registration by maximization of mutual information. Medical Image Analysis 1(1), 35–51 (1996)
13. Wu, J., Murphy, M.J., Weiss, E., Sleeman IV, W.C., Williamson, J.: Development of a population-based model of surface segmentation uncertainties for uncertainty-weighted deformable image registrations. Medical Physics 37(2), 607–614 (2010)
14. Wrz, S., Rohr, K.: Physics-based elastic registration using non-radial basis functions and including landmark localization uncertainties. Computer Vision and Image Understanding 111(3), 263–274 (2008)

Tracking by Detection for Interactive Image Augmentation in Laparoscopy[*]

Jae-Hak Kim[1,2], Adrien Bartoli[1], Toby Collins[1], and Richard Hartley[3]

[1] ISIT, Faculté de Médecine, Université d'Auvergne, France
[2] LASMEA, Université Blaise Pascal, France
[3] CECS, The Australian National University, Australia

Abstract. We present a system for marking, tracking and visually augmenting a deformable surgical site by the robust automatic detection of natural landmarks (image features) in laparoscopic surgery. In our system, the surgeon first selects a frame containing an organ of interest, and this is used by our system both to detect every instance of the organ in a laparoscopic video feed, and to recover the nonrigid deformations. The system then augments the video with customizable visual information such as the location of hidden or weakly visible structures (cysts, vessels, etc), or planned incision points, acquired from pre-operative or intra-operative data. Frame-rate organ detection is performed via a novel procedure that matches the current frame to the reference frame. Because laparoscopic images are known to be extremely difficult to match, we propose to use Shape-from-Shading and conformal flattening to cancel out much of the variation in appearance due to perspective foreshortening, and we then apply robust matching to the flattened surfaces. Experiments show robust tracking and detection results on a laparoscopic procedure with the uterus as target organ. As our system detects the organ in every frame, it is not impaired by target loss, contrary to most previous methods.

Keywords: tracking, detection, laparoscopy, conformal mapping, deformable surface.

1 Introduction

In laparoscopic surgery, one of the difficulties for surgeons is to correctly identify the surgical site, such as the location of hidden structures and planned incision points, in the camera's image. This is especially significant in tumor resection, when the tumor is occluded behind tissue. To resolve this, surgeons and radiologists currently use pre-operative data such as Magnetic Resonance Imaging (MRI), Computed Tomography (CT) or Ultrasound (US) images to help locate the target structure in the image.

[*] This research has been supported by Prof. Richard Hartley's Chair of Excellence grant from Région Auvergne, France.

B.M. Dawant et al. (Eds.): WBIR 2012, LNCS 7359, pp. 246–255, 2012.
© Springer-Verlag Berlin Heidelberg 2012

It is estimated that there are 1,300 to 2,700 wrong-site surgeries annually in the United States [12]. Similar problems may arise in laparoscopy because it can be difficult for the surgeons to find the target site correctly, mainly due to disorientation and the difficulty of mentally matching the laparoscopic view with the pre-operative images. Solving the medical imaging problem of automatically overlaying laparoscopic images with surgical target locations is an open, yet highly important research goal. Not only would the solution benefit surgeons, but also patients in reducing the likelihood of surgical errors and complications.

We present a new system to mark and track the surgical site in laparoscopic images. The surgical site is first marked by the surgeon in the 2D input images and in the reconstructed 3D surface video at an early stage of the laparoscopy. Then, our system automatically detects the location of the surgical site during surgery, and overlays the laparoscopic frames and reconstructed 3D surface video with visual information. Detecting the location of the surgical site requires robust feature matching and registration methods on nonrigid deformable surfaces. For this feature matching and tracking, a new approach using Shape-from-Shading (SfS) and conformal mapping is proposed and two robust methods are introduced for mapping a polygon boundary of the uterus in the reference image into the other frames by estimating a similarity transformation. Also, augmentation of the laparoscopic video using affine Moving Least Squares (affine-MLS) is proposed. We carried out experiments on in-vivo laparoscopic images captured by a Karl Storz laparoscopy system. Our method shows robust feature matching, tracking and augmentation results in laparoscopy.

Steps of Our Proposed System. Our proposed system takes steps such as marking and tracking surgical sites, then augmenting the surgical target. First, surgeons and radiologists examine pre-operative data such as MRI, CT and US images and determine the surgical site. However, the surgical site is only known in this pre-operative data in this stage. When a laparoscope is placed into a patient's body, surgeons and radiologists can see the surgical target and identify the exact location of the surgical site by referring to the pre-operative data. This identified location needs to be maintained during the surgery and it is our primary outcome to detect it at runtime. To locate and track the identified location of the target surgical site, a surgeon pauses a streaming video from the laparoscopy system, and draws a polygon around the surgical target, for instance, an ellipse surrounding a uterus. The 3D surface of the surgical target reconstructed by our system is then viewed by the surgeon in order to locate the surgical site in 3D. Next, the surgeon marks the surgical site on the 3D surface, for instance, a 3D arrow, which is stored in our system for tracking in the following frames. At this stage, anatomical landmarks can be used to register the pre-operative data to the reference laparoscopic image. This process of pausing and editing for augmentation in a laparoscopic image can be repeated by the surgeon as many times as needed during the surgical procedure. From this minor interaction by surgeons in the first image, our system computes the positions of the surgical target in the rest of the images and displays the surgical sites along with visual information such as boundaries of organs and 3D arrows in the 2D image or 3D view. As the system remembers the location of the surgical sites and allows surgeons to find them quickly, surgeons are now free to view monitor and check a patient's database then easily continue the surgery without referring to, or re-examining the pre-operative data to repeatedly identify the surgical site.

Surgical Site Tracking in Laparoscopic Images. Feature matching is a necessary first step, however, it is not straightforward as the target organ is often deformable and many state-of-the-art feature-matching algorithms [8] in computer vision are designed only for rigid objects. Our motivation comes from the assumption that it is possible to map a reconstructed 3D shape into another representation in a space which can be easier for feature matching. For mapping to another space, a conformal mapping is applied to the known 3D shape. Conformal mapping is a popular method in computer graphics [6] as it can be used to assign a texture onto a surface. This conformal mapping flattens out the 3D shape onto a plane while preserving angles locally. This is a nice property, as given two conformally mapped flattened surfaces they should be related by a local similarity transformation. In other words, two neighbouring points on a flattened mesh can be transformed to two corresponding points on another flattened mesh by a scale, rotation and translation. (Note that the similarity transformation is valid only locally but not globally.) Therefore, feature matching is done on the flattened images instead of the original input images, and we · used Pizarro and Bartoli's feature matching algorithm [10] to incorporate the local similarity, which is based on the SIFT [7] descriptor.

Once a set of matching points and the initial position of the organ are given, tracking becomes a problem of finding the approximation by a global similarity transformation. We assume that a set of local similarity transformations can be approximated by a global similarity transformation, which means the deformation on the surface changes only a small part of the shape of the surface. Also, the positions of the surgical targets tracked and overlaid on the original image are obtained by using affine Moving Least Squares [11].

2   Related Work

Mountney *et al.* [8] evaluated various feature descriptors on Minimally Invasive Surgery (MIS) images and showed many feature descriptors do not work well. Although they provide an approach to selecting the best method among their evaluated algorithms and a Bayesian fusion method to increase accuracy and performance, it is preferable to have a single algorithm to find matches instead of running various feature descriptors since computing various feature descriptors for Bayesian fusion consumes most of the computation time for a practical MIS application. Su *et al.* [14] used augmented reality for stereo-laparoscopic images, however, this is limited to a rigid surface and stereo camera based laparoscopy is required to recover the 3D structure of the surface. Schaefer *et al.* [11] introduced affine-MLS for image deformation. They showed that a proper deformation can be estimated from given key points on the surface mesh by a similarity transformation. Augmented Reality (AR) has been used in neurosurgery, otolaryngology and maxillofacial surgery [13]. Nicolau *et al.* claim that AR systems applied to MIS can increase the surgeon's intra-operative vision by providing virtual transparency of the patient, but they also emphasized that AR systems are not robust enough since deformation of organs and human movement make registration difficult [9].

3   Proposed Method

The general framework of our system is shown in Fig 1. Given a laparoscopic image $\mathcal{I}_0$ as a reference frame, an image point $\mathbf{p}_0$ is a projection of a 3D point

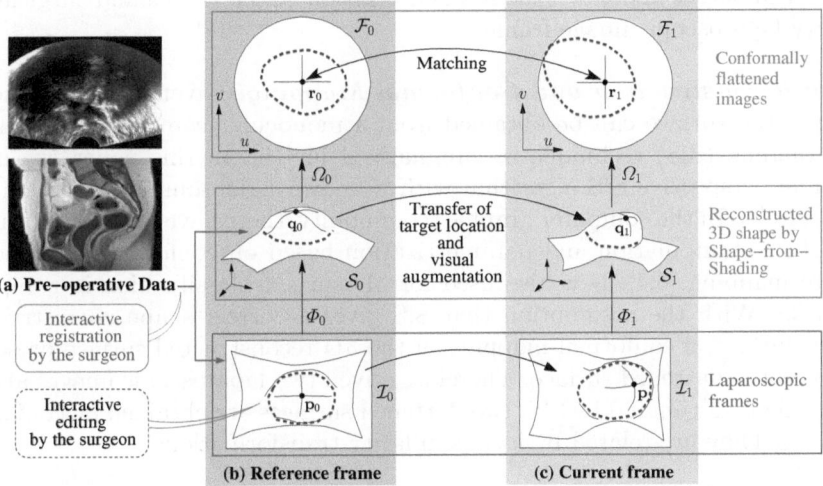

Fig. 1. System Overview. Three columns showing (a) Pre-operative Data, (b) The Reference Frame and (c) The Current Frame. In a manual-preprocessing phase, registration is achieved interactively between (a) and (b). Then any surgical target planned from (a), for instance regions of interest or planned incision paths to be visualised in the laparoscopic images, can be transformed onto (b) via the interactive registration. The second phase involves tracking the surgical target, transferring the target location and augmenting visual information in subsequent laparoscopic images. The correspondence between (b) and (c) is achieved automatically using our robust matching method. This results in a set of robust feature matches. Determining the positions of the targets in (c) can then be achieved by mapping their locations in (b) to (c) via feature-based warping. Points $\mathbf{p}_0$ and $\mathbf{p}_1$ in two laparoscopic images $\mathcal{I}_0$ and $\mathcal{I}_1$ are back-projected by Φ to the surfaces $\mathcal{S}_0$ and $\mathcal{S}_1$ as 3D points $\mathbf{q}_0$ and $\mathbf{q}_1$, respectively. These 3D points are mapped to points $\mathbf{r}_0$ and $\mathbf{r}_1$ on planar surfaces $\mathcal{F}_0$ and $\mathcal{F}_1$ by a conformal mapping Ω. Blue dotted lines indicate the boundary of the uterus, which is determined by surgeons and radiologists from pre-operative data such as MRI, CT or US in the reference image $\mathcal{I}_0$. The boundary and marked point in the reference frame $\mathcal{I}_0$ are tracked to the next frame $\mathcal{I}_1$ automatically. Our goal for augmentation is thus to determine and visualise the bounding region in $\mathcal{I}_1$, by performing image matching between $\mathcal{F}_0$ and $\mathcal{F}_1$.

$\mathbf{q}_0$ on the surface $\mathcal{S}_0$. This projection can be represented by Φ^{-1}. Therefore, the 3D point $\mathbf{q}_0$ is $\mathbf{q}_0 = \Phi_0(\mathbf{p}_0)$. It can be mapped to a point $\mathbf{r}_0$ on a flat surface $\mathcal{F}_0$ by a conformal mapping Ω_0. As a result, $\mathbf{r}_0 = \Omega_0(\mathbf{q}_0) = \Omega_0(\Phi_0(\mathbf{p}_0))$. Given another frame image $\mathcal{I}_1$ and a point $\mathbf{p}_1$, in a similar way we may obtain the point $\mathbf{r}_1$ on a planar surface $\mathcal{F}_1$ as $\mathbf{r}_1 = \Omega_1(\mathbf{q}_1) = \Omega_1(\Phi_1(\mathbf{p}_1))$. Assuming that image pixel points $\mathbf{p}_0$ and $\mathbf{p}_1$ are a corresponding match, then the points $\mathbf{r}_0$ and $\mathbf{r}_1$ on the flat surfaces should be a pair of matching points in local isotropy. In other words, $\mathbf{r}_0$ and $\mathbf{r}_1$ are related by a similarity transformation locally. This is a key motivation that constructs our system for tracking by detection in laparoscopic images. Surgeons and radiologists use pre-operative data such as MRI, CT or US to locate the uterus and surgical site. Then the position of the surgical site is marked on the reference image $\mathcal{I}_0$ and 3D mesh surface $\mathcal{S}_0$. Afterwards our system will detect and track the marked position of the uterus and surgical site in every laparoscopic image frame.

Shape Reconstruction and Conformal Mapping. Given an image, the 3D shape of the surface can be obtained from a monocular camera by the Shape-from-Shading (SfS) technique as summarized in [15]. In this paper, we use a real-time perspective SfS algorithm with a known light source calibration, described in [1]. In the computer graphics community, there have been many studies on surface manipulation and parametrization based on conformal mapping for texture mapping [6,4]. It is also used for 3D surface classification in computer vision [3]. With the assumption that SfS gives a correct shape reconstruction for the surface, a conformal mapping of the 3D reconstructed surface preserves angles on the flattened surface. Therefore, given two laparoscopic images and an surface shape estimated by SfS, two flattened surfaces are obtained by conformal mapping. They are related by local similarity transformations.

Feature Matching and Outlier Removal. For every incoming video frame, we estimate the 3D surface $\mathcal{S}_1$ using the same SfS method as for $\mathcal{S}_0$, and flatten it to give us image $\mathcal{F}_1$. We then detect features in $\mathcal{F}_1$ using SIFT, to give a query feature set $\mathcal{G}_1$. We then perform robust, nonrigid matching between $\mathcal{G}_0$ and $\mathcal{G}_1$ using Pizarro and Bartoli's feature matching algorithm [10]. It works by matching features using descriptor similarity, and determines a high-probability inlier set based on spatial agreement with respect to local warp models. However, it is not completely outlier-free. We suppose that the boundary warp of the organ between $\mathcal{F}_0$ and $\mathcal{F}_1$ can be coarsely approximated by a similarity transform. This contrasts with the transformation of the boundary from image $\mathcal{I}_0$ and $\mathcal{I}_1$, which, since these images comprise viewpoint changes, are likely to be more complex than a similarity transform. We have tested two robust similarity transformation estimation methods based on Horn's absolute orientation [5]. The first is to use matched features with RANSAC (Random Sample Consensus) [2] and the second is to optimise a robust pseudo-huber norm cost function. Both methods allow us to detect outliers (based on their matches conflicting with the similarity transform) which are then removed (we use a prediction error threshold). Once the boundary of the organ is estimated in $\mathcal{F}_1$ its shape in $\mathcal{I}_1$ is estimated as follows: first the vertices of the boundary in $\mathcal{F}_1$ are mapped into 3D space on $\mathcal{S}_1$ by barycentric interpolation. Then, they are projected onto $\mathcal{I}_1$ using the camera's projection function Φ to give the boundary of the organ in $\mathcal{I}_1$.

Surgical Target Mapping. Finally, we determine the positions of the surgical targets in $\mathcal{I}_1$ as follows. First, we transform the inlier matches from $\mathcal{F}_1$ to $\mathcal{I}_1$. We then use affine-MLS [11] to smoothly warp the target positions located on $\mathcal{I}_0$ to $\mathcal{I}_1$, driven by the feature correspondences. This involves a single free parameter, the affine-MLS bandwidth, which we have set to $\sigma = 150$ pixels in all of our tests. Once in position, the locations of the surgical targets are marked and presented to the surgeon, overlaid on top of the original input frame.

4 Experiments

We have carried out experiments on an image sequence in which a uterus is to be cut by a surgeon in order to remove a myoma (uterine fibroid) inside the uterus. As the myoma is not visible, surgeons and radiologists examine pre-operative data such as MRI and CT to determine the location of the surgical site, which will be the point of first-cut. An image sequence is captured by a Karl Storz laparoscopy system and the size of image is 1048×576 pixels at 25 FPS. The number of captured frames is 2661 (1 min and 46 seconds). Samples of the image sequence are shown in Fig 2-(Top Row). From the input images, our SfS algorithm estimates the shape of the uterus as shown in Fig 2-(Middle Row).

Then, conformal mapping is applied to the shape to obtain a flattened image at each frame as shown in Fig 2-(Bottom Row). These flattened images are used for finding feature matches. These matches are used to estimate a global similarity transformation for mapping the polygon boundary of the uterus at the reference frame to the following image frames as shown in Fig 3.

Assuming that the surgeon selects frame 489 as a reference image, a polygon is drawn by the surgeon around the boundary of the uterus. The polygon is then transfered to other images when the video is resumed by the surgeon. Several frames of this result are shown in Fig 4 and Fig 5.

In Fig 6, the incision path and surgical site are shown as 3D arrows and a green curve, which are aligned on the surface of the uterus and augmented over all frames. The 3D arrows are orthogonal to the surface of the uterus recovered from SfS. Therefore, they provide useful information for surgeons to decide the orientation of the blade to enter the uterus. In this experiment, we used an open arc in Fig 6-(Bottom-right) as our planned incision path This was manually marked by burning on the surface of the uterus, then overlaid in each subsequent view in the sequence by mapping using the correspondence via affine-MLS [11]. A selection of augmented frames from the sequence is shown in Fig 6. A video result is available at `http://youtu.be/LiZKmcV_fRg`. With our system, this redundant burn mark is no longer necessary.

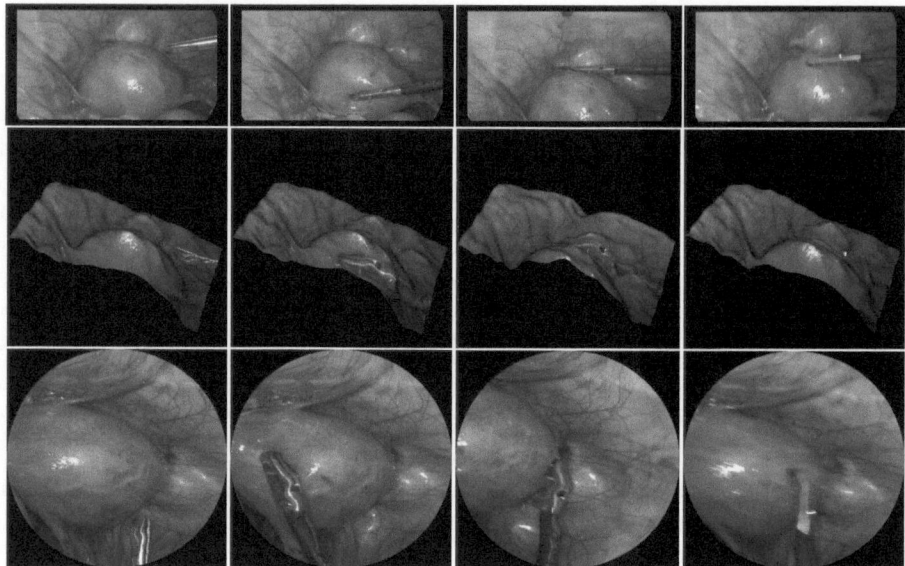

Fig. 2. Samples of input images, 3D surface reconstruction and conformal mapping. (Top Row) Frames number 489, 630, 733 and 790 (Left to Right). At frame 489, the uterus (an ellipsoid-like shape) is completely visible and it is a best candidate as a reference frame. At frame 630, the uterus is occluded by a surgical tool and it is deformed when pressed. At frame 733, only a half of the uterus is visible. At frame 790, the image is blurred by fast motion of the camera. (Middle Row) 3D surface shape from SfS at frame 480, 630, 730 and 790. (Bottom Row) Flattened image by conformal mapping of the 3D shape at frame 480, 630, 730 and 790.

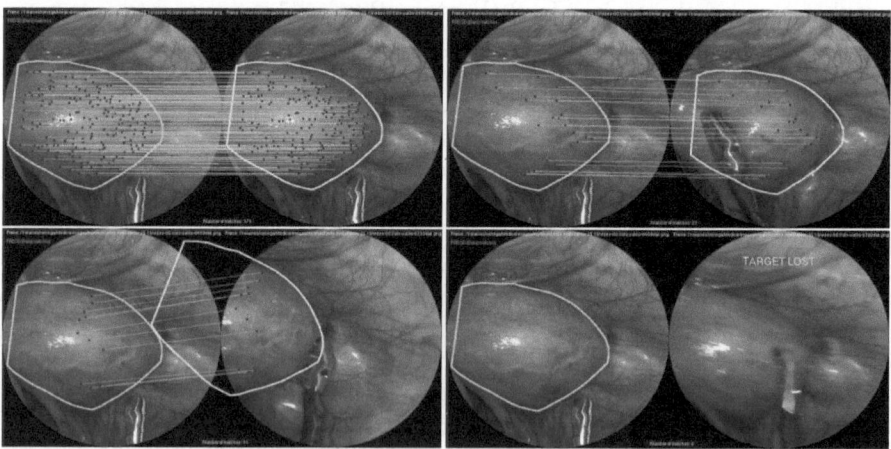

Fig. 3. Feature matching and tracking between flattened images. (Top-left) In frames 489 and 490, a total of 179 matches are found and the cyan polygon in reference frame 489 is mapped to a yellow polygon in the next frame 490. (Top-right) Matches and tracking between frame 489 and 630. In total 22 matches are found. (Bottom-left) 11 matches are found between frame 489 and 733. (Bottom-right) Tracking failed as no matches are found between frame 489 and 790.

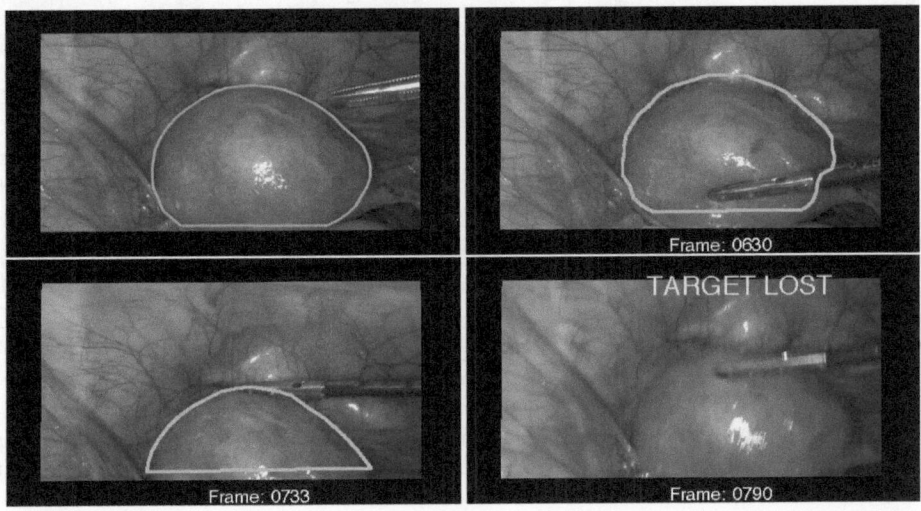

Fig. 4. Frames with uterus tracking. (Top-Left) Reference frame 489 with a green polygon drawn on the boundary of the uterus. (Top-Right) At frame 630, tracking of the uterus is shown as a green polygon. (Bottom-Left) At frame 730, tracking is still successful for the half visible uterus. (Bottom-Right) At frame 799, tracking fails because of blurring in the image.

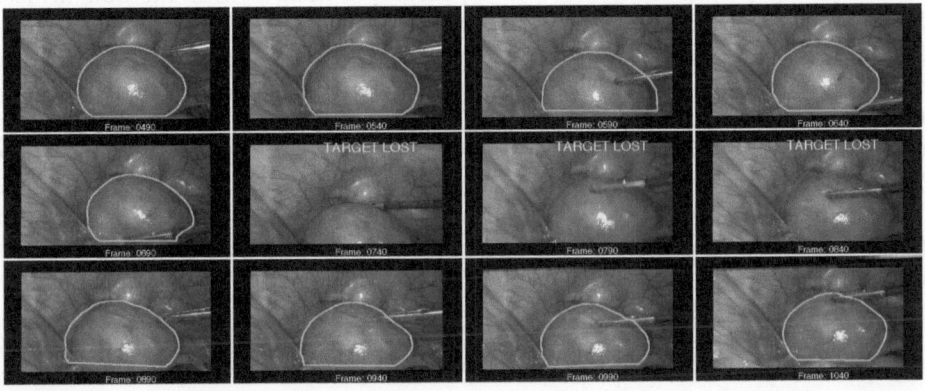

Fig. 5. Tracking the uterus. Results of tracking a uterus from laparoscopic images are shown. The boundary of the tracked uterus is indicated as a green polygon and a message (target lost) is given when the system is searching for the uterus at the current frame. Note that our system fails to track the uterus at frame 740, however tracking resumes and finds the uterus successfully at frames 890 and 1,040.

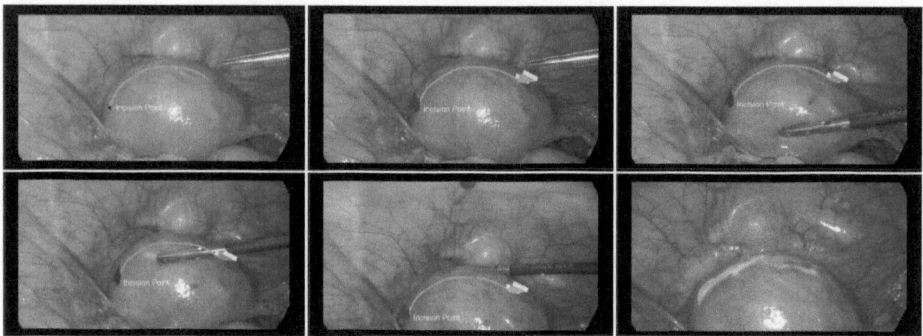

Fig. 6. 3D augmentation in laparoscopy. (Top row and bottom first two columns) These are sample images of 3D augmentation in laparoscopic images. A red (left) 3D arrow indicates the incision point, A yellow (right) 3D arrow shows the ending point, and a green curve shows the surgical site for the surgeon's first-cut. Our system augments this 3D visual information by tracking the uterus over all frames. (Bottom-right) At frame 2173, a surgeon made a burn mark on the surface of the uterus. This is not necessary in our system. The video is available at the link: http://youtu.be/hvzE9VIAjPI.

5   Conclusion

In this paper, we presented a new method for tracking and augmenting surgical targets in laparoscopic images. The system allows surgeons to mark the surgical site using pre-operative data in laparoscopic images. Our method utilizes Shape-from-Shading to recover the 3D shape of the surface, and the 3D shape is flattened by a conformal mapping which preserves angles on the surface. Feature matching is carried out on the flattened images and a global similarity transformation is applied to obtain a mapped boundary of the surgical target and outliers are removed. The surgical target registration by an affine Moving Least Squares warp made the surgical target can be localized in a laparoscopic image. Real experiments conducted on a uterus in laparoscopic images show robust tracking of the uterus and consistent surgical target augmentation. The method obviates the necessity to mark the surgical site physically on the organ surface

References

1. Collins, T., Bartoli, A.: Towards live monocular 3d laparoscopy using shading and specularity information. In: IPCAI (2012)
2. Fischler, M., Bolles, R.: Random sample consensus: a paradigm for model fitting with applications to image analysis and automated cartography. Communications of the ACM 24(6) (June 1981)
3. Gu, X., Yau, S.: Surface classification using conformal structures. In: Proceedings. Ninth IEEE International Conference on Computer Vision, vol. 1, pp. 701–708 (2003)

4. Haker, S., Angenent, S., Tannenbaum, A., Kikinis, R., Sapiro, G., Halle, M.: Conformal surface parameterization for texture mapping. IEEE Transactions on Visualization and Computer Graphics 6(2), 181–189 (2000)
5. Horn, B.K.P.: Closed-form solution of absolute orientation using unit quaternions. JOSA A 4(4), 629–642 (1987)
6. Lévy, B., Petitjean, S., Ray, N., Maillot, J.: Least squares conformal maps for automatic texture atlas generation. In: ACM SIGGRAPH Conference Proceedings (April 2002)
7. Lowe, D.: Distinctive image features from scale-invariant keypoints. International Journal of Computer Vision 60(2), 91–110 (2004)
8. Mountney, P., Lo, B., Thiemjarus, S., Stoyanov, D., Zhong-Yang, G.: A Probabilistic Framework for Tracking Deformable Soft Tissue in Minimally Invasive Surgery. In: Ayache, N., Ourselin, S., Maeder, A. (eds.) MICCAI 2007, Part II. LNCS, vol. 4792, pp. 34–41. Springer, Heidelberg (2007)
9. Nicolau, S., Solar, L., Mutter, D., Marescaux, J.: Augmented reality in laparoscopy surgical oncology. Surgical Oncology 20, 189–201 (2011)
10. Pizarro, D., Bartoli, A.: Feature-based deformable surface detection with self-occlusion reasoning. International Journal of Computer Vision (2011) (published online April 27, 2011)
11. Schaefer, S., McPhail, T., Warren, J.: Image deformation using moving least squares. ACM Transactions on Graphics (TOG) 25(3), 533–540 (2006)
12. Seiden, S.C., Barach, P.: Wrong-side/wrong-site, wrong-procedure, and wrong-patient adverse events: Are they preventable? Archives of Surgery 141(9), 931–939 (2006)
13. Shuhaiber, J.H.: Augmented reality in surgery. ARCH SURG 139, 170–174 (2004)
14. Su, L.M., Vagvolgyi, B.P., Agarwal, R., Reiley, C.E., Taylor, R.H., Hager, G.D.: Augmented reality during robot-assisted laparoscopic partial nephrectomy: Toward real-time 3d-ct to stereoscopic video registration. Journal of Urology 73(4), 896–900 (2009)
15. Zhang, R., Tsai, P., Cryer, J., Shah, M.: Shape-from-shading: a survey. IEEE Transactions on Pattern Analysis and Machine Intelligence 21(8), 690–706 (1999)

On Combining Algorithms
for Deformable Image Registration

Sascha E.A. Muenzing[1], Bram van Ginneken[2], and Josien P.W. Pluim[1]

[1] Image Sciences Institute, University Medical Center Utrecht, The Netherlands
[2] Diagnostic Image Analysis Group, Radboud University Nijmegen Medical Center,
The Netherlands
{sascha,josien}@isi.uu.nl, b.vanginneken@rad.umcn.nl

Abstract. We propose a meta-algorithm for registration improvement by combining deformable image registrations (MetaReg). It is inspired by a well-established method from machine learning, the combination of classifiers. MetaReg consists of two main components: (1) A strategy for composing an improved registration by combining deformation fields from different registration algorithms. (2) A method for regularization of deformation fields post registration (UnfoldReg). In order to compare and combine different registrations, MetaReg utilizes a landmark-based classifier for assessment of local registration quality. We present preliminary results of MetaReg, evaluated on five CT pulmonary breathhold inspiration and expiration scan pairs, employing a set of three registration algorithms (NiftyReg, Demons, Elastix). MetaReg generated for each scan pair a registration that is better than any registration obtained by each registration algorithm separately. On average, 10% improvement is achieved, with a reduction of 30% of regions with misalignments larger than 5mm, compared to the best single registration algorithm.

Keywords: Deformable image registration, meta-algorithm, combination, pattern recognition.

1   Introduction

Accurate registration of medical images is key to medical image analysis. Recently an evaluation study on pulmonary intra-patient CT registration has evaluated and ranked state-of-the-art registration algorithms on a common data set [11]. Although many of those algorithms achieve excellent results on average, e.g. for the currently top five ranked algorithms average landmark registration errors are no more than 0.83mm, no single algorithm outperforms all others on every scan pair and every region within the images. (cp. empire10.isi.uu.nl/mainResults: category rankings on average and per scan pair).

In this paper we propose a meta-algorithm for deformable image registration (MetaReg) that composes an improved registration by combining locally superior regions from different registrations. In order to compare different registrations, MetaReg utilizes a landmark-based classifier for assessment of local

B.M. Dawant et al. (Eds.): WBIR 2012, LNCS 7359, pp. 256–265, 2012.

registration quality. Based on this assessment, deformation fields are partitioned and quality categories are assigned to each partition. Next, a voting scheme is applied to compose an improved registration by selecting superior partitions of the deformation fields generated by different registration algorithms. Finally, UnfoldReg is applied, primarily to unfold regions where different deformation field partitions are joined.

Deformable Image Registration. Registration of a moving image $I_M(\mathbf{x})$: $\Omega_M \subset \mathbb{R}^D \mapsto \mathbb{R}$ to a fixed image $I_F(\mathbf{x}) : \Omega_F \subset \mathbb{R}^D \mapsto \mathbb{R}$, both of dimension D, is the problem of finding a displacement $\mathbf{u}(\mathbf{x})$ that makes $I_M(\mathbf{x} + \mathbf{u}(\mathbf{x}))$ spatially aligned to $I_F(\mathbf{x})$. We define the obtained transformation field $\mathbf{T}(\mathbf{x}) = \mathbf{x} + \mathbf{u}(\mathbf{x})$ and the registered image $I_R(\mathbf{x}) = I_M(\mathbf{x}) \circ \mathbf{T}(\mathbf{x})$. The optimal transformation is found by optimizing a distance or similarity measure, such as the normalized mutual information (NMI). If the underlying transformation model allows local deformations, i.e. nonlinear fields $\mathbf{T}(\mathbf{x})$, then we call it deformable image registration (DIR).

2   Materials

The MetaReg algorithm has several input components: image data, registration algorithms and a method to locally assess registration quality. These components are considered interchangeable (i.e. can be replaced by other choices) and they are therefore described here.

2.1   Image Data

Five patients (male, ages 51-75yrs) were chosen randomly from a lung cancer screening database, each with a breathhold inspiration and a breathhold expiration CT scan, made in the same session. The inspiration scan was created using a low-dose protocol (30mAs) whereas the expiration scan was ultra-low-dose (20mAs), both with a slice spacing of 0.70 mm and pixel spacing between 0.63mm and 0.77mm.

2.2   Registration Algorithms

To compose an improved registration result by combining the best outcomes of various methods, registrations by several methods are required. We have chosen the following three registration algorithms for this study, because they performed well in EMPIRE10 [11], are publicly available, and have very different approaches. Other methods can of course be included.

NiftyReg [7] contains a global and local registration algorithm. The global registration is based on a block-matching technique and the local registration is based on a B-Spline deformation model. The objective function is composed of the normalized mutual information as a metric and optionally, the bending energy and the squared Jacobian determinant as penalty terms.

Elastix [4] is a toolbox that consists of algorithms for image registration. We employed in our experiments an affine and a nonrigid B-Spline registration algorithm along with a normalized correlation criterion as similarity measure and a parameter-free stochastic gradient optimizer.

Demons [15] is a non-parametric registration algorithm that can be seen as an optimization procedure on the entire space of displacement fields. We employed in our experiments a diffeomorphic version of demons along with a second-order minimization technique to optimize a normalized intensity similarity measure.

2.3   Local Registration Quality Assessment

We employ an extended version of the method for automatic detection of registration errors described in [8]. The method is based on supervised learning of local alignment patterns, which are captured by statistical image features at automatically detected landmarks.

For supervised learning a training database S is established. It combines information from three datasets: a) reference landmark matchings, b) reference image registrations, and c) statistical image features. The set of reference landmark matchings consists of landmarks l_F on the fixed image I_F and their corresponding location l_M in the moving image I_M. Landmarks l_F are automatically detected whereas landmarks l_M are matched manually. The landmark detection method is based on [5]. This method proved reliable in covering the anatomy of lungs in CT images. Landmarks are automatically detected in the lung region based on their distinctiveness, i.e. the dissimilarity to their surrounding region. The detection method is regulated to produce an even distribution of landmarks throughout the lungs. The generated landmarks are typically located at vessel bifurcations. The set of reference image registrations consists of several transformation fields **T** obtained by different automatic registration algorithms. Typically, an affine registration, and a coarse and fine level deformable registration is suitable to obtain a reference of local alignment variations, of both, correctly and wrongly aligned image structures. The set of statistical image features (FS) contains for each landmark l_F corresponding feature values that are computed based on nine different image feature types. Gaussian, correlation, and entropy features are calculated from the intensity images (I_F and I_R), and deformation features are computed on the transformation field (**T**).

Based on the database S, a classifier cascade is trained to classify local alignment patterns into three quality categories: correct (CA), poor (PA), and wrong alignment (WA). The quality categories are based on the landmark registration error (LRE), i.e. the amount of misalignment between a registered landmark position $\mathbf{T}(l_F)$ and the corresponding reference matching l_M, which is defined as follows: $CA \doteq \{LRE \leq 2\text{ mm}\}$, $PA \doteq \{2 < LRE < 5\text{ mm}\}$, $WA \doteq \{LRE \geq 5\text{ mm}\}$.

To automatically classify a previously unseen registration, first a set of l_P landmarks is automatically detected on I_F. Second, image features are extracted according to FS for each landmark l_P. Finally, the trained classifier is employed to predict for each landmark sample one of the above defined quality categories. That way, an assessment of local image registration quality is obtained. In the following we refer to the entity of this supervised Registration Error Detection method by RED.

3   Methods

A graphical overview of MetaReg is given in Figure 1. It visualizes from top to bottom the main computing steps of the MetaReg algorithm, from the input of a set of transformations from different registration algorithms to the output of a combined registration. In the following we first briefly formulate the basic idea of MetaReg and then explain step by step the stages illustrated in Figure 1.

Given a set of registration algorithms $\psi_1, \psi_2, \ldots, \psi_N$ and their corresponding deformation fields $\mathbf{u}_1, \mathbf{u}_2, \ldots, \mathbf{u}_N$ for a particular scan pair $sp = \{I_F, I_M\}$, we aim to find a combination $\Psi := \sum_{n=1}^{N} \mathbf{a}_n \mathbf{u}_n(\mathbf{x})$ such that Ψ outperforms any single ψ_n. $\mathbf{a}_n$ denotes the weight coefficient with which $\mathbf{u}_n$ is combined. That means we aim to exploit the locally different behavior of base registration algorithms ψ_n to improve the accuracy and the reliability of the combined registration algorithm, MetaReg. The weight coefficients $\mathbf{a}_n$ are determined by assessment of the local registration quality of each deformation field $\mathbf{u}_n$. For this assessment we utilize the RED system described in Section 2.3.

3.1   RED Partitioning

RED obtains automatically local estimates of registration quality by comparing local alignment patterns between the fixed image I_F and the registered moving image I_R at landmarks l_P. Next we perform a Voronoi decomposition of the deformation field $\mathbf{u}_n$ based on the landmarks l_P. That is, $\mathbf{u}_n$ is partitioned into regions such that the partition s_i contains all those points of $\mathbf{u}_n$ that are closer to landmark l_i than to any other landmark l_j. We calculate the Voronoi decomposition based on the distance of the landmarks l_P in the fixed image I_F employing an algorithm that approximates the Euclidean distance with voxel accuracy [2,1]. This Voronoi decomposition serves as a dense and closed estimate of registration quality assessment, i.e. every voxel of the ROI is assigned a quality category: CA,PA or WA. We define $\mathbf{u}_n \text{RED}_p$ as the registration quality at partition s_p generated by base registration algorithm ψ_n.

3.2   Voting

A voting scheme is needed to select for each partition s_p the best performing registration algorithm(s) ϕ_n. We select the partition s_p of $\mathbf{u}_n$ by assigning the weight coefficient $\mathbf{a}_n(\mathbf{x}) = 1, \forall \mathbf{x} : \mathbf{x} \in s_p(\mathbf{x})$. All weight coefficients are initialized with $\mathbf{a}_n = 0$.

We opt for following voting strategy: Compare all registrations $\mathbf{u}_n$ for the partition s_p and select the registration $\mathbf{u}_i$ which registration quality $\mathbf{u}_i \text{RED}_p$ is superior to all other $\mathbf{u}_n \text{RED}_p$. If there is more than one registration $\mathbf{u}_n$ with $\mathbf{u}_i \text{RED}_p$, then select all those $\mathbf{u}_n$.

3.3 Combining

In the above voting scheme we determined weight coefficients $\mathbf{a}_n$ for all $\mathbf{u}_n$. We are now able to generate the combined registration $\Psi = \sum_{n=1}^{N} \mathbf{a}_n \mathbf{u}_n(\mathbf{x}) / \sum_{n=1}^{N} \mathbf{a}_n$, where the division by $\sum_{n=1}^{N} \mathbf{a}_n$ results in averaged deformation field vectors at those voxels $\mathbf{x}$ with ties in the vote. Although the domain of Ψ is completely defined for each $\mathbf{x} \in I_F$, we further aim to obtain a bijective mapping Ψ. By imposing this property it can be ensured that the established Ψ contains no physical impossible mappings.

3.4 UnfoldReg

We developed a method (UnfoldReg) for unfolding deformation fields post registration. UnfoldReg is based on an algorithm for scattered data approximation that uses a multi-resolution uniform B-spline approximation scheme [14,5]. We refer to [14] for details of this algorithm.

In UnfoldReg we employ this algorithm for scattered data approximation as reconstruction algorithm. We compute the Jacobian map $JM(\mathbf{x}) = |J(\mathbf{T}(\mathbf{x}))|$ (J denotes the Jacobian matrix) for $\Psi(\mathbf{x})$, and construct a confidence map $CM(\mathbf{x})$, where we assign $CM(\mathbf{x}) = 0, \forall \mathbf{x} : JM(\mathbf{x}) \leq 0$. Further we expand these folding areas by applying a morphological dilation with a spherical kernel of radius 3 voxels. The confidence map $CM(\mathbf{x})$ is then used along with deformation field $\Psi(\mathbf{x})$ as input for the approximation algorithm. All voxels $\mathbf{x}$ of $\Psi(\mathbf{x})$ with $CM(\mathbf{x}) = 0$ are disregarded, and a reconstruction of the entire $\Psi(\mathbf{x})$ is obtained based on the remaining data. We use a linear B-Spline kernel function along with a multi-resolution scheme of 7 spatial resolutions. The reconstructed deformation field is again analyzed and processed as described above. This procedure is performed in an iterative scheme until all foldings are removed. Further, we monitor the unfolding progress and if foldings could not be removed in a consecutive iteration, then these folding voxels are dilated by an increased radius, thereby giving more space to unfold the deformation field. Foldings of large magnitude require more space to unfold than smaller ones. The iterative scheme evolves the deformation field gradually into a folding-free approximation of the original deformation field. In addition we assign staged confidence values (0.1,0.2,0.5,0.75) at voxels where two partitions from different registrations were joined (voting borders). Compare Figure 1 (n) (o).

4 Experiments

This section describes the application of the proposed MetaReg algorithm on a set of five pulmonary CT breath-hold inspiration-expiration scan pairs. The RED classifier was trained on this data. Each scan pair was registered with three different registration algorithms (NiftyReg, Demons and Elastix). MetaReg was then applied to the five scan pairs using the three resulting transformations and the trained RED classifier.

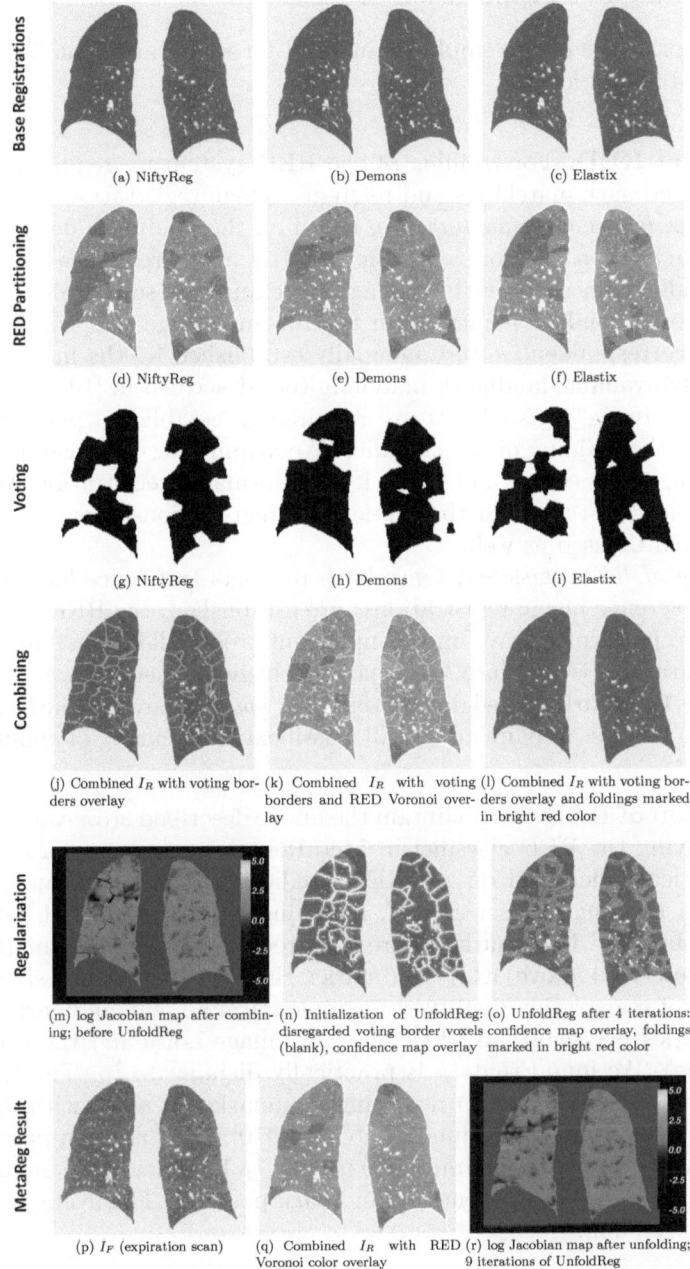

Fig. 1. Visualization of the main steps of the MetaReg shown exemplarily at transverse plane views of scan pair 5. RED color overlay: green, yellow and red color denote correct, poor and wrong alignment, respectively. Voting shows masks where black color marks selected regions.

4.1   Training and Application of RED

The main principle of the employed method for registration quality assessment is described in Section 2.3.

Training of RED. For training of the RED system we require a dataset of: reference landmark matchings and reference image registrations.

Reference landmark matchings are based on the landmark detection method described in Section 2.3. For each scan pair a set of 100 reference landmarks l_F is automatically defined on the fixed image I_F (expiration scan), and then matched with the corresponding points l_M in the moving image (inspiration scan). All landmark correspondences were manually established by the first author using the publicly available landmark matching tool described in [10].

Reference image registrations are required to establish a pool of alignment samples for the training of the classifier. We acquire for each scan pair an affine registration, and a coarse and a fine level deformable registration. We used the NiftyReg package to obtain these reference registrations, however, Demons or Elastix could be used as well.

Training of RED classifier. Once both datasets (reference landmark matchings and reference image registrations) are established, the RED system can be trained. We performed leave-one-scanpair-out cross-validation. This means, the learning dataset S is split into k mutually exclusive subsets S_k, $k \in 1, .., 5$ so that S_k contains landmark related data of scan pair sp_k exclusively. The RED classifier achieves on these scan pairs an overall classification accuracy of about 78%.

Application of RED. We maintain the above described cross-validation set-up when applying the RED classifier in MetaReg. A separate set of l_P landmarks is automatically detected on I_F. RED predictions on l_P of scan pair sp_k are based on a training dataset $S \setminus S_k$, including landmark related data from all scan pairs but sp_k. Landmarks l_P are acquired by the same landmark detection method (described above) as l_F landmarks. However, to obtain a spatially dense prediction of registration quality, we sampled around 500 landmarks (the exact number varies per scan pair, depending on image noise and the occurrence of emphysema). We found that l_F is practically disjunct to l_P. This is due to an increased sampling density for detecting landmarks l_P, along with the selection scheme of the automatic landmark detection [10]. Over all scan pairs, the averaged mean distance of l_F landmarks to nearest l_P landmarks is 6.8mm, with only in scan pairs 4 and 5 one identical landmark position. The averaged maximum distance is 12.9mm.

4.2   Configuration and Application of DIR Algorithms

For all three registrations algorithms employed in our experiments, a specific parametrization and registration set-up had been investigated and published in the context of an pulmonary intra-patient CT registration workshop [11].

Table 1. NiftyReg. Evaluated based on (a) reference data, and (b) RED predictions.

(a) Reference Evaluation

scan pair	min	max	mean	std	>5	>10	>20	fold-ing	over-lap
1	0.00	15.58	1.61	1.81	4	1	0	0	0
2	0.00	21.27	1.97	3.09	10	3	1	0	0
3	0.00	15.17	1.53	2.20	7	2	0	0	0
4	0.00	16.20	2.60	2.89	10	4	0	0	0
5	0.00	34.19	3.93	6.91	17	11	6	0	0
avg	0.00	20.48	**2.33**	3.38	48	21	7	0	0

(b) RED

scan pair	CA	PA	WA	# LMs
1	296	79	71	446
2	452	41	41	534
3	388	60	94	542
4	166	124	76	366
5	373	49	70	492
Sum	1675	353	352	2380
%	**70**	**15**	**15**	—

Table 2. Demons. Evaluated based on (a) reference data, and (b) RED predictions.

(a) Reference Evaluation

scan pair	min	max	mean	std	>5	>10	>20	fold-ing	over-lap
1	0.00	11.39	1.76	1.93	6	2	0	0	0
2	0.00	22.09	2.07	3.56	9	5	1	0	0
3	0.00	15.75	1.50	1.96	3	1	0	0	0
4	0.00	15.44	2.50	2.66	13	3	0	0	0
5	0.00	14.38	1.88	2.57	9	3	0	0	0
avg	0.00	15.81	**1.94**	2.53	40	14	1	0	0

(b) RED

scan pair	CA	PA	WA	# LMs
1	258	105	83	446
2	428	60	46	534
3	405	58	79	542
4	181	100	85	366
5	364	75	53	492
Sum	1636	398	346	2380
%	**69**	**17**	**14**	—

Table 3. Elastix. Evaluated based on (a) reference data, and (b) RED predictions.

(a) Reference Evaluation

scan pair	min	max	mean	std	>5	>10	>20	fold-ing	over-lap
1	0.00	18.51	2.12	2.80	8	3	0	0	7
2	0.00	19.52	2.33	2.82	10	2	0	4486	761
3	0.00	12.84	1.55	2.06	5	1	0	8	3196
4	0.00	16.74	2.33	2.39	7	1	0	0	825
5	0.00	19.85	2.26	3.24	13	5	0	50	1
avg	0.00	17.49	**2.12**	2.66	43	13	0	909	958

(b) RED

scan pair	CA	PA	WA	# LMs
1	215	151	81	446
2	328	123	83	534
3	318	95	129	542
4	156	136	75	366
5	319	88	85	492
Sum	1335	593	452	2380
%	**56**	**25**	**19**	—

These configuration settings were empirically established and were shown to perform particularly well on this data. We therefore refer in the following to these publications for a detailed description.

NiftyReg. We employed the NiftyReg registration package (version 1.3) for our experiments, and used the particular registration set-up and parametrization proposed in [6].

Elastix. We employed elastix (version 4.3) for our experiments, and used the particular registration set-up and parametrization proposed in [13].

Table 4. Combined Registrations. Evaluated based on (a) reference data, and (b) RED predictions.

(a) Reference Evaluation

scan pair	LRE min	max	mean	std	>5	>10	>20	fold-ing	over-lap
1	0.00	12.62	1.59	1.78	4	2	0	0	0
2	0.00	21.54	1.83	3.25	7	4	1	0	0
3	0.00	13.47	1.30	1.78	3	1	0	0	0
4	0.00	14.77	2.12	2.15	7	1	0	0	0
5	0.00	20.41	1.89	2.97	8	4	1	0	0
avg	0.00	16.56	**1.75**	2.39	29	12	2	0	0

(b) RED

scan pair	prediction CA	PA	WA	# LMs
1	318	76	52	446
2	470	34	30	534
3	428	44	70	542
4	239	85	42	366
5	434	31	27	492
Sum	1889	270	221	2380
%	**80**	**11**	**9**	—

Demons. We employed the diffeomorphic demons for our experiments, and used the particular registration set-up and parametrization proposed in [9].

5   Evaluation and Results

We evaluated the MetaReg algorithm using the reference landmark set l_F and the landmarks l_P. On l_F we compute the landmark registration error (LRE). To assess the number of larger misalignments, we list the number of landmarks with misalignment larger than 5mm,10mm and 20mm. For comparison the quality predictions made by RED on l_P are shown in the accompanying tables.

In addition to the landmark-based measures, which primarily evaluate the alignment accuracy of the interior of the lungs, we also compute a boundary measure to assess the registration accuracy at the lung boundaries. For the boundary evaluation we count the number of overlapping voxels, based on the following overlap measure: $|M_{FROI} - (M_{FROI} \circ \mathbf{T})| \otimes SE$, where $\otimes$ denotes a morphological dilation operator and SE is its structuring element with spherical radius of 2 voxels. That way we allow two voxels tolerance to both inside and outside the ROI to account for possible inaccuracies of the lung segmentations [12]. Further, the number of foldings is listed, that is the number of voxels within the lung mask for which $|J(\mathbf{T})| \leq 0$ (J denotes the Jacobian matrix). Note, that classification bias in RED is avoided by the use of a rotation training set (leave-one-scanpair-out). And DIR bias towards l_F landmarks is avoided by using separate landmark sets l_P. Moreover, the employed DIR algorithms do not involve any landmark matching, optimization is purely intensity-based.

6   Conclusion

MetaReg generated for each scan pair a registration that is better than any registration obtained by each registration algorithm separately. On average, 10% improvement is achieved compared to best single registration algorithm (Demons).

More significantly, registrations combined by MetaReg contain about 30% fewer regions with misalignments larger than 5mm, compared to the best single registration algorithm.

References

1. Danielsson, P.E.: Euclidean Distance Mapping. Computer Graphics and Image Processing 14, 227–248 (1980)
2. Ibáñez, L., Schroeder, W., Ng, L., Cates, J.: The ITK Software Guide. Kitware, Inc. (2005)
3. Kittler, J., Hatef, M., Duin, R.P.W., Matas, J.: On combining classifiers. IEEE Trans. on Pattern Analysis and Machine Intelligence 20(3), 226–239 (1998)
4. Klein, S., Staring, M., Murphy, K., Viergever, M., Pluim, J.: elastix: a toolbox for intensity-based medical image registration. IEEE Transactions on Medical Imaging 29(1), 196–205 (2010)
5. Lee, S., Wolberg, G., Shin, S.: Scattered data interpolation with multilevel b-splines. Trans. on Visualization and Computer Graphics 3(3), 228–244 (1997)
6. Modat, M., McClelland, J., Ourselin, S.: Lung registration using the NiftyReg package. Medical Image Analysis for the Clinic - A Grand Challenge 2010, 33–42 (2010)
7. Modat, M., Ridgway, G.R., Taylor, Z.A., Lehmann, M., Barnes, J., Hawkes, D.J., Fox, N.C., Ourselin, S.: Fast free-form deformation using graphics processing units. Computer Methods and Programs in Biomedicine 98(3), 278–284 (2010)
8. Muenzing, S.E.A., Murphy, K., van Ginneken, B., Pluim, J.P.W.: Automatic detection of registration errors for quality assessment in medical image registration. In: Proceedings of the SPIE, vol. 7259, pp. 72590K–72590K–9 (2009)
9. Muenzing, S.E.A., van Ginneken, B., Pluim, J.P.W.: Knowledge-driven regularization of the deformation field for PDE based nonrigid registration algorithms. Medical Image Analysis for the Clinic - A Grand Challenge 2010, 127–136 (2010)
10. Murphy, K., van Ginneken, B., Klein, S., Staring, M., de Hoop, B., Viergever, M., Pluim, J.P.W.: Semi-automatic construction of reference standards for evaluation of image registration. Medical Image Analysis 15, 71–84 (2011)
11. Murphy, K., et al.: Evaluation of registration methods on thoracic CT: The EM-PIRE10 challenge. IEEE Trans. on Medical Imaging 30, 1901–1920 (2011)
12. van Rikxoort, E., de Hoop, B., Viergever, M., Prokop, M., van Ginneken, B.: Automatic lung segmentation from thoracic computed tomography scans using a hybrid approach with error detection. Medical Physics 36(7), 2934–2947 (2009)
13. Staring, M., Klein, S., Reiber, J., Niessen, W., Stoel, B.: Pulmonary Image Registration With elastix Using a Standard Intensity-Based Algorithm. Medical Image Analysis for the Clinic - A Grand Challenge 2010 (2010)
14. Tustison, N., Gee, J.: N-d c^k b-spline scattered data approximation. The Insight Journal (2005)
15. Vercauteren, T., Pennec, X., Perchant, A., Ayache, N.: Non-parametric Diffeomorphic Image Registration with the Demons Algorithm. In: Ayache, N., Ourselin, S., Maeder, A. (eds.) MICCAI 2007, Part II. LNCS, vol. 4792, pp. 319–326. Springer, Heidelberg (2007)

A Unified Image Registration Framework for ITK*

Brian B. Avants[1], Nicholas J. Tustison[2], Gang Song[1], Baohua Wu[1],
Michael Stauffer[1], Matthew M. McCormick[3], Hans J. Johnson[4],
James C. Gee[1], and The Insight Software Consortium[5]

[1] Penn Image Computing and Science Lab,
Dept. of Radiology
University of Pennsylvania, Philadelphia, PA, 19104
[2] Dept. of Radiology and Medical Imaging,
University of Virginia, Charlottesville, VA 22903
[3] Department of Psychiatry
The University of Iowa, IA 52242
[4] Kitware, Inc.,
Clifton Park, NY 12065
[5] http://www.insightsoftwareconsortium.org

Abstract. Publicly available scientific resources help establish evaluation standards, provide a platform for teaching and may improve reproducibility. Version 4 of the Insight ToolKit (ITK[4]) seeks to establish new standards in publicly available image registration methodology. In this work, we provide an overview and preliminary evaluation of the revised toolkit against registration based on the previous major ITK version (3.20). Furthermore, we propose a nomenclature that may be used to discuss registration frameworks via schematic representations. In total, the ITK[4] contribution is intended as a structure to support reproducible research practices, will provide a more extensive foundation against which to evaluate new work in image registration and also enable application level programmers a broad suite of tools on which to build.

1 Introduction

As image registration methods mature—and their capabilities become more widely recognized—the number of applications increase [20,22,21,16,5,6,3,19,15,13,8,17]. Consequently, image registration transitioned from being a field of active research, and few applied results, to a field where the main focus is translational. Image registration is now used to derive quantitative biomarkers from images [11], plays a major role in business models and clinical products (especially in radiation oncology) [6], has led to numerous new findings in studies of brain and behavior (e.g. [4]) and is a critical component in applications in pathology, microscopy, surgical planning and more [21,16,9,5,6,19,13,17]. Despite the increasing relevance of image registration across application domains, there are relatively few reference algorithm implementations available to the community.

One source of benchmark methodology is the Insight ToolKit (ITK) [24,1], which marked a significant contribution to medical image processing when it first emerged

---

* This work is supported by National Library of Medicine sponsored ARRA stimulus funding.

B.M. Dawant et al. (Eds.): WBIR 2012, LNCS 7359, pp. 266–275, 2012.

over 10 years ago. Since that time, ITK has become a standard-bearer for image processing algorithms and, in particular, for image registration methods. In a review of ITK user interests, image registration was cited as the most important contribution of ITK (personal communication). Numerous papers use ITK algorithms as standard references for implementations of Demons registration and mutual information-based affine or B-Spline registration [22,21,9,5,6]. Multiple toolkits extend ITK registration methods in unique ways. Elastix provides very fast and accurate B-Spline registration [14,17]. The diffeomorphic demons is a fast/efficient approximation to a diffeomorphic mapping [23]. ANTs provides both flexibility and high average performance [2]. The Brains-Fit algorithm is integrated into slicer for user-guided registration [13]. Each of these toolkits has both strengths and weaknesses [14,17] and was enabled by an ITK core.

The Insight ToolKit began a major refactoring effort in 2010. The refactoring aimed to both simplify and extend the techniques available in version 3.x with methods and ideas from a new set of prior work [12,7,20,16,19,2]. To make this technology more accessible, ITK^4 unifies the dense registration framework (displacement field, diffeomorphisms) with the low-dimensional (B-Spline, Affine, rigid) framework by introducing composite transforms, deformation field transforms and specializations that allowed these to be optimized efficiently. A sub-goal set for ITK^4 was to simplify parameter setting by adding helper methods that use well-known principles of image registration to automatically scale transform components and set optimization parameters. ITK^4 transforms are also newly applicable to objects such as vectors and tensors and will take into account covariant geometry if necessary. Finally, ITK^4 reconfigures the registration framework to use multi-threading in as many locations as possible. The revised registration framework within ITK is more thoroughly integrated across transform models, is thread-safe and provides broader functionality than in prior releases.

The remainder of the document will provide an overview of the new framework via the context of a potential general nomenclature. We also establish performance benchmarks for the current ITK^4 registration. Finally, we discuss future developments in the framework.

2   Nomenclature

The nomenclature below designates an image registration algorithm pictorially. This nomenclature is intended to be a descriptive, but also technically consistent, system for visually representing algorithms and applications of registration. Ideally, any standard algorithm can be written in the nomenclature below.

A physical point: $x \in \Omega$ where Ω is the domain, usually of an image.

An image: $I\colon \Omega^d \to \mathbb{R}^n$ where n is the number of components per pixel and d is dimensionality. A second image is J.

Domain map: $\phi\colon \Omega_I \to \Omega_J$ where $\to$ may be replaced with any mapping symbol below.

Affine mapping: $\leftrightarrow$ a low-dimensional invertible transformation: affine, rigid, translation, etc.

Affine mapping: $\to$ designates the direction an affine mapping is applied.

Deformation field: $\rightsquigarrow$ deformation field mapping J to I. May not be invertible.

Spline-based mapping: $\vec{b}$ e.g. B-Spline field mapping J to I.

Diffeomorphic mapping: $\rightsquigarrow$ these maps should have an accurate inverse that is computed in the algorithm or can be computed from the results.

Composite mapping: $\phi = \phi_1(\phi_2(x))$ is defined by $\rightsquigarrow\rightarrow$ where ϕ_2 is of type $\rightsquigarrow$.

Not invertible: $\leftrightarrow$ indicates a mapping that is not invertible.

Image warping: For example, $\rightarrow J$ represents applying affine transform $\rightarrow$ on image J. $\rightarrow J = J(A(x))$.

Similarity measure: $\overset{\approx}{s}$ or $\approx_s$ indicates the metric s that compares images.

We would then write a standard Demons registration application that maps one image, J, into the space of I (presumably a template) as:

$$I \rightsquigarrow\rightarrow J \quad \text{which symbolizes} \quad I \approx J(A(\phi(x))),$$

with A an affine mapping and ϕ a generic deformation. The notation means that the algorithm first optimizes an affine mapping, $\rightarrow$, between J and I. This is followed by a deformation in the second stage, $\rightsquigarrow$, from $\rightarrow J$ to I. In terms of transformation composition, we would write $\rightsquigarrow\rightarrow J = J_w(x) = J(\phi_{\text{Affine}}(\phi_{\text{Demons}}(x)))$ where J_w is the result of warping J to I. The ϕ are the specific functions corresponding to the schematic arrows. Note, also, that the tail of the arrow indicates the transform's domain. The arrowhead indicates its range. Finally, we denote the similarity metric as $\approx$ which indicates a sum of squared differences (the default similarity metric). ITK^4 supports metrics such as mutual information, $\overset{\approx}{\text{mi}}$, or cross-correlation, $\overset{\approx}{\text{cc}}$. We will use this nomenclature to write schematics for registration applications in the following sections.

3   Overview of the Unified Framework

The key ideas for ITK^4 registration are:

1. Registration maps can be applied or optimized through the *itkCompositeTransform* which chains transforms together as in Figure 1.
2. Each ITK^4 transform has either global support (affine transform) or local (or compact) support (a displacement field transform). If any map in a composite transform has global support then the composite transform has global support.
3. ITK^4 metrics are applicable to both types of transforms and may optimize over dense or sparse samples from Ω. Metrics may be multi-channel (e.g. for registering RGB or tensor images).
4. The optimization framework is multi-threaded and memory efficient to allow high-dimensional transformations to be optimized quickly on multi-core systems.
5. The ITK^4 optimization framework comes with parameter setting tools that automatically select parameter scales and learning rates for gradient-based optimization schemes. These parameter setting tools use physical units to help provide the user with intuition on the meaning of parameters.

Below we will discuss (1) gradient-based optimization within the framework, (2) techniques to estimate optimization parameters for arbitrary metric and transformation combinations and (3) a generalized diffeomorphic matching approach.

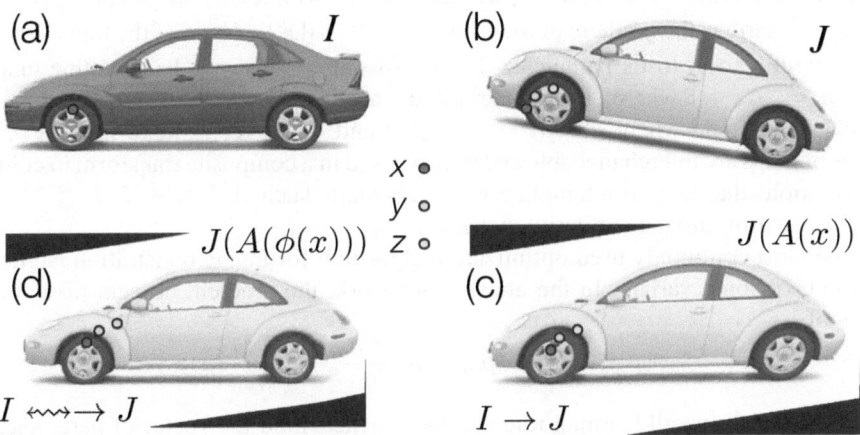

Fig. 1. Define x in Ω_I and z in Ω_J as the same material point but existing in different domains. The point y is in a domain that is intermediate between Ω_I and Ω_J. The standard approach in the ITKv4 registration framework is to map image J (b) to image I (a) by first identifying the linear transformation, $\rightarrow$, between the images, shown in (c). Second, we remove the shape (diffeomorphic) differences (d). Consequently, we have a composite mapping, computed via the mutual information similarity metric, that identifies $I(x) \approx_{\text{mi}} J(A(\phi(x))) = J_{\text{Affine}}(y) = J(z)$. The image $J_{\text{Affine}}(y)$ represents J after application of the affine transformation A i.e. $J(A(x))$.

3.1 Optimization Framework

The general ITK^4 optimization criterion is summarized as:

$$\text{Find mapping } \phi(x,p) \in \mathcal{T} \text{ such that } M(I, J, \phi(x,p)) \text{ is minimized.} \qquad (1)$$

While, for functional mappings, this formulation is not strictly correct, the practical implementation of even high-dimensional continuous transformations involves parameterization. The space $\mathcal{T}$ restricts the possible transformations over which to optimize the mapping ϕ. The arguments to ϕ are its parameters, p, and the spatial position, x. Note that, in ITK^4, the image I may also contain a mapping, although it is not directly optimized in most cases. As will be seen later in the document, this mapping may also be used within large deformation metrics.

The similarity metric, M, is perhaps the most critical component in image registration. Denote a parameter set as $p = (p_1, p_2 \ldots p_n)$. The metric (or comparison function between images) is then defined by $M(I, J, \phi(x,p))$. For instance, $M = \|I(x) - J(\phi(x,p))\|^2$ i.e. the sum of squared differences (SSD) metric. Its gradient with respect to parameter p_i is (using the chain rule),

$$M_{p_i} = \frac{\partial M}{\partial p_i} = \frac{\partial M}{\partial J} \frac{\partial J(\phi(x,p))}{\partial \phi} \frac{\partial \phi}{\partial p_i}^T |_x . \qquad (2)$$

This equation provides the metric gradient specified for sum of squared differences (at point x) but similar forms arise for the correlation and mutual information [10].

Both are implemented in ITK[4] for transformations with local and global support. The $\frac{\partial J(\phi(x,p))}{\partial \phi}$ term is the gradient of J at $\phi(x)$ and $\frac{\partial \phi}{\partial p_i}$ is the Jacobian of the transformation taken with respect to its parameter. The transform $\phi(x,p)$ may be an affine map i.e. $\phi(x,p) = Ax + t$ where A is a matrix and t a translation. Alternatively, it may be a displacement field where $\phi(x,p) = x + u(x)$ and u is a vector field. In ITK[4], both types of maps are interchangeable and may be used in a composite transform to compute registrations that map to a template via a schematic such as $I \approx\to J$, $I \overset{\approx}{\underset{\text{mi}}{}} \overset{\leftrightsquigarrow}{b} \to J$, $I \overset{\approx}{\underset{\text{cc}}{}} \leftrightsquigarrow\to J$ or, mixing similarity metrics, $I \approx_{\text{cc}}\leftrightsquigarrow\approx_{\text{mi}}\to J_i$.

The most commonly used optimization algorithm for image registration is gradient descent, or some variant. In the above framework, the gradient descent takes on the form of

$$\phi(p_{\text{new}}, x) = \phi(p_{\text{old}} + \lambda \, [\frac{\partial M}{\partial p_1}, \cdots , \frac{\partial M}{\partial p_n}], x),$$

where λ is the overall learning rate and the brackets hold the vector of parameter updates. Note that, as in previous versions of ITK, a naive application of gradient descent will not produce a smooth change of parameters for transformations with mixed parameter types. For instance, a change Δ to parameter p_i will produce a different magnitude of impact on ϕ if p_i is a translation rather than a rotation. Thus, we develop an estimation framework that sets "parameter scales" (in ITK parlance) which, essentially, customize the learning rate for each parameter. The update to ϕ via its gradient may also include other steps (such as Gaussian smoothing) that project the updated transform back to space $\mathcal{T}$. Multi-threading is achieved in the gradient computation, transformation update step and (if used) the regularization by dividing the parameter set into computational units that correspond to contiguous sub-regions of the image domain.

3.2 Parameter Scale Estimation

We choose to estimate parameter scales by analyzing the result of a small parameter update on the change in the magnitude of physical space deformation induced by the transformation. The impact from a unit change of parameter p_i may be defined in multiple ways, such as the maximum shift of voxels or the average norm of transform Jacobians [12].

Denote the unscaled gradient descent update to p as Δp. The goal is to rescale Δp to $q = s \cdot \Delta p$, where s is a diagonal matrix $\text{diag}(s_1, s_2 \ldots s_n)$, such that a unit change of q_i will have the same impact on deformation for each parameter $i = 1...n$. As an example, we want $\|\phi(x, p_{\text{new}}) - \phi(x, p_{\text{old}})\| = constant$ regardless of which of the i parameters is updated by the unit change. The unit is an epsilon value, e.g. 1.e-3.

Rewrite $[\frac{\partial M}{\partial p_1}, \cdots , \frac{\partial M}{\partial p_n}]$ as $\frac{\partial M}{\partial J} \frac{\partial J(\phi(x,p))}{\partial \phi} [\frac{\partial \phi}{\partial p_1}, \cdots , \frac{\partial \phi}{\partial p_n}]$. To determine the relative scale effects of each parameter, p_i, we can factor out the constant terms on the outside of the bracket. Then the modified gradient descent step becomes $\text{diag}(s)\frac{\partial \phi}{\partial p}$. We identify the values of $\text{diag}(s)$ by explicitly computing the values of $\|\phi(x, p_{\text{new}}) - \phi(x, p_{\text{old}})\|$ with respect to an ϵ change. A critical variable, practically, is which x to choose for evaluation of $\|\phi(x, p_{\text{new}}) - \phi(x, p_{\text{old}})\|$. The corners of the image domain work well for affine transformations. In contrast, local regions of small radius (approximately 5) work well for transformations with local support. Additional work is needed to verify

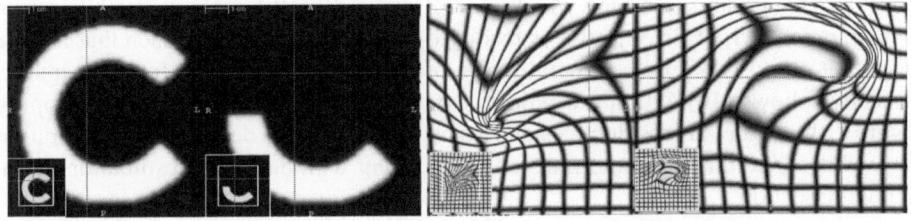

Fig. 2. An ITK diffeomorphic mapping of the type $I \leftrightsquigarrow J$. The "C" and 1/2 "C" example illustrate the large deformations that may be achieved with time varying velocity fields. In this case, the moving (deforming) image is the 1/2 "C". The right panels illustrate the deformed grid for the transformation of the "C" to 1/2 "C" (middle right) and its inverse mapping (far right) which takes the 1/2 "C" to the reference space. The unit time interval is discretized into 15 segments in order to compute this mapping. 15*5 integration steps were used in the Runge-Kutta *ode* integration over the velocity field. A two core MacBook Air computed this registration in 110 seconds. The images each were of size 150×150.

optimal parameters for this new ITK[4] feature. However, a preliminary evaluation is performed in the results section. The new parameter scale estimation effectively reduces the number of parameters that the user must tune from $k + 1$ (λ plus the scales for each parameter type where there are k types) to only 1, the learning rate.

The learning rate, itself, may not be intuitive for a user to set. The difficulty—across problem sets—is that a good learning rate for one problem may result in a different amount of change per iteration in another problem. Furthermore, the discrete image gradient may become invalid beyond one voxel. Thus, it is good practice to limit a deformation step to one voxel spacing [12]. We therefore provide the users the ability to specify the learning rate in terms of the *maximum physical space change per iteration*. As with the parameter scale estimation, the domain over which this maximum change is estimated impacts the outcome and similar practices are recommended for both cases. This feature is especially useful for allowing one to tune gradient descent parameters without being concerned about which similarity metric is being used. That is, it effectively rescales the term $\lambda \partial M / \partial p$ to have a consistent effect, for a given λ, regardless of the metric choice.

3.3 Diffeomorphic Mapping with Arbitrary Metrics

Beg proposed the Large Deformation Diffeomorphic Metric Mapping (LDDMM) algorithm [16] which minimizes the sum of squared differences criterion between two images. LDDMM parameterizes a diffeomorphism through a time varying velocity field that is integrated through an *ode*. In ITK[4], we implement an alternative to LDDMM that also uses a time varying field and an *ode* but minimizes the following objective function:

$$E(\mathbf{v}) = M(I, J, \phi_{1,0}) + w \int_0^1 \|\mathcal{L}v_t\|^2 dt . \tag{3}$$

This is an instance of equation 1 where w is a scalar weight and $\phi_{1,0}$ is a standard integration of the time-varying velocity field v_t which is regularized by linear operator $\mathcal{L}$.

ITK^4 uses Gaussian smoothing which is the Green's kernel for generalized Tikhonov regularization [18]. This objective is readily optimized using an approach that is similar to that proposed by Beg. Generalization of the LDDMM gradient for other metrics basically follows [10] with a few adjustments to accomodate diffeomorphic mapping. Figure 2 shows an ITK result on a standard example for large deformation registration. We will evaluate this diffeomorphic mapping, along with parameter estimation, in the following section.

4   Evaluation

We first investigate the ability of our automated parameter estimation to facilitate parameter tuning across metrics. We then compare ITK^4 with an open-source ITK^3 registration application. In the future, the latest evaluation numbers will be available at: ITKv4 latest evaluation results.

Parameter Estimation across Metrics. ITK^4 provides similarity metrics that may be applied for both deformable and affine registration. In a previous section, we provided a parameter estimation strategy that is applicable to both deformable and affine transformations with arbitrary metrics. Denote images I, J, K, where the latter two are "moving" images, and K is an intensity-inverted version of J. We then evaluate the following schema,

$$I \approx_{\leftsquigarrow\rightarrow} J, \qquad I \approx_{cc}{\leftsquigarrow\rightarrow} K, \qquad I \approx_{mi}{\leftsquigarrow\rightarrow} K$$

where, for each schematic, we use the corresponding metric for both affine and diffeomorphic mapping. Furthermore, we keep the same parameters for each registration by exploiting parameter scale estimators. Figure 3 shows the candidate images for this test.

As shown in figure 3, very similar results are achieved for each schematic without additional parameter tuning. To determine this quantitatively, we perform registration for each schematic and then compare the Dice overlap of a ground-truth three-tissue segmentation. For each result, we have the Dice overlap of dark tissue (cerebrospinal fluid, CSF), medium intensity tissue (gray matter) and bright tissue (white matter). For the mean squares metric, we have: 0.588, 0.816 and 0.90; for CC, we have: 0.624, 0.786, 0.882; for MI, we have: 0.645, 0.779, 0.858. Mutual information does best for the CSF while mean squares does best for other tissues. CC performs in the mid-range for all classes of tissue. Thus, a single set of tuned parameters provides a reasonable result for an affine plus diffeomorphic mapping across three different metrics. While improvement might be gained by further tuning for each metric, this result shows that our parameter estimation method achieves the goal of reducing user burden.

Comparison against ITK^3. We compare the ITK^4 registration against an ITK^3 registration suite BrainsFit (nitrc.org multimodereg). We present preliminary, encouraging evaluation results for this approach to gradient descent with both affine and deformable registration in Figure 4. The dataset consists of ten elderly and demented subjects with manual labels of brain parenchyma. Of importance is that the ventricles are not included in the parenchyma. Large deformation is required to match ventricles and, as such, this evaluation provides some insight into the benefit of the new ITK^4 diffeomorphic matching.

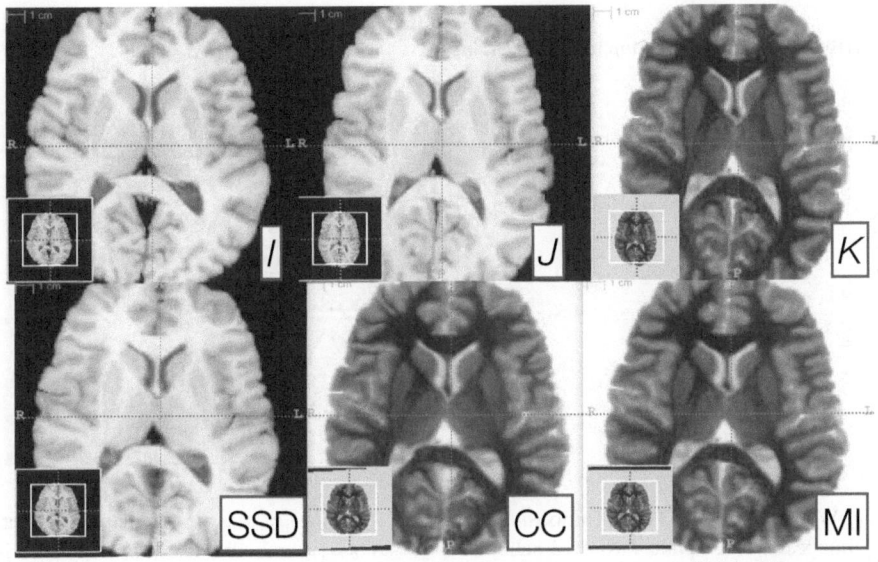

Fig. 3. Three references images, I (left), J (middle top), and K (right top), are used to illustrate the robustness of our parameter scale estimation for setting consistent parameters across both metrics and transform types. K is the negation of J and is used to test the correlation and mutual information registrations. We optimized, by hand, the step-length parameters for one metric (the sum of squared differences) for both the affine and deformable case. Thus, two parameters had to be optimized. We then applied these same parameters to register I and K via both correlation and mutual information. The resulting registrations (bottom row) were all of similar quality. Further, the same metric is used for both affine and diffeomorphic mapping by exploiting the general optimization process given in equation 1.

5   Discussion and Future Work

ITK is a community built and maintained toolkit and is a public resource for repro-ducible methods. The updated ITK[4] registration framework provides a novel set of user-friendly parameter setting tools and benchmark implementations of both standard and advanced algorithms. Robustness with respect to parameter settings has long been a goal of image registration and ITK[4] takes valuable steps toward the direction of au-tomated parameter selection. By the time of the workshop, we intend to have a more extensive series of benchmark performance studies completed on standard datasets and hope that presentation of this work will provide a valuable foundation for future work. The number of possible applications exceeds what can possibly be evaluated via the ITK core. Community involvement is needed in order to increase the number of possi-ble registration applications and metric / transform / optimizer / data combinations that have been evaluated. At the same time, documentation, usability and examples must be provided by the development team in order to improve user involvement. Future work will enhance the depth and breadth of this documentation as well as seek to optimize

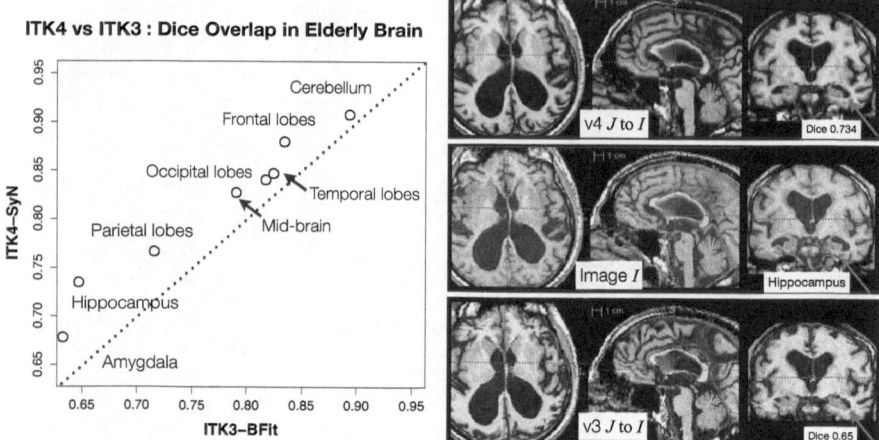

Fig. 4. We compare an ITKv4 composite schema as $I \approx_{cc} \rightsquigarrow \approx_{mi} \rightarrow J_i$ for mapping a set of $\{J_i\}$ images to a template I to a v3 schema: $I \approx_{mi} \rightsquigarrow_b \approx_{mi} \rightarrow J_i$. We use this schematic in a registration-based segmentation of multiple brain structures in an elderly population as a benchmark for algorithm performance, similar to [14]. Example large-deformation results from the dataset are at right. The largest improvement in performance is within hippocampus, where a 13% improvement in v4 is gained. Overlap improvement from v3 to v4, quantified via paired t-test, is significant. The example pair of images will be included in v4 for regression testing.

the current implementations for speed and memory. With this effort, the user community will be capable of efficiently implementing novel applications and even algorithms based on the ITK^4 framework.

References

1. Ackerman, M.J., Yoo, T.S.: The visible human data sets (VHD) and insight toolkit (ITk): experiments in open source software. In: AMIA Annu. Symp. Proc., p. 773 (2003)
2. Avants, B.B., Tustison, N.J., Song, G., Cook, P.A., Klein, A., Gee, J.C.: A reproducible evaluation of ANTs similarity metric performance in brain image registration. Neuroimage 54(3), 2033–2044 (2011)
3. Baloch, S., Davatzikos, C.: Morphological appearance manifolds in computational anatomy: groupwise registration and morphological analysis. Neuroimage 45(1 suppl.), S73–S85 (2009)
4. Bearden, C.E., van Erp, T.G.M., Dutton, R.A., Tran, H., Zimmermann, L., Sun, D., Geaga, J.A., Simon, T.J., Glahn, D.C., Cannon, T.D., Emanuel, B.S., Toga, A.W., Thompson, P.M.: Mapping cortical thickness in children with 22q11.2 deletions. Cereb. Cortex 17(8), 1889–1898 (2007)
5. Chen, M., Lu, W., Chen, Q., Ruchala, K.J., Olivera, G.H.: A simple fixed-point approach to invert a deformation field. Med. Phys. 35(1), 81–88 (2008)
6. Cheung, M.R., Krishnan, K.: Interactive deformation registration of endorectal prostate mri using itk thin plate splines. Acad. Radiol. 16(3), 351–357 (2009)

7. Christensen, G.E., Rabbitt, R.D., Miller, M.I.: Deformable templates using large deformation kinematics. IEEE Trans. Image Process 5(10), 1435–1447 (1996)
8. Fedorov, A., Li, X., Pohl, K.M., Bouix, S., Styner, M., Addicott, M., Wyatt, C., Daunais, J.B., Wells, W.M., Kikinis, R.: Atlas-guided segmentation of vervet monkey brain MRI. Open Neuroimag. J. 5, 186–197 (2011)
9. Floca, R., Dickhaus, H.: A flexible registration and evaluation engine (f.r.e.e.). Comput Methods Programs Biomed. 87(2), 81–92 (2007)
10. Hermosillo, G., Chefd'Hotel, C., Faugeras, O.: A variational approach to multi-modal image matching. Intl. J. Comp. Vis. 50(3), 329–343 (2002)
11. Jack Jr., C.R., Knopman, D.S., Jagust, W.J., Shaw, L.M., Aisen, P.S., Weiner, M.W., Petersen, R.C., Trojanowski, J.Q.: Hypothetical model of dynamic biomarkers of the Alzheimer's pathological cascade. Lancet Neurol. 9(1), 119–128 (2010)
12. Jenkinson, M., Smith, S.: A global optimisation method for robust affine registration of brain images. Med. Image Anal. 5(2), 143–156 (2001)
13. Kikinis, R., Pieper, S.: 3d slicer as a tool for interactive brain tumor segmentation. In: Conf. Proc. IEEE Eng. Med. Biol. Soc. 2011, pp. 6982–6984 (August 2011)
14. Klein, S., Staring, M., Murphy, K., Viergever, M.A., Pluim, J.P.W.: elastix: a toolbox for intensity-based medical image registration. IEEE Trans. Med. Imaging 29(1), 196–205 (2010)
15. Metz, C.T., Klein, S., Schaap, M., van Walsum, T., Niessen, W.J.: Nonrigid registration of dynamic medical imaging data using nd + t b-splines and a groupwise optimization approach. Med. Image Anal. 15(2), 238–249 (2011)
16. Miller, M.I., Beg, M.F., Ceritoglu, C., Stark, C.: Increasing the power of functional maps of the medial temporal lobe by using large deformation diffeomorphic metric mapping. Proc. Natl. Acad. Sci. U.S.A. 102(27), 9685–9690 (2005)
17. Murphy, K., van Ginneken, B., et al.: Evaluation of registration methods on thoracic ct: the empire10 challenge. IEEE Trans. Med. Imaging 30(11), 1901–1920 (2011)
18. Nielsen, M., Florack, L., Deriche, R.: Regularization, scale-space, and edge detection filters. J. Math. Imaging Vis. 7, 291–307 (1997)
19. Peyrat, J.M., Delingette, H., Sermesant, M., Xu, C., Ayache, N.: Registration of 4d cardiac ct sequences under trajectory constraints with multichannel diffeomorphic demons. IEEE Trans. Med. Imaging 29(7), 1351–1368 (2010)
20. Rueckert, D., Sonoda, L.I., Hayes, C., Hill, D.L., Leach, M.O., Hawkes, D.J.: Nonrigid registration using free-form deformations: application to breast mr images. IEEE Trans. Med. Imaging 18(8), 712–721 (1999)
21. Shelton, D., Stetten, G., Aylward, S., Ibez, L., Cois, A., Stewart, C.: Teaching medical image analysis with the insight toolkit. Med. Image Anal. 9(6), 605–611 (2005)
22. van Dalen, J.A., Vogel, W., Huisman, H.J., Oyen, W.J.G., Jager, G.J., Karssemeijer, N.: Accuracy of rigid CT-FDG-PET image registration of the liver. Phys. Med. Biol. 49(23), 5393–5405 (2004)
23. Vercauteren, T., Pennec, X., Perchant, A., Ayache, N.: Diffeomorphic demons: efficient nonparametric image registration. Neuroimage 45(1 suppl.), S61–S72 (2009)
24. Yoo, T.S., Ackerman, M.J., Lorensen, W.E., Schroeder, W., Chalana, V., Aylward, S., Metaxas, D., Whitaker, R.: Engineering and algorithm design for an image processing api: a technical report on itk–the insight toolkit. Stud. Health Technol. Inform. 85, 586–592 (2002)

A Novel Framework
for Metric-Based Image Registration

Qian Xie[1], Sebastian Kurtek[1], Gary E. Christensen[2], Zhaohua Ding[3],
Eric Klassen[4], and Anuj Srivastava[1]

[1] Department of Statistics, Florida State University
[2] Department of Electrical and Computer Engineering, University of Iowa
[3] Institute of Imaging Science, Vanderbilt University
[4] Department of Mathematics, Florida State University

Abstract. The registrations of functions and images is a widely-studied problem
that has seen a variety of solutions in the recent years. Most of these solutions
are based on objective functions that fail to satisfy two most basic and desired
properties in registration: (1) invariance under identical warping: since the registration between two images is unchanged under identical domain warping, the
cost function evaluating registrations should also remain unchanged; (2) inverse
consistency: the optimal registration of image A to B should be the same as that
of image B to A. We present a novel registration approach that uses the L^2 norm,
between certain vector fields derived from images, as an objective function for
registering images. This framework satisfies symmetry and invariance properties.
We demonstrate this framework using examples from different types of images
and compare performances with some recent methods.

1 Introduction

The problem of image registration is one of the most widely studied problems in medical image analysis. Given a set of observed images, the goal is to register points across
the domains of these images. This problem has many names: registration, matching,
correspondence, re-parameterization, warping, deformation, etc but the basic problem
is essentially the same – which pixel/voxel on an image matches which pixel/voxel on
the other image. Although this problem has been studied for almost two decades, there
continue to be some fundamental limitations in the popular solutions that make them
suboptimal, difficult to evaluate and limited in scope.

To explain this issue consider images on a domain $\mathcal{D}$ taking the form $f : \mathcal{D} \to \mathbb{R}^n$. A
pairwise registration between any two images f_1, f_2 is defined as finding a mapping γ,
typically a diffeomorphism from $\mathcal{D}$ to itself, such that $f_1(s)$ and $f_2(\gamma(s))$ are optimally
matched to each other (under a chosen criterion) for all $s \in \mathcal{D}$. Registration problems are
commonly posed as variational problems, with the most common form of an objective
function being

$$\int_{\mathcal{D}} \|f_1(s) - f_2 \circ \gamma(s)\|^2 ds + \lambda \mathcal{R}(\gamma), \ \gamma \in \Gamma \ , \tag{1}$$

where $\|\cdot\|$ is the Euclidean norm, $\mathcal{R}$ is a regularization penalty on γ commonly involving
its first or second derivatives, Γ is a set of diffeomorphisms, and λ is a positive constant.
Several variations of this objective function have also been used, where the first term

B.M. Dawant et al. (Eds.): WBIR 2012, LNCS 7359, pp. 276–285, 2012.

is replaced by mutual information [12], minimum description length [5], etc., and/or the second term is replaced by the length of a geodesic in the warping space (as in the LDDMM approach [3]). Another idea is to impose regularization externally using a Gaussian smoothing (diffeomorphic demons [11]) of images. Some methods optimize the objective function over a proper subset $\Gamma_0 \subset \Gamma$ (e.g. the set of volume-preserving diffeos), some on Γ, and some on larger group Γ_b that contains Γ (e.g. the one including non-diffeomorphic mappings also).

Although the numerical techniques for optimization in Eqn. 1 have become quite mature over the last ten years, these objective functions themselves have several fundamental shortcomings. We start with an important question: What should be the properties of an objective function for use in registering images? The answer to this question is difficult since we may desire different results in different contexts. In fact, one can argue that we may never have a "perfect" objective function that matches human intuition and vision. Still there is a basic set of properties that seems essential in a registration framework; some of them have been discussed previously in [4,9] and others. In the following let $L(f_1, f_2 \circ \gamma)$ denote the objective function for matching f_1 and f_2 by optimizing over γ (here γ is assumed to be applied to f_2). The most important property that we need in L is **invariance to identical warping**, defined as follows. For any $f_1, f_2 \in \mathcal{F}$, and $\gamma \in \Gamma$, this invariance implies that $L(f_1, f_2) = L(f_1 \circ \gamma, f_2 \circ \gamma)$. In case L is a proper metric, then this property is nothing but action of Γ on $\mathcal{F}$, where the action is given by $(f, \gamma) \to f \circ \gamma$, by isometries. Also, assuming that Γ is a group, this property implies that $L(f_1, f_2 \circ \gamma) = L(f_1 \circ \gamma^{-1}, f_2)$. Note that some papers that do not use the full group Γ but some finite-dimensional subset (e.g. spline-based warping functions) will not satisfy this property.

Why is this property important? Consider the two functions f_1 and f_2 shown in the left panel of Fig. 1. Even though the two functions are different, their peaks and valleys are nicely aligned. The middle panel shows an example of warping function γ and the right panel shows the warped versions $f_1 \circ \gamma$ and $f_2 \circ \gamma$. It is interesting to note that the peaks and valleys in the warped functions are still aligned. Furthermore, the full correspondence between the two functions is unchanged despite the warping. In fact, one can show that an identical warping of any two functions keeps their registration unchanged and, hence, any good objective function must have this invariance to identical warping.

There is another important property that is termed **inverse consistency** ([4,2]). This property implies that the optimal registration between two functions remains the same even if they are treated in the reverse order. That is, if $\gamma^* \in \arg\min_{\gamma \in \Gamma} L(f_1, f_2 \circ \gamma)$, then $\gamma^{*-1} \in \arg\min_{\gamma \in \Gamma} L(f_2, f_1 \circ \gamma)$. It can be shown that if we have invariance to identical warping and an additional symmetry condition ($L(f_1, f_2) = L(f_2, f_1)$), then we have inverse consistency. The symmetry condition is usually satisfied by most objective functions but the invariance condition is the one that many of them fail to meet. Without the invariance to identical warping, we will not have inverse consistency in general. So, once again that the property turns out to be paramount in registration.

We note that many of the popular objective functions ([10,12,5,11,3,9]) do not satisfy these two basic properties.

There is an additional property of interest. A majority of post-matching analyses compare registered images, and apply statistical techniques such as PCA for modeling and analysis. The question is: What should be the metric for this post-registration

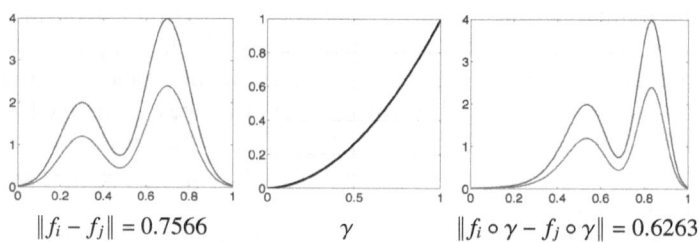

$$\|f_i - f_j\| = 0.7566 \qquad \gamma \qquad \|f_i \circ \gamma - f_j \circ \gamma\| = 0.6263$$

Fig. 1. An identical deformation of domains preserves the registration of functions

analyses? In many current systems, one performs registration using an objective function and then chooses a separate metric to perform analysis. Ideally, one would like a framework so that it can *align, compare, average, and model* multiple images in a **unified** framework that leads to efficient algorithms and consistent estimators. The objective function presented in this paper not only satisfies the invariance and the inverse consistency properties listed above but also forms an extrinsic metric on the quotient space for image comparison. Therefore, we have called our framework a metric-based method for registration and comparison of images.

2   Proposed Framework

In this section we lay out the framework for joint image registration and comparison under an objective function which induces an extrinsic distance. This method applies to mathematical objects whose range space has dimension at least as much as that of their domain, for $f : \mathcal{D} \to \mathbb{R}^n$, where $n \geq m, m = \dim(\mathcal{D})$. In case of 2D images, this means that pixels have at least two coordinates which is the case for colored images, or multimodal images. To register gray-scale images, we have a way to get away from this constraint, which will be discussed in Chap. 4.

Let $\mathcal{F} = \{f : \mathcal{D} \to \mathbb{R}^n \,|\, f \in C^\infty(\mathcal{D}), \|f\| = 1\}$ and $\Gamma = \{\gamma : \mathcal{D} \to \mathcal{D} \,|\, \gamma \in \text{Diff}(\mathcal{D})\}$, where $\|\cdot\|$ denotes the standard $\mathbb{L}^2$ norm and $\text{Diff}(\mathcal{D})$ is the diffeomorphism group on $\mathcal{D}$. The action of Γ on $\mathcal{F}$ is defined as follows.

Definition 1. *For an $f \in \mathcal{F}$, define the right action $\mathcal{F} \times \Gamma \to \mathcal{F}$ by $(f, \gamma) = f \circ \gamma$.*

Note that for any two $f_1, f_2 \in \mathcal{F}$, and a $\gamma \in \Gamma$, we usually have $\|f_1 - f_2\| \neq \|f_1 \circ \gamma - f_2 \circ \gamma\|$ and invariance consition is not satisfied. Thus, we do not work with the images directly. Instead, we will use a novel mathematical representation of images, called a q-map, that has been motivated by recent work in shape analysis of surfaces [7]. Here we adapt it for analyzing images.

Definition 2. *For an $f \in \mathcal{F}$, define a mapping $Q : \mathcal{F} \to \mathbb{L}^2$ such that $Q(f)(s) = \sqrt{a(s)} f(s), \forall s \in \mathcal{D}$ where $a(s)$ is the multiplication factor of f at s given by $|J_f(s)|_{\text{area}}$. For any $n \times m$ matrix A $(n \geq m)$, $|A|_{\text{area}}$ is defined as $|A|_{\text{area}} = \sqrt{\sum_{B:B \text{ is } m \times m \text{ submatrix of } A} |B|^2}$ and where $|B|$ denotes determinant of B.*

For any $f \in \mathcal{F}$, we will refer to $q = Q(f)$ as its q-map. Assuming the original set of images to be smooth, the set of all q-maps is a subset of $\mathbb{L}^2$. The corresponding action of Γ on $\mathbb{L}^2$ is given as follows.

Definition 3. *Define the right action* $\mathbb{L}^2 \times \Gamma \to \mathbb{L}^2$ *by* $(q, \gamma) = \sqrt{J_\gamma}(q \circ \gamma)$, *where* J_γ *denotes the Jacobian of* γ.

Note that, for an image f, $Q(f \circ \gamma) = (Q(f), \gamma)$. We define $[q] = \{(q, \gamma) | \gamma \in \Gamma\}$ to be the set (or an orbit) of all warpings of a q-map. Since all elements of $[q]$ can be obtained using warpings of the same image (and then forming the q-map), we deem them equivalent from the perspective of registration. One would like a registration cost function that equals zero when evaluated on any two elements of an orbit. Let $\mathbb{L}^2/\Gamma$ be the (quotient) set of all such orbits. The most important property of this mathematical representation is the following.

Proposition 1. *The re-parametrization group* Γ *acts on* $\mathbb{L}^2$ *by isometries under the* $\mathbb{L}^2$ *norm, i.e.* $\forall q_1, q_2 \in \mathbb{L}^2, \forall \gamma \in \Gamma, \|(q_1, \gamma) - (q_2, \gamma)\| = \|q_1 - q_2\|$.

Upon a close inspection, this proposition is exactly the same as the property of invariance to identical warping in Sect. 1. In view of this isometry, the $\mathbb{L}^2$ norm between the q-maps is a proper measure of the registration between any two images since it remains the same if the registration is unchanged. This leads to a quantity that will serve as both the registration objective function and an extrinsic distance between registered images.

Definition 4. *Define an objective function between any two images* f_1 *and* f_2, *represented by their q-maps* q_1 *and* q_2, *as* $L(f_1, f_2; \gamma) \equiv \|q_1 - (q_2, \gamma)\|$.

The registration is then solved by minimizing the objective function:

$$\gamma^* = \arg\inf_{\gamma \in \Gamma} L(f_1, f_2; \gamma) \ . \tag{2}$$

The objective function L introduced as above satisfies the properties of invariance to identical warping and inverse consistency. Therefore, we are able to compare images with the value of objective function at the optimal γ, which gives a solution to registering two images. We point out that there are some unresolved mathematical issues concerning to existence of a unique global solution for γ^*, especially its existence inside Γ rather than being on its boundary. We leave this for a future discussion and focus on a numerical approach that estimates γ^*.

3 Implementation

3.1 Gradient Method for Optimization Over Γ

The optimization problem over Γ stated in Eqn. 2 forms the crux of our registration framework and we will use a gradient descent method to solve it. Since Γ is a group, we use the gradient to solve for the incremental warping γ, on top of the previous cumulative warping γ_0, as follows. (In this way the required gradient is an element of $T_{\gamma_{id}}(\Gamma)$ and one needs to understand only that space.) We define a cost function with respect to γ as $E[\gamma] = \|q_1 - \phi(\gamma)\|^2$, where $\tilde{q}_2 = (q_2, \gamma_0)$ and $\phi : \Gamma \mapsto [q_2]$ is defined to be $\phi(\gamma) = (\tilde{q}_2, \gamma)$. Given a unit vector $b \in T_{\gamma_{id}}(\Gamma)$, the directional derivative of E at γ_{id} in the direction of b is $\langle q_1 - \phi(\gamma_{id}), \phi_*(b) \rangle b$, where ϕ_* is the differential of ϕ at γ_{id}. It has an explicit form which is the same as that derived for parameterized surfaces in [7]. In order to compute the gradient of E and to update γ_0 we need to specify an orthonormal basis for $T_{\gamma_{id}}(\Gamma)$.

3.2   Basis on $T_{\gamma_{id}}(\Gamma)$

In this paper, we investigate registration of 2D images with domain as $\mathcal{D} = [0,1]^2$ but the framework applied to other domains as well. In this case Γ contains all boundary preserving diffeomorphisms on $[0,1]^2$. The tangent space of Γ at identity γ_{id} is $T_{\gamma_{id}}(\Gamma) = \{b : [0,1]^2 \to [0,1]^2 \mid b$ *is a smooth tangent vector field on* $[0,1]^2\}$.

We begin by constructing an orthonormal basis for $\mathbb{L}^2([0,1],\mathbb{R})$ and then extend it to the 2D case. It is known that $\mathcal{B}_{\mathbb{L}^2}^{1D} = \{\sqrt{2}\sin(2\pi nt) \mid n \geq 1\} \cup \{\sqrt{2}\cos(2\pi nt) \mid n \geq 1\} \cup \{1\}$ forms an orthonormal basis for $\mathbb{L}^2([0,1],\mathbb{R})$ under the $\mathbb{L}^2$ metric.

We seek an orthonormal basis for $\mathbb{L}^2([0,1],\mathbb{R})$ under the Palais metric due to some nice properties of this Riemannian metric ([8]). The Palais metric is defined as $\langle f, g \rangle = f(0)g(0) + \int_0^1 f'(t)g'(t)dt$ for $f, g \in \mathbb{L}^2([0,1],\mathbb{R})$. Under this metric an orthonormal basis of $\mathbb{L}^2([0,1],\mathbb{R})$ can be defined as $\mathcal{B}_{Pal}^{1D} = \left\{\frac{\sin(2\pi nt)}{\sqrt{2}\pi n} \mid n \geq 1\right\} \cup \left\{\frac{\cos(2\pi nt)-1}{\sqrt{2}\pi n} \mid n \geq 1\right\} \cup \{t\} \cup \{1\}$. It is important to note that the set $\tilde{\mathcal{B}}_{Pal}^{1D} = \left\{\frac{\sin(2\pi nt)}{\sqrt{2}\pi n} \mid n \geq 1\right\} \cup \left\{\frac{\cos(2\pi nt)-1}{\sqrt{2}\pi n} \mid n \geq 1\right\}$ provides an orthonormal basis of functions that vanish at $t \in \{0,1\}$. The subspace of functions that vanish at $t \in \{0,1\}$ has codimension two (due to the two imposed conditions). This means that in order to define a full orthonormal basis of $\mathbb{L}^2([0,1],\mathbb{R})$, we must add two additional elements that give linearly independent pairs of values at $t \in \{0,1\}$. We will refer to the additional elements as $\mathring{\mathcal{B}}_{Pal}^{1D}$.

We will use Cartesian product of $\mathring{\mathcal{B}}_{Pal}^{1D}$ (with elements $\mathring{b}$) and $\tilde{\mathcal{B}}_{Pal}^{1D}$ (with elements $\tilde{b}$) to construct an orthonormal basis for $[0,1]^2$. First, consider two parameters $u \in [0,1]$ and $v \in [0,1]$ that define the domain $[0,1]^2$. Begin by constructing an orthonormal basis for functions on $[0,1]^2$ that vanish at the boundaries using all possible products of elements of $\tilde{\mathcal{B}}_{Pal}^{1D}$: $\tilde{\mathcal{B}}_{Pal}^{2D} = \{\tilde{b}_i(u)\tilde{b}_j(v), 0\}_{i,j \geq 1} \cup \{0, \tilde{b}_i(u)\tilde{b}_j(v)\}_{i,j \geq 1}$. In addition, we need basis elements that are tangential to the boundaries. These can be formed using the additional basis elements $\mathring{\mathcal{B}}_{Pal}^{1D}$. Define this set as: $\mathring{\mathcal{B}}_{Pal}^{2D} = \{\tilde{b}_i(u)\tilde{b}_j(v), 0\}_{i \geq 1; j=1,2} \cup \{0, \mathring{b}_i(u)\tilde{b}_j(v)\}_{i=1,2; j \geq 1}$. Then, the union $\mathcal{B}_{Pal}^{2D} = \tilde{\mathcal{B}}_{Pal}^{2D} \cup \mathring{\mathcal{B}}_{Pal}^{2D}$ provides a basis for $T_{\gamma_{id}}(\Gamma)$ under the Palais metric given by the inner product:

$$\langle\!\langle f, g \rangle\!\rangle = \langle f(0,0), g(0,0) \rangle_{\mathbb{R}^n} + \int \int \langle \nabla f(u,v), \nabla g(u,v) \rangle_{\mathbb{R}^{2n}} du\, dv \ .$$

4   Experimental Results

In this section, we will present some experimental results for grayscale images and multimodal images to demonstrate the use of the framework introduced in this paper. However, in case of grayscale images, with $n = 1$, our method does not apply directly since the dimension of range is less than the dimension of the domain. Instead, we apply it on gradient images g formed using $g = \nabla f : [0,1]^2 \to \mathbb{R}^2$ and $\nabla f = (f_u, f_v)$ for $(u,v) \in [0,1]^2$. Image gradients are a type of edge measure and are often used in their own right as robust spatial features for image registration. We will use the gradient field as a *feature* to establish optimal registrations and compute distances between gray-scale images. In other words, we register and compare two images by registering their gradient images. One can obtain the original image from a gradient image using PDEs [1]. (Note that this idea of using gradients to form vector-valued images will apply to volume images also, although we will restrict ourselves to 2D images for simplicity of presentation.) In order to register two images, we can use the registered gradients and get back to images ([1]). However, this approach may lead to changes in image intensities by applying diffeomorphisms. An alternative is to consider gradients as an image feature and directly use the optimal γ to register the images. This is the method applied in this paper. We will compare our method to the diffeomorphic demons method ([6]).

4.1 Synthetic Data

As a test to evaluate the framework we proposed, we first use it to register synthetic grayscale image pairs. The images f_1 and f_2 are registered twice by first taking f_1 as the template image and estimating γ_{21} that optimally deforms f_2. Similarly, f_2 is used as the template to get γ_{12}. We show the two converged energies, $\|(q_1, \gamma_{12}) - q_2\|$ and $\|q_1 - (q_2, \gamma_{21})\|$, associated with the the optimal γ_{12} and γ_{21} to verify the symmetry.

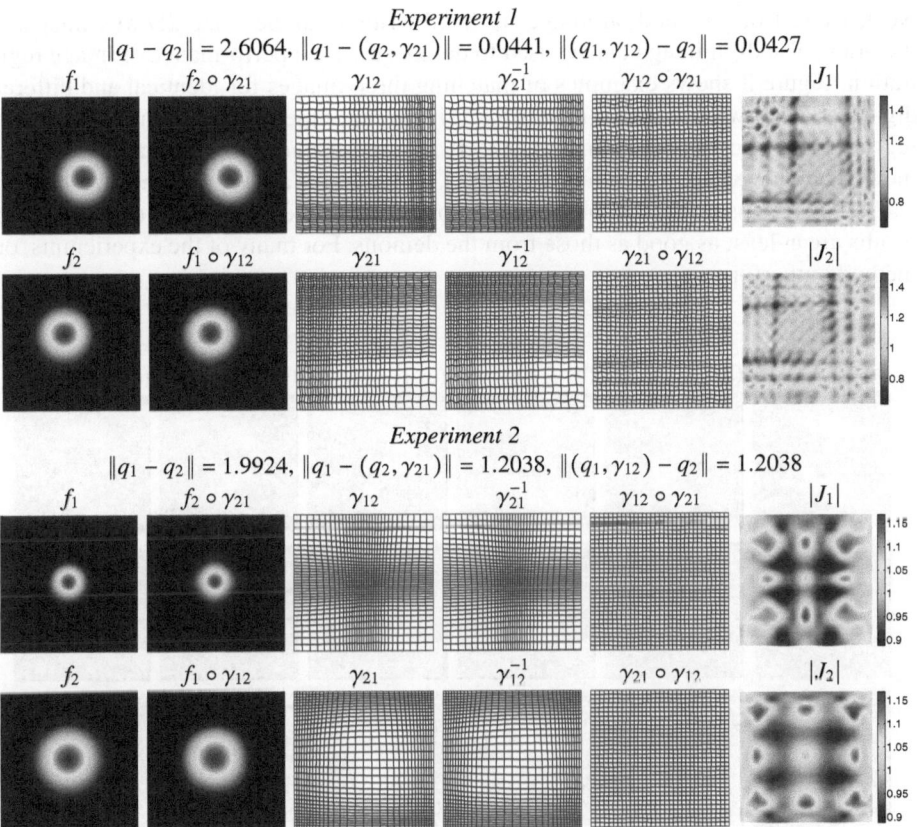

Fig. 2. Results of registration: synthetic images

The cumulative diffeomorphisms $\gamma_{21} \circ \gamma_{12}$ and $\gamma_{12} \circ \gamma_{21}$ are also used to demonstrate the symmetry of the proposed metric. In our method, γ_{12} and γ_{21} are expected to be inverses of each other.

The results for registering two datasets are shown in Fig. 2. We show the original images f_1 and f_2 with the warped images $f_2 \circ \gamma_{21}$ and $f_1 \circ \gamma_{12}$, that match with f_1 and f_2, respectively. The diffeomorphisms, γ_{12} and γ_{21} learnt to register the images are also presented. By composing them in different orders, we expect the resulting diffeomorphisms to be the identity map. In order to better visualize that the composed diffeomorphisms are close to identity, their Jacobian maps are also given. If the compositions are the exact identity map, the Jacobian images should be constant images with value 1. We observe that the composed diffeomorphisms $\gamma_{21} \circ \gamma_{12}$ and $\gamma_{12} \circ \gamma_{21}$ are close to the identity map. Although there are cases when γ_{12} and γ_{21} are not exact inverses of each other, the resulting distances are still approximately symmetric. Possible explanations include errors due to numerical interpolation of grids or γ^* being a local solution instead of a global minimizer.

4.2 Image Registration

Next, we test our method on images of hand written numbers and 2D MR images of the brain. The digit image data is used to demonstrate the performance of image registration. Figure 3 shows examples of matching three images for identical and different digit(s). Each row contains the results for a single experiment. The original images to be registered are shown in columns (a) and (d). The registration results obtained using our method are presented in columns (b) and (e). Columns (c) and (f) are the corresponding warped images using the demons method. For the experiments in Fig. 3, our registration results are at least as good as those from the demons. For many of the experiemnts, our method outperforms the other.

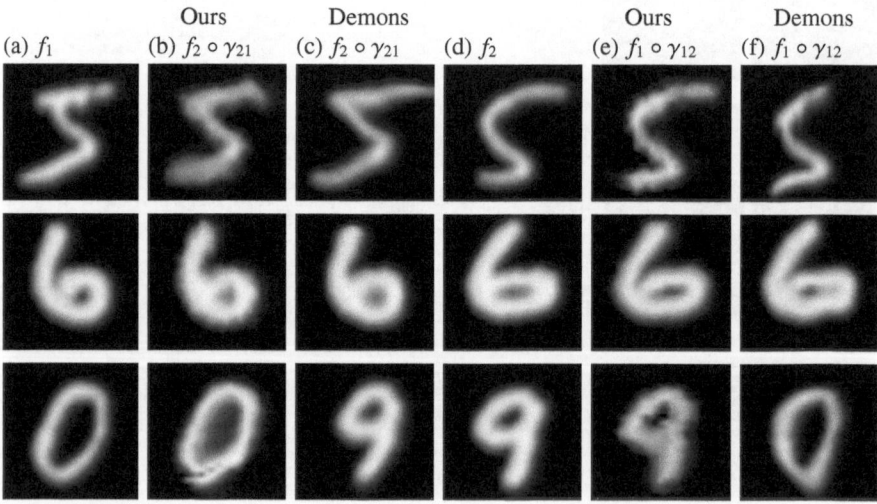

Fig. 3. Three experiments for registering digits. Each row represents an experiment

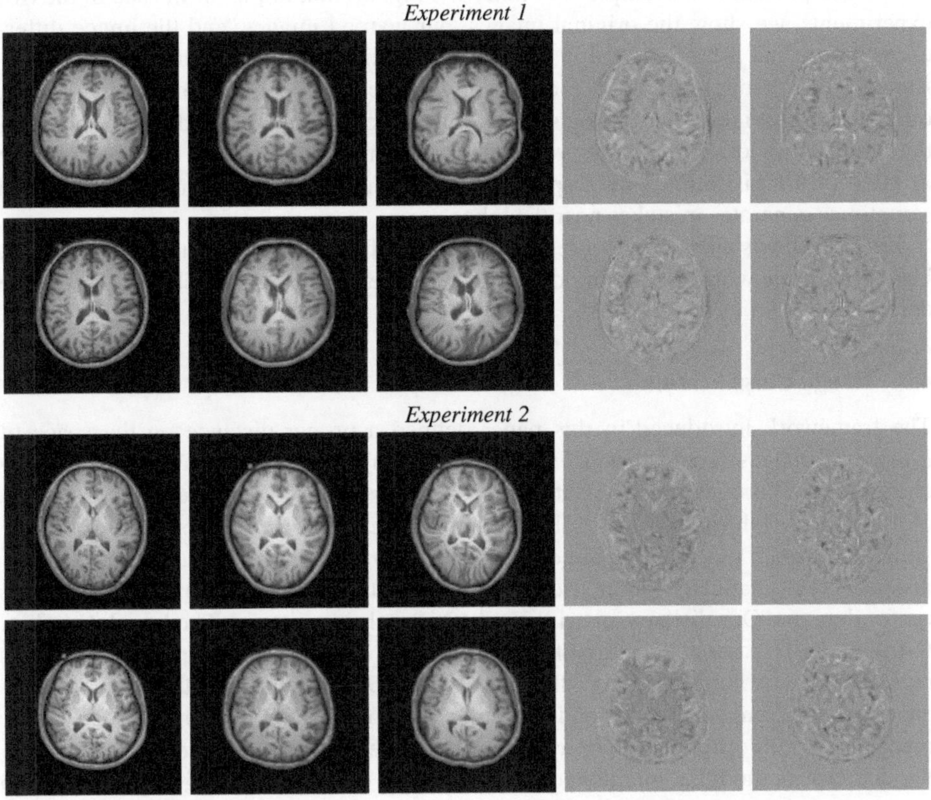

Experiment 1

Experiment 2

Fig. 4. Results for registering brain images. Column (a) contains two given images. The registered images from our method and diffeomorphic demons are shown in columns (b) and (c), respectively. Column (d) gives the image differences after registration using our method and column (e) contains the image differences after registration using Demons.

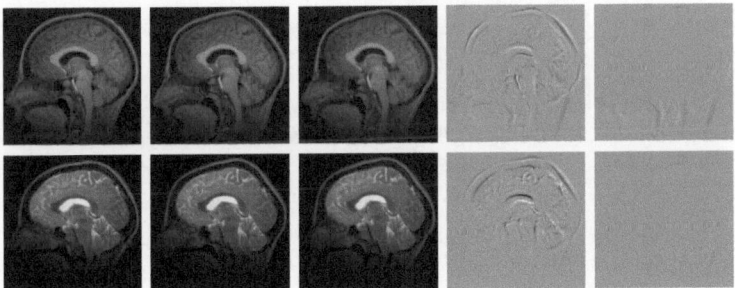

Fig. 5. Results for registering brain images from two modalities. First two columns contain given images, with the first row from T1 and the second from T2. The registered images are shown in the third column. The last two columns give the image differences before and after registration.

We also present two examples of brain MRI registration in Fig. 4. In each of the two experiments, we show the original images, our warped images, and the image differences before and after registration to illustrate our method. At the same time, the registered images from using the demons are used for comparison. For these experiments, our method provides a decent registration for the ventricular part and the boundary of the brain; most lobes remain approximately the same. The demons does not provide as good of a registration with respect to the ventricles and/or the boundaries. It also sometimes generates mistakes near the lobes.

Figure 5 shows an example of registering a pair of brain images from two modalities. Under our framework, the two modalities are registered simultaneously using the same deformation.

4.3 Image Classification

The framework introduced in this paper defined a proper distance on the space of q-maps of images. These distances can be used for pattern analysis of images, using clustering or classification. The dataset used for classification purpose contains images of digits from 0 through 9 and each digit has ten images. The distance matrices for L^2 without warping, our method and demons are shown in Fig. 6 from (a) to (c). The L^2 distance is automatically symmetric. We observe that the distance matrix is not symmetric for demons. Our distance matrix is approximately symmetric. The boxplots in Fig. 6 (d) are used to assess the amount of asymmetry for the distance matrices. The boxes represent the absolute values for all entries in $|D - D'|/D$. These are the relative differences between diagonal entries and are supposed to be zero for a symmetric matrix. Our method provides differences closer to zero and therefore more symmetric compared to the demons method. As mentioned previously, the differences being not exactly zero may be due to computational issues such as local minima. The leave-one-out nearest-neighbor (LOO-NN) method is utilized to classify the digits based on distance matrices. The classification rates are shown in Fig. 6.

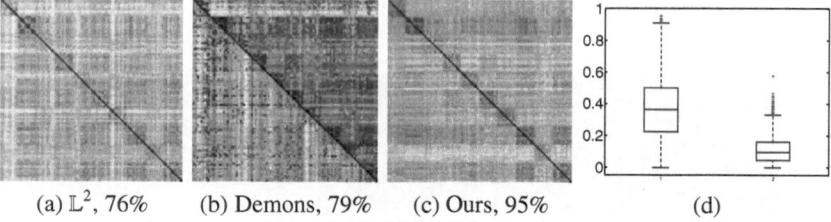

(a) L^2, 76%   (b) Demons, 79%   (c) Ours, 95%   (d)

Fig. 6. Classification results

5 Discussion

We proposed a unified framework to register and compare images jointly. Our distance provides a symmetric metric between image gradients and thus a good measure of registration without ambiguity. The forward and backward matching diffeomorphisms are inverses of each other when global solutions are reached. With this framework, our method gives better results for registration, comparison and classification of images compared to the demons method. Future work will involve studying mathematical properties such as injectivity of the Q map.

Acknowledgement. This research is supported in part by the Office of Naval Research under N00014-09-1-0664 and in part by the National Science Foundation under Grant DMS-0915003.

References

1. Agrawal, A., Raskar, R., Chellappa, R.: An algebraic approach to surface reconstructions from gradient fields? In: Intenational Conference on Computer Vision, ICCV (2006)
2. Avants, B., Grossman, M., Gee, J.: Symmetric diffeomorphic image registration: Evaluating automated labeling of elderly and neurodegenerative cortex and frontal lobe. Biomedical Image Registration 4057, 50–57 (2006)
3. Beg, M., Miller, M., Trouvé, A., Younes, L.: Computing large deformation metric mappings via geodesic flows of diffeomorphisms. Int. J. Comput. Vision 61, 139–157 (2005)
4. Christensen, G., Johnson, H.: Consistent image registration. IEEE Transactions on Medical Imaging 20(7), 568–582 (2001)
5. Davies, R., Twining, C., Cootes, T., Waterton, J., Taylor, C.: A minimum description length approach to statistical shape modeling. IEEE Transactions on Medical Imaging 21(5), 525–537 (2002)
6. Kroon, D., Slump, C.: MRI modalitiy transformation in demon registration. In: IEEE International Symposium on Biomedical Imaging: From Nano to Macro, ISBI 2009, pp. 963–966 (2009)
7. Kurtek, S., Klassen, E., Ding, Z., Jacobson, S., Jacobson, J., Avison, M., Srivastava, A.: Parameterization-invariant shape comparisons of anatomical surfaces. IEEE Transactions on Medical Imaging 30(3), 849–858 (2011)
8. Palais, R.: Morse theory on Hilbert manifolds. Topology 2, 299–340 (1963)
9. Tagare, H., Groisser, D., Skrinjar, O.: Symmetric non-rigid registration: A geometric theory and some numerical techniques. Journal of Mathematical Imaging and Vision 34, 61–88 (2009)
10. Taquet, M., Macq, B., Warfield, S.: A generalized correlation coefficient: application to DTI and multi-fiber DTI. In: MMBIA 2012 (2012)
11. Vercauteren, T., Pennec, X., Perchant, A., Ayache, N.: Diffeomorphic demons: Efficient non-parametric image registration. NeuroImage 45(1, supplement 1), S61–S72 (2009)
12. Viola, P., Wells III, W.M.: Alignment by maximization of mutual information. In: Proceedings of Fifth International Conference on Computer Vision, pp. 16–23 (June 1995)

Non-rigid Image Registration
Using Gaussian Mixture Models

Sangeetha Somayajula[1,*], Anand A. Joshi[2], and Richard M. Leahy[2]

[1] Dept. of Informatics IT, Merck Research Laboratories, Boston MA
[2] Signal and Image Processing Institute, University of Southern California, Los Angeles CA

Abstract. Non-rigid mutual information (MI) based image registration is prone to converge to local optima due to Parzen or histogram based density estimation used in conjunction with estimation of a high dimensional deformation field. We describe an approach for non-rigid registration that uses the log-likelihood of the target image given the deformed template as a similarity metric, wherein the distribution is modeled using a Gaussian mixture model (GMM). Using GMMs reduces the density estimation step to that of estimating the parameters of the GMM, thus being more computationally efficient and requiring fewer number of samples for accurate estimation. We compare the performance of our approach (GMM-Cond) with that of MI with Parzen density estimation (Parzen-MI), on inter-subject and inter-modality (CT to MR) mouse images. Mouse image registration is challenging because of the presence of a rigid skeleton within non-rigid soft tissue, and due to major shape and posture variability in inter-subject registration. The results show that GMM-Cond has higher registration accuracy than Parzen-MI in terms of sum of squared difference in intensity and dice coefficients of overall and skeletal overlap. The GMM-Cond approach is a general approach that can be considered a semi-parametric approximation to MI based registration, and can be used an alternative to MI for high dimensional non-rigid registration.

1 Introduction

Longitudinal and inter-subject imaging studies are often performed to study changes in anatomy and function in a subject over a period of time, or across populations. Non-rigid registration is required to normalize anatomical changes such as posture variability in longitudinal studies or anatomical variability across populations in inter-subject studies. Several non-rigid registration algorithms have been developed, a review of which can be found in [7].

Mutual information (MI) measures the amount of information shared between two random variables and can be used as a similarity metric in image registration. It has been successfully applied to multi-modality rigid registration [21] and some approaches to non-rigid registration using MI have also been proposed in [5], [15]. However, MI is a non-convex function of the registration parameters and the registration could converge to an inaccurate local optimum. The problem of converging to local optima is exacerbated in the non-rigid registration case because of the increased dimensionality of the

---

* Work done while at University of Southern California.

B.M. Dawant et al. (Eds.): WBIR 2012, LNCS 7359, pp. 286–295, 2012.

deformation field compared to the rigid case. Additionally, MI between the reference image (target) and the image to be registered (template) is a function of the joint density of their intensities, which is unknown. Typically a non-parametric approach such as Parzen windowing is used to estimate the entire joint density from the images [14]. This approach requires appropriate choice of the Parzen window width, which is usually taken as a design parameter and kept fixed over the entire sample. This has the drawback that for long-tailed distributions the density estimate tends to be noisy at the tails, and increasing the window width to deal with this might lead to oversmoothing the details in the distribution [4]. The former scenario would result in a cost function that has more local optima, while the latter could lead to inaccurate registration results. The non-parametric approach also requires a large number of samples to accurately estimate the distribution.

Maximizing MI is closely related to maximizing the joint probability of the target and template images, or the conditional probability of the target given the template image [6], [8], [13]. An interpretation of MI as a special case of maximum likelihood estimation is given in [13]. In [6] a maximum *a posteriori* (MAP) framework for non-rigid registration is used wherein a Parzen-like conditional density estimate is computed and used as the likelihood term. In [23] multinomial joint intensity distributions were used in a MAP framework for registration and a relationship with joint entropy was derived for the uniformative prior case. In [8] a registered training set was used to model the joint intensity distribution using Parzen density estimation and Gaussian mixture models (GMMs), and the estimated distribution was used to perform rigid registration of a test set. Approximating the joint density using multiple Gaussians was described in [18] as an approach to increasing the robustness of a joint entropy based regularizer for limited angle transmission tomography image reconstruction.

In this paper we describe an approach for non-rigid registration that uses the log-likelihood of the target image given the deformed template as a similarity metric for non-rigid registration, wherein the distribution is modeled using a GMM. Gaussian distributions are commonly used in image segmentation to represent the distribution of intensities corresponding to a particular tissue type in MR or CT images [2], [12],[16]. In [2], [12] a unified MAP framework was described for brain segmentation, artifact correction, and non-linear registration with spatial prior maps obtained from a probabilistic atlas. We focus on registration and use GMMs to model the joint intensity distribution of the two MR/CT images to be registered, since their distributions are typically characterized by localized blobs. Using GMMs reduces the density estimation step to that of estimating the parameters of the GMM, which consist of the mean, covariance, and weight of each Gaussian. For images that have a few distinct regions of intensity such as mouse CT images, the number of parameters to be estimated is small and can be robustly estimated from fewer samples compared to the non-parametric approach. Our approach of using the log-likelihood of the target given the template in conjunction with a GMM can be viewed as a semi-parametric alternative to MI based registration when dealing with the high dimensional non-rigid registration case.

We compare the performance of our conditional likelihood metric with GMM parameterization, with that of MI with non-parametric density estimation. We will henceforth refer to these methods as the GMM-Cond and the Parzen-MI methods respectively.

We evaluate these methods using mouse CT and MR images. Registration of mice and other small animals is challenging because of the presence of rigid skeleton within non-rigid soft tissue. Additionally, inter-subject whole body mouse images may have considerable shape and postural differences. Registration approaches specific to small animal registration were described in [3], [10], [11], [17], [19], and [22]. Specifically, in [17] and [22] MI was used as a similarity metric for intra-modality mouse CT registration. We evaluate the GMM-Cond approach on inter-modality, inter-subject mouse registration.

2   Methods and Results

Let the target and template images be I_1 and I_2, and their intensity at position $\mathbf{x}$ be $i_1(\mathbf{x})$ and $i_2(\mathbf{x})$ respectively. Let the transformation that maps the template to the target be $T(\mathbf{x}) = \mathbf{x} - \mathbf{u}(\mathbf{x})$, where $\mathbf{u}$ is the displacement field. The deformed template is then represented by $I_2^{\mathbf{u}}$, whose intensities are given by $i_2(\mathbf{x} - \mathbf{u}(\mathbf{x}))$. We define the similarity metric $D_{\mathbf{u}}(I_1, I_2)$ between the target and deformed template as the log likelihood of the target given the deformed template. Assuming that the voxel intensities in I_1 and I_2 are independent identically distributed random variables with joint density $p(i_1, i_2)$, the similarity metric is given by,

$$D_{\mathbf{u}}(I_1, I_2) = \log p(I_1 | I_2^{\mathbf{u}}) = \sum_{\mathbf{x}} \log \frac{p(i_1(\mathbf{x}), i_2(\mathbf{x} - \mathbf{u}(\mathbf{x})))}{p(i_2(\mathbf{x} - \mathbf{u}(\mathbf{x})))}. \tag{1}$$

We assume a Gaussian mixture model for the joint density $p(i_1, i_2)$. Let the number of components of the Gaussian mixture model be K, the mixing proportions be π_k, and $g(i_1, i_2 | m_k, \Sigma_k)$ be a Gaussian with mean m_k and covariance Σ_k, where $k = 1, 2, \cdots, K$. Let the unknown deterministic GMM parameters for each component k be represented as $\theta_k = (\pi_k, m_k, \Sigma_k)$, and let $\Theta = [\theta_1, \theta_2, \cdots, \theta_K]$ be the vector of all unknown parameters. Then, the joint density is given by

$$p(i_1, i_2 | \Theta) = \sum_{k=1}^{K} \pi_k g(i_1, i_2 | m_k, \Sigma_k), \tag{2}$$

where $\pi_k > 0$ and $\sum_{k=1}^{K} \pi_k = 1$.

We use the Laplacian of the displacement field as a regularizing term to penalize deformations that are not smooth. We parameterize the displacement field using the discrete cosine transform (DCT) basis. The DCT bases are eigenfunctions of the discrete Laplacian, so using the DCT representation of the displacement field in conjunction with Laplacian regularization simplifies the regularization term to a diagonal matrix [1]. Let $\beta_i(\mathbf{x})$, $i = 1, 2, \cdots, N_b$, represent the DCT coefficients that parameterize the deformation field and let γ_i, $i = 1, 2, \cdots, N_b$ be the corresponding eigen values of the discrete Laplacian matrix $\mathbf{L}$. Then the norm $||\mathbf{Lu}(\mathbf{x})||^2 = \sum_{i=1}^{N_b} \gamma_i^2 \beta_i^2$. The objective function is then given by,

$$\max_{\mathbf{u}, \Theta} \sum_{\mathbf{x}} \log p(i_1(\mathbf{x}) | i_2(\mathbf{x} - \mathbf{u}(\mathbf{x})), \Theta) - \mu \sum_{i=1}^{N_b} \gamma_i^2 \beta_i^2, \tag{3}$$

where μ is a hyperparameter that controls the weight on the regularizing term.

To simplify the problem, we replace the combined optimization with respect to the deformation field and GMM parameters with an iterative two step procedure. Here, the GMM parameters are first estimated from the target and deformed template images through maximum likelihood estimation, and the deformation field is then computed given the estimated GMM parameters. The two step optimization is given by

$$\hat{\Theta}(\hat{\mathbf{u}}^m) = \arg\max_{\Theta} \sum_{\mathbf{x}} \log p(i_1(\mathbf{x}), i_2(\mathbf{x} - \hat{\mathbf{u}}^m(\mathbf{x}))|\Theta) \tag{4}$$

$$\hat{\mathbf{u}}^{m+1} = \arg\max_{\mathbf{u}} \sum_{\mathbf{x}} \log p(i_1(\mathbf{x})|i_2(\mathbf{x} - \mathbf{u}(\mathbf{x})), \hat{\Theta}(\hat{\mathbf{u}}^m)) - \mu \sum_{i=1}^{N_b} \gamma_i^2 \beta_i^2, \tag{5}$$

where $\hat{\mathbf{u}}^m$ represents the estimated deformation field at overall optimization iteration m. The estimation of GMM parameters is described in the next section. The estimation of the deformation field in Equation 5 given the GMM parameters is performed using conjugate gradient (CG) optimization with Armijo line search.

2.1   Estimation of Parameters of Gaussian Mixture Model

The maximum likelihood estimate of the GMM parameters $\hat{\Theta}$ in Equation 4 can be obtained by the expectation maximization (EM) algorithm [9]. Let the data sample at voxel j corresponding to the position $\mathbf{x}_j$ be $S_j^{\mathbf{u}} = [i_1(\mathbf{x}_j), i_2(\mathbf{x}_j - \mathbf{u}(\mathbf{x}_j))]^T$, where $j = 1, 2, \cdots, N$, and N is the number of voxels in each image. The component of the GMM from which S_j arises is taken as the hidden variable in the EM algorithm. The EM update equations are given in Equations 6 - 9.

$$\tau_{jk}^i = \frac{\pi_k^i g(S_j^{\mathbf{u}}, m_k^i(\mathbf{u}), \Sigma_k^i(\mathbf{u}))}{\sum_{h=1}^{K} \pi_h^i(\mathbf{u}) g(S_j^{\mathbf{u}}, m_h^i(\mathbf{u}), \Sigma_h^i(\mathbf{u}))} \tag{6}$$

$$\pi_k^{i+1}(\mathbf{u}) = \frac{1}{N} \sum_{j=1}^{N} \tau_{jk}^i \tag{7}$$

$$m_k^{i+1}(\mathbf{u}) = \frac{\sum_{j=1}^{N} \tau_{jk}^i S_j^{\mathbf{u}}}{\sum_{j=1}^{N} \tau_{jk}^i} \tag{8}$$

$$\Sigma_k^{i+1}(\mathbf{u}) = \frac{\sum_{j=1}^{N} \tau_{jk}^i (S_j^{\mathbf{u}} - m_k^{i+1}(\mathbf{u}))(S_j^{\mathbf{u}} - m_k^{i+1}(\mathbf{u}))^T}{\sum_{j=1}^{N} \tau_{jk}^i}, \tag{9}$$

where $\pi_k^i(\mathbf{u})$, $m_k^i(\mathbf{u})$, and $\Sigma_k^i(\mathbf{u})$ are the GMM parameter estimates at EM iteration i and deformation field $\mathbf{u}$. The objective function to be optimized in Equation 4 is a non-convex function of Θ, so a good initial estimate is needed to converge to a global optimum. We use the k-nearest neighbors algorithm [14] to identify cluster centers in the joint histogram of the target and template images, and the number of samples that fall into a particular cluster. The cluster centers and the proportion of samples in a cluster relative to the total number of samples were used as the initializations m_k^0 and p_k^0 respectively, and Σ_k^0 was assumed to be identity for all k. The number of clusters was chosen to visually match the initial histogram of the two images. Assuming a reasonable initial global alignment, the number of clusters was then kept constant throughout the registration process.

Figure 1 shows the GMM estimate of the joint pdf of intensities of the target and template images shown in Figure 2 (a) and (b). The joint histogram of the intensities of these two images is shown in Figure 1 (a), and the pdf estimated using GMM is shown in Figure 1 (b) with the component means overlaid. The number of components was chosen to be $K = 7$ to match the joint histogram.

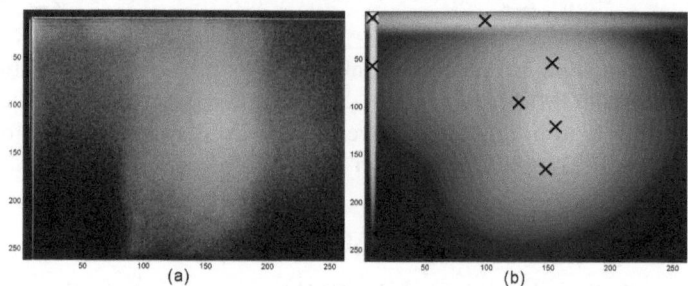

Fig. 1. Estimation of joint pdf of images in Fig. 2 (a) and (b) : (a) Joint histogram of images, (b) GMM estimate (the component means shown with 'x' marks)

2.2 Relation to Mutual Information

Let the random variables corresponding to the intensities of I_1 and $I_2^{\mathbf{u}}$ be ζ_1 and ζ_2 respectively. Mutual information between ζ_1 and ζ_2 is defined as ,

$$D(\zeta_1, \zeta_2) = \int p(z_1, z_2) \log \frac{p(z_1, z_2)}{p(z_1)(z_2)} dz_1 dz_2 = E(\log \frac{p(z_1, z_2)}{p(z_1)p(z_2)}). \quad (10)$$

MI between two random variables can be interpreted as the reduction in uncertainty of one random variable given the other. Using MI as a similarity metric for registration aims to find a deformation that makes the joint density of the target and deformed template images maximally clustered, thus implying that the uncertainty of one image given the other is minimized [21].

An alternative formulation can be obtained by approximating the expectation in Equation 10 by a sample mean where the intensity at each voxel in the target and deformed template images constitutes the random sample. Hence we get

$$\hat{D}(\zeta_1, \zeta_2) = \frac{1}{N} \sum_{\mathbf{x}} \log \frac{p(i_1(\mathbf{x}), i_2(\mathbf{x} - \mathbf{u}(\mathbf{x})))}{p(i_1(\mathbf{x}))p(i_2(\mathbf{x} - \mathbf{u}(\mathbf{x})))}$$

$$= \frac{1}{N} \sum_{\mathbf{x}} \log \frac{p(i_1(\mathbf{x}), i_2(\mathbf{x} - \mathbf{u}(\mathbf{x})))}{p(i_2(\mathbf{x} - \mathbf{u}(\mathbf{x})))} - \frac{1}{N} \sum_{\mathbf{x}} \log p(i_1(\mathbf{x})). \quad (11)$$

Since the target is fixed and independent of $\mathbf{u}(\mathbf{x})$, dropping the terms containing the marginal density $p(i_1)$, we get the approximate MI based similarity metric as

$$\hat{D}(\zeta_1, \zeta_2) = \frac{1}{N} \sum_{\mathbf{x}} \log \frac{p(i_1(\mathbf{x}), i_2(\mathbf{x} - \mathbf{u}(\mathbf{x})))}{p(i_2(\mathbf{x} - \mathbf{u}(\mathbf{x})))}. \tag{12}$$

Thus, computing the deformation field that maximizes mutual information is approximately equivalent to maximizing the conditional density of the target given the template image as defined in Equation 1. In [13] a similar relationship between maximum likelihood and conditional entropy was derived. The pdf $p(i_1, i_2)$ in Equation 12 is unknown, and needs to be estimated. The pdf can be estimated using a non-parametric approach such as Parzen windowing or a GMM based approach can be taken to parametrize the pdf and estimate those parameters.

The Parzen window estimate of a pdf at random variable values z_1, z_2 is defined by [14]

$$p(z_1, z_2) = \frac{1}{N} \sum_{j=1}^{N} g\left(\frac{z_1 - i_1(j)}{\sigma}\right) g\left(\frac{z_2 - i_2^{\mathbf{u}}(j)}{\sigma}\right), \tag{13}$$

where $g(\frac{z_2}{\sigma})$ is a Gaussian window of width σ, which is usually taken as a design parameter. Note that this can be considered as a Gaussian mixture model with as many Gaussians as the number of samples ($K = N$), with mean given by the sample $m_k = [i_1(k), i_2^{\mathbf{u}}(k)]^T$, fixed standard deviation $\Sigma_k = \begin{bmatrix} \sigma^2 & 0 \\ 0 & \sigma^2 \end{bmatrix}$, and equal weighting probabilities $\pi_k = \frac{1}{N}$. However, we expect the GMM-Cond approach to have two advantages over the Parzen-MI approach

1. The density estimation requires estimation of $6K$ GMM parameters that can be robustly estimated from the given images for small K. In contrast, the Parzen-MI approach computes the entire $N_{bin} \times N_{bin}$ pdf from the samples, where N_{bin} is the number of bins at which the pdf is computed
2. Estimation of the displacement field may be more robust to trapping in local minima because of the much lower dimensionality with which the joint density is parameterized.

We expect to gain computationally as well as in robustness from this reduction in dimensionality of the problem. However, if the joint density does not fit a GMM, the number of mixture components might be large, approaching a Parzen window estimate.

2.3   Results

We perform validation studies of our method using multi-modality (CT and MR) inter-subject mouse images. Mouse CT images typically consist of mainly soft tissue versus bone contrast, and can be assumed to follow a GMM. Though mouse MR images have a larger number of intensity levels than the CT, the number of components required in the GMM is not prohibitively large. We consider two mice that were imaged using both MR and CT (referred to as MR1 and CT1, MR2 and CT2) and two other mice that were imaged using only CT (referred to as CT3 and CT4). This gives 6 possible inter-modality, inter-subject registrations (CT1-MR2, CT3-MR2, CT4-MR2, CT2-MR1,CT3-MR1, CT4-MR1). The MR images were obtained on a Biospec 7T system at a resolution of $0.23 \times 0.17 \times 0.50$ mm. The CT images corresponding to the MR were acquired on a Siemens Inveon system and the others were obtained from a microCT system, at a resolution of $0.2 \times 0.2 \times 0.2$ mm. We first perform a 12 parameter affine registration of the CT images to the MR image using the AIR software [20]. We downsampled the MR and affinely registered CT images to size $128 \times 128 \times 64$ to reduce computation. The downsampled MR and affinely registered CT images were then used as the target and template images respectively for non rigid registration. We compare our semi-parametric GMM-Cond approach to non-parametric Parzen-MI approach in the context of high-dimensional non-rigid registration, rather than comparing to existing registration algorithms that address mouse registration with application specific constraints such as skeletal rigidity. The goal is to evaluate GMM-Cond as a general framework for non-rigid inter-modality registration in small animal studies.

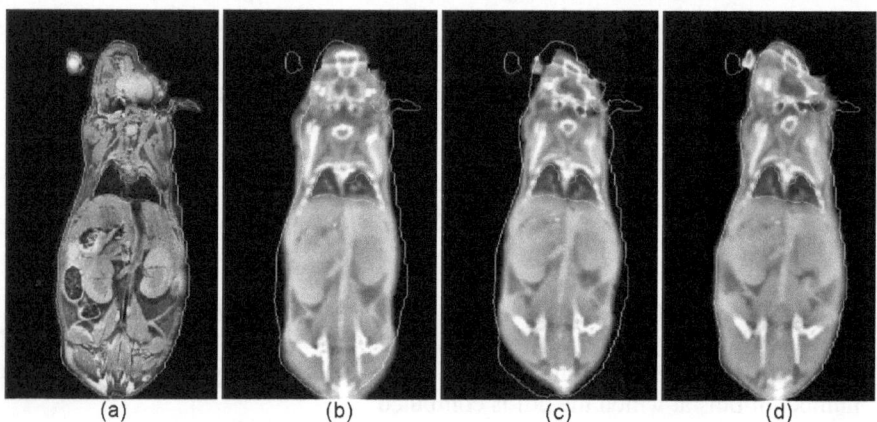

Fig. 2. Multi-modality inter-subject registration: Coronal view of (a) target MR image with outline of body and lungs, (b) template CT image affinely registered to MR, (c) Parzen-MI registered image, and (d) GMM-Cond registered image. Images (b)-(d) are shown with target body and lung outlines

For both methods, we used $15 \times 15 \times 15$ DCT bases to represent the displacement field. We choose the weight μ on the regularizing term such that the determinant of the Jacobian of the displacement field is positive. For the Parzen-MI registration we followed a hierarchical approach, first aligning the images that were smoothed with a Gaussian of width 3 voxels, and used the displacement field thus obtained to initialize the registration of the original images. We observed that directly aligning the original images causes the algorithm to reach an inaccurate local minimum in a few iterations. A Parzen window width of $\sigma = 5$ was used to compute the distribution at every iteration. For the GMM-Cond approach, we used 5 overall iterations between the density estimation and deformation field estimation. Each displacement field estimation involved 50 iterations of the CG algorithm. Coronal view of the registered images for one dataset along with the target and template images are shown in Figure 2. We used $K = 7$ components in the GMM for this dataset. The outline of the body and lungs of the target image was overlaid in green on all the images. We applied the displacement field resulting from both registration algorithms to the higher resolution images for display purposes. We quantify the performance of the registration through three measures:

1. Overall overlap: The target and template images can be segmented into mouse and background regions. The overall overlap of the target and deformed template can then be measured by computing the dice coefficients of the region labeled as mouse in the two images.
2. Overlap of skeleton: The skeleton can be segmented in the target and template images by thresholding. The dice coefficients of the skeleton in the target and deformed template images give a measure of overlap in the skeleton.
3. Mean squared difference (MSD) between intensities: The target MR image has a corresponding CT image acquired with it. The normalized mean squared difference between intensities of the CT corresponding to the target, and the deformed template images gives a measure of registration accuracy.

The average and standard deviation values of the three measures for the 6 inter-subject CT to MR registrations are given in Table 1.

It can be seen from the images and the outline overlay that the GMM-Cond method shows better overall shape and lung alignment compared to the MI-Parzen and AIR methods. On average, the GMM-Cond method has higher dice coefficients for the skeleton as well as overall shape, and lower normalized MSD between intensities than the MI-Parzen and AIR registration methods, indicating better alignment. It is promising that the GMM-Cond shows improved performance for the inter-subject, multi-modality registration considered, since these images have considerable difference in intensities, overall shape, and skeletal structure.

Table 1. Quantitative measures of overlap

Affine	Parzen-MI	GMM-Cond
Mean ± SD of dice coefficients for overall overlap		
0.84 ± 0.03	0.87 ± 0.04	0.91 ± 0.03
Mean ± SD of dice coefficients for overlap of skeleton		
0.24 ± 0.07	0.31 ± 0.07	0.34 ± 0.04
Mean ± SD of squared difference between intensities		
0.56 ± 0.07	0.50 ± 0.07	0.44 ± 0.11

3 Discussion

We used the conditional density of the target given the deformed template as a similarity metric for non-rigid registration, wherein the conditional density is modeled as a Gaussian mixture model. A DCT representation of the deformation field was used in conjunction with a Laplacian regularizing term to reduce computation. We compared the performance of our approach with that of Parzen-MI based approach using multi-modality MR/CT mouse images.

The GMM-Cond approach showed higher registration accuracy than the Parzen-MI approach in terms of dice coefficients and mean squared difference between intensities of the target and registered images. The GMM parametrization is not only computationally more efficient than the Parzen method, but also improves performance by reducing the overall dimensionality of the estimation problem, and through more robust and accurate density estimation. Additionally, the only design parameter that needs to be chosen is the number of clusters in the GMM, which can be obtained from the initial joint histogram.

The performance of the GMM-Cond method is promising as it performs better than the Parzen MI approach for multi-modality whole body images with postural variations. This indicates that this is a robust approach that can potentially be applied to multi-modality non-rigid registration problems. It can be used as an alternative to MI based registration when dealing with high dimensional deformation fields. The GMM-Cond approach can be viewed as a general framework that can be used in conjunction with other models for the deformation field, and with additional constraints specific to the application (e.g., rigidity constraints for the skeleton in mouse images). It should be noted however, that if the joint density of the images does not follow a GMM, a large number of clusters would be required to fit the data, thus increasing the number of parameters to be estimated and might not perform better than Parzen-MI in that case. We expect this approach to be particularly useful in applications where the images have a few distinct regions of intensity such as mouse CT images.

Acknowledgments. This work was supported by grants NIH/NIBIB P41 EB015922, P41 RR013642 and R01 NS074980

References

1. Ashburner, J., Friston, K.: Nonlinear spatial normalization using basis functions. Human Brain Mapping 7(4), 254–266 (1999)
2. Ashburner, J., Friston, K.J.: Unified segmentation. NeuroImage 26(3), 839–851 (2005)
3. Baiker, M., Staring, M., Löwik, C.W.G.M., Reiber, J.H.C., Lelieveldt, B.P.F.: Automated Registration of Whole-Body Follow-Up MicroCT Data of Mice. In: Fichtinger, G., Martel, A., Peters, T. (eds.) MICCAI 2011, Part II. LNCS, vol. 6892, pp. 516–523. Springer, Heidelberg (2011)
4. Silverman, B.W.: Density estimation for Statistics and Data analysis. Chapman and Hall (1986)
5. D'Agostino, E., Maes, F., Vandermeulen, D., Suetens, P.: A viscous fluid model for multimodal non-rigid image registration using mutual information. Medical Image Analysis 7(4), 565–575 (2003)
6. Zhang, J., Rangarajan, A.: Bayesian multimodality non-rigid image registration via conditional density estimation. In: Information Proc. in Med. Imaging, pp. 499–511 (2003)
7. Krum, W., Griffin, L.D., Hill, D.L.G.: Non-rigid image registration: Theory and practice. Br. Journ. Radiol. 1(77), S140–S153 (2004)

8. Leventon, M.E., Grimson, W.E.L.: Multi-modal Volume Registration Using Joint Intensity Distributions. In: Wells, W.M., Colchester, A.C.F., Delp, S.L. (eds.) MICCAI 1998. LNCS, vol. 1496, pp. 1057–1066. Springer, Heidelberg (1998)
9. MacLachlan, G., Peel, D.: Finite Mixture Models. Wiley (2000)
10. Kovacevic, N., Hamarneh, G., Henkelman, M.: Anatomically Guided Registration of Whole Body Mouse MR Images. In: Ellis, R.E., Peters, T.M. (eds.) MICCAI 2003. LNCS, vol. 2879, pp. 870–877. Springer, Heidelberg (2003)
11. Papademetris, X., Dione, D.P., Dobrucki, L.W., Staib, L.H., Sinusas, A.J.: Articulated Rigid Registration for Serial Lower-Limb Mouse Imaging. In: Duncan, J.S., Gerig, G. (eds.) MICCAI 2005, Part II. LNCS, vol. 3750, pp. 919–926. Springer, Heidelberg (2005)
12. Pohl, K.M., Fisher, J., Grimson, W.E.L., Kikinis, R., Wells, W.M.: A Bayesian model for joint segmentation and registration. NeuroImage 31(1), 228–239 (2006)
13. Roche, A., Malandain, G., Ayache, N., Prima, S.: Towards a Better Comprehension of Similarity Measures Used in Medical Image Registration. In: Taylor, C., Colchester, A. (eds.) MICCAI 1999. LNCS, vol. 1679, pp. 555–566. Springer, Heidelberg (1999)
14. Duda, R.O., Hart, P.E., Stork, D.G.: Pattern Classification, 2nd edn. Wiley (2001)
15. Rueckert, D., Sonoda, L.I., Hayes, C., Hill, D.L., Leach, M.O., Hawkes, D.J.: Nonrigid registration using free-form deformations: application to breast mr images. IEEE Trans. Med. Imaging 18(8), 712–721 (1999)
16. Shattuck, D.W., Sandor-Leahy, S.R., Schaper, K.A., Rottenberg, D.A., Leahy, R.M.: Magnetic resonance image tissue classification using a partial volume model. NeuroImage 13(5), 856–876 (2001)
17. Somayajula, S., Joshi, A.A., Leahy, R.M.: Mutual information based non-rigid mouse registration using a scale-space approach. In: 5th IEEE Intl. Symposium on Biomedical Imaging, pp. 1147–1150 (2008)
18. Van de Sompel, D., Brady, M.: Regularising limited view tomography using anatomical reference images and information theoretic similarity metrics. Medical Image Analysis 16(1), 278–300 (2012)
19. Wang, H., Stout, D., Chatziioannou, A.: Estimation of mouse organ locations through registration of a statistical mouse atlas with micro-ct images. IEEE Transactions on Medical Imaging 31(1), 88–102 (2012)
20. Woods, R.P., Grafton, S.T., Watson, J.D.G., Sicotte, N.L., Mazziotta, J.C.: Automated image registration: I. General methods and intrasubject, intramodality validation. Journal of Computed Assisted Tomography 22, 139–152 (1998)
21. Wells, W., Viola, P., Atsumi, H., Nakajima, S., Nakajima, S., Kikinis, R.: Multimodal volume registration by maximization of mutual information. Med. Image Analysis 1(1), 35–51 (1996)
22. Li, X., Peterson, T.E., Gore, J.C., Dawant, B.M.: Automatic Inter-subject Registration of Whole Body Images. In: Pluim, J.P.W., Likar, B., Gerritsen, F.A. (eds.) WBIR 2006. LNCS, vol. 4057, pp. 18–25. Springer, Heidelberg (2006)
23. Zöllei, L., Jenkinson, M., Timoner, S.J., Wells, W.M.: A Marginalized MAP Approach and EM Optimization for Pair-Wise Registration. In: Karssemeijer, N., Lelieveldt, B. (eds.) IPMI 2007. LNCS, vol. 4584, pp. 662–674. Springer, Heidelberg (2007)

Registration for Correlative Microscopy Using Image Analogies

Tian Cao[1], Christopher Zach[3], Shannon Modla[4], Debbie Powell[4], Kirk Czymmek[4], and Marc Niethammer[1,2]

[1] UNC Chapel Hill
[2] BRIC
[3] Microsoft Research Cambridge
[4] University of Delaware

Abstract. Correlative microscopy is a methodology combining the functionality of light microscopy with the high resolution of electron microscopy and other microscopy technologies for the same biological specimen. In this paper, we propose an image registration method for correlative microscopy, which is challenging due to the distinct appearance of biological structures when imaged with different modalities. Our method is based on image analogies and allows to transform images of a given modality into the appearance-space of another modality. Hence, the registration between two different types of microscopy images can be transformed to a mono-modality image registration. We use a sparse representation model to obtain image analogies. The method makes use of representative corresponding image training patches of two different imaging modalities to learn a dictionary capturing appearance relations. We test our approach on backscattered electron (BSE) Scanning Electron Microscopy (SEM)/confocal and Transmission Electron Microscopy (TEM)/confocal images and show improvements over direct registration using a mutual-information similarity measure to account for differences in image appearance.

1   Introduction

Correlative microscopy integrates different microscopy technologies including conventional light-, confocal- and electron transmission microscopy [1] for the improved examination of biological specimens. E.g., fluorescent markers can be used to highlight regions of interest combined with an electron-microscopy image to provide high-resolution structural information of the regions. To allow such joint analysis requires the registration of multi-modal microscopy images. This is a challenging problem due to (large) appearance differences between the image modalities. Fig. 1 shows an example of correlative microscopy for a confocal/TEM image pair.

A solution for registration for correlative microscopy is to perform landmark-based alignment, which can be greatly simplified by adding fiducial markers [2]. Fiducial markers cannot easily be added to some specimen, hence an alternative

B.M. Dawant et al. (Eds.): WBIR 2012, LNCS 7359, pp. 296–306, 2012.
© Springer-Verlag Berlin Heidelberg 2012

image-based method is needed. This can be accomplished in some cases by appropriate image filtering. This filtering is designed to only preserve information which is indicative of the desired transformation, to suppress spurious image information, or to use knowledge about the image formation process to convert an image from one modality to another. E.g., multichannel microscopy images of cells can be registered by registering their cell segmentations [3]. However, such image-based approaches are highly application-specific and difficult to devise for the non-expert.

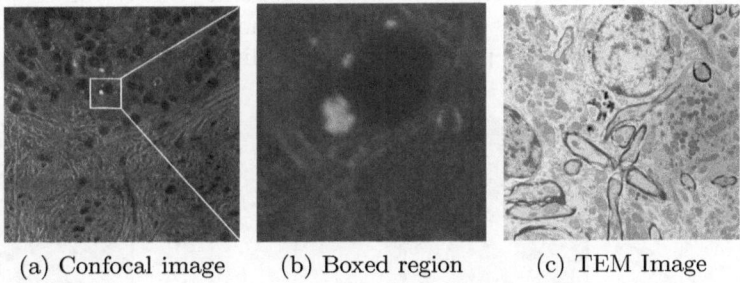

(a) Confocal image   (b) Boxed region   (c) TEM Image

Fig. 1. Example of Correlative Microscopy. The goal is to align (b) to (c).

In this paper we therefore propose a method inspired by early work on texture synthesis in computer graphics using image analogies [4]. Here, the objective is to transform the appearance of one image to the appearance of another image (for example transforming an expressionistic into an impressionistic painting). The transformation rule is learned based on example image pairs. For image registration this amounts to providing a set of (manually) aligned images of the two modalities to be registered from which an appearance transformation rule can be learned. A multi-modal registration problem can then be converted into a mono-modal one. The learned transformation rule is still highly application-specific, however it only requires manual alignment of sets of training images which can easily be accomplished by a non-expert in image registration.

Arguably, transforming image appearance is not necessary if using an image similarity measure which is invariant to the observed appearance differences. In medical imaging, mutual information (MI) [5] is the similarity measure of choice for multi-modal image registration. We show for two correlative microscopy example problems that MI registration is indeed beneficial, but that registration results can be improved by combining MI with an image analogies approach. To obtain a method with better generalizability than standard image analogies [4] we devise an image-analogies method using ideas from sparse coding [6], where corresponding image-patches are represented by a learned basis (a dictionary). Dictionary elements capture correspondences between image patches from different modalities and therefore allow to transform one modality to another modality.

This paper is organized as follows: Sec. 2 describes the image analogies method with sparse coding and our numerical solutions approach. Image registration results are shown and discussed in Sec. 3. The paper concludes with a summary of results and an outlook on future work in Sec. 4.

2   Image Analogies

The objective for image analogies [4] is to create an image B' from an image B with a similar relation in appearance as a training image set (A, A'). Fig. 2 shows an image analogies example. The standard image analogies algorithm [4] achieves the mapping between B and B' by looking up best-matching patches for each image location between A and B which then imply the patch appearance for B' from the corresponding patch A' (A and A' are assumed to be aligned). These best patches are smoothly combined to generate the overall output image B'. To avoid costly lookups and to obtain a more generalizable model with noise-reducing properties we propose a sparse coding image analogies approach.

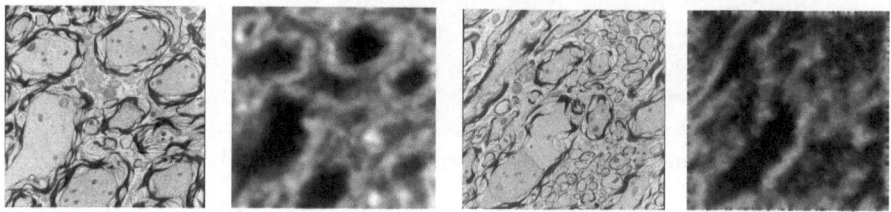

A: training TEM A': training confocal B: input TEM B': output confocal

Fig. 2. Result of Image Analogy: Based on a training set (A, A') an input image B can be transformed to B' which mimics A' in appearance

2.1   Sparse Representation Model

Sparse representation is a technique to reconstruct a signal as a linear combination of a few basis signals from a typically over-complete dictionary. A dictionary is a collection of basis signals. The number of dictionary elements in an over-complete dictionary exceeds the dimension of the signal space (here the dimension of an image patch). Suppose a dictionary D is pre-defined. To sparsely represent a signal x the following optimization problem is solved [7]:

$$\hat{\alpha} = \arg\min_{\alpha} \parallel \alpha \parallel_0, \quad \text{s.t.} \parallel x - D\alpha \parallel_2 \leq \epsilon, \tag{1}$$

where α is a sparse vector that explains x as a linear combination of columns in dictionary D with error ϵ and $\parallel \cdot \parallel_0$ indicates the number of non-zero elements in the vector α. Solving (1) is an NP-hard problem. One possible solution of this problem is based on a relaxation that replaces $\parallel \cdot \parallel_0$ by $\parallel \cdot \parallel_1$, where $\parallel \cdot \parallel_1$ is the L^1 norm of a vector, resulting in the optimization problem [7],

$$\hat{\alpha} = \arg\min_{\alpha} \parallel \alpha \parallel_1, \quad \text{s.t.} \parallel x - D\alpha \parallel_2 \leq \epsilon. \tag{2}$$

The equivalent Lagrangian form of (2) is

$$\hat{\alpha} = \arg\min_{\alpha} \lambda \parallel \alpha \parallel_1 + \parallel x - D\alpha \parallel_2^2, \tag{3}$$

which is a convex optimization problem that can be solved efficiently [6, 8]. We adapt this formulation for our sparse coding image analogy method and learn the dictionary D directly from aligned sets of training images.

2.2   Image Analogies with Sparse Representation Model

For image registration of correlative microscopy images, given two training images A and A' from different modalities, we can transform image B to the other modality by synthesizing B'. Consider the sparse, dictionary-based image denoising/reconstruction, u, given by minimizing

$$E(u, \{\alpha_i\}) = \gamma \int \frac{1}{2}(Lu - f)^2 dx + \frac{1}{N}\left(\sum_{i=1}^{N} \frac{1}{2} \parallel R_i u - D\alpha_i \parallel_V^2 + \lambda \parallel \alpha_i \parallel_1 \right), \quad (4)$$

where f is the given (potentially noisy) image, D is the dictionary, $\{\alpha_i\}$ are the patch coefficients, R_i selects the i-th patch from the image reconstruction u, γ, $\lambda > 0$ are balancing constants, L is a linear operator (e.g., describing a convolution), and the norm is defined as $\parallel x \parallel_v^2 = x^T V x$, where $V > 0$ is positive definite. Unlike most work in sparse coding, we are not computing alphas independently per patch first, and then average the result [7]. Instead we jointly optimize for the coefficients and the reconstructed/denoised image. Formulation (4) can be extended to image analogies by minimizing

$$E(u^{(1)}, u^{(2)}, \{\alpha_i\}) = \gamma \int \frac{1}{2}(L^{(1)}u^{(1)} - f^{(1)})^2 + \frac{1}{2}(L^{(2)}u^{(2)} - f^{(2)})^2 dx$$
$$+ \frac{1}{N}\left(\sum_{i=1}^{N} \frac{1}{2} \parallel R_i \begin{pmatrix} u^{(1)} \\ u^{(2)} \end{pmatrix} - \begin{pmatrix} D^{(1)} \\ D^{(2)} \end{pmatrix} \alpha_i \parallel_V^2 + \lambda \parallel \alpha_i \parallel_1 \right), \quad (5)$$

where we have a set of two images $\{f^{(1)}, f^{(2)}\}$, their reconstructions $\{u^{(1)}, u^{(2)}\}$ and corresponding dictionaries $\{D^{(1)}, D^{(2)}\}$. Note that there is only one set of coefficients α_i per patch, which indirectly relates the two reconstructions. This is similar to estimating a super-resolution image from a low-resolution one [7].

Patch-based (non-sparse) denoising has also been proposed for the denoising of fluorescence microscopy images [9]. A conceptually similar approach using sparse coding and image patch transfer has been proposed to relate different magnetic resonance images in [10]. However, this approach does not address dictionary learning or spatial consistency considered in the sparse coding stage. Our approach addresses both and learns the dictionaries $D^{(1)}$ and $D^{(2)}$ jointly.

2.3   Sparse Coding

Assuming that the two dictionaries $\{D^{(1)}, D^{(2)}\}$ are given, the objective is to minimize (5). However, unlike for image denoising, when computing image analogies only one of the images, $f^{(1)}$, is given and we are seeking a reconstruction of both, a denoised version of $u^{(1)}$ and $f^{(1)}$ as well as the corresponding analogous denoised image $u^{(2)}$ (without the knowledge of $f^{(2)}$). Hence, for sparse coding (5) simplifies to

$$
\begin{aligned}
E(u^{(1)}, u^{(2)}, \{\alpha_i\}) = \gamma \int \frac{1}{2} (L^{(1)} u^{(1)} - f^{(1)})^2 dx \\
+ \frac{1}{N} (\sum_{i=1}^{N} \frac{1}{2} \parallel R_i \begin{pmatrix} u^{(1)} \\ u^{(2)} \end{pmatrix} - \begin{pmatrix} D^{(1)} \\ D^{(2)} \end{pmatrix} \alpha_i \parallel_V^2 + \lambda \parallel \alpha_i \parallel_1),
\end{aligned}
\tag{6}
$$

which is a denoising of $f^{(1)}$ inducing a denoised reconstruction of the sought for image $u^{(2)}$. The problem is convex (for given $D^{(i)}$) which allows to compute a globally optimal solution. Sec. 2.6 describes our numerical solution approach.

2.4 Dictionary Learning

Given sets of training patches $\{p_i^{(1)}, p_i^{(2)}\}$ We want to estimate the dictionaries themselves as well as the coefficients $\{\alpha_i\}$ for the sparse coding. The problem is non-convex (bilinear in D and α_i). The standard solution approach [7] is alternating minimization, i.e., solving for α_i keeping $\{D^{(1)}, D^{(2)}\}$ fixed and vice versa. Two cases need to be distinguished: (i) L locally invertible and (ii) L not locally-invertible (e.g., due to convolution).

We only consider local dictionary learning here with L and V set to identities[1]. We assume that the training patches $\{p^{(1)}, p^{(2)}\} = \{f^{(1)}, f^{(2)}\}$ are unrelated, non-overlapping patches. Then the dictionary learning problem decouples from the image reconstruction and requires minimization of

$$
\begin{aligned}
E_d(D, \{\alpha_i\}) = \sum_{i=1}^{N} \frac{1}{2} \parallel \begin{pmatrix} f_i^{(1)} \\ f_i^{(2)} \end{pmatrix} - \begin{pmatrix} D^{(1)} \\ D^{(2)} \end{pmatrix} \alpha_i \parallel^2 + \lambda \parallel \alpha_i \parallel_1 \\
= \sum_{i=1}^{N} \frac{1}{2} \parallel f_i - D\alpha_i \parallel^2 + \lambda \parallel \alpha_i \parallel_1 .
\end{aligned}
\tag{7}
$$

The image analogy dictionary learning problem is identical to the one for image denoising. The only difference is a change in dimension for the dictionary and the patches (which are stacked up for the corresponding image sets).

2.5 Numerical Solution

Sparse Coding. We use the simultaneous-direction method of multipliers (SDMM) [8, 11] which allows us to simplify the optimization problem, by breaking it into easier subparts. To apply SDMM, we write the image analogy problem as

---

[1] Our approach can also be applied to L which are locally not invertible. However, this complicates the dictionary learning.

$$\overbrace{\qquad}^{:=f_D^{(1)}(v^{(1)})} \quad \overbrace{\qquad}^{:=f_D^{(2)}(v^{(2)})}$$
$$E = \frac{\gamma_1}{2} \parallel v^{(1)} - f^{(1)} \parallel_2^2 + \frac{\gamma_2}{2} \parallel v^{(2)} - f^{(2)} \parallel_2^2$$

$$\overbrace{\qquad\qquad\qquad\qquad\qquad}^{:=f_i^{(p)}\left(\begin{pmatrix} v_i^{(1)} \\ v_i^{(2)} \end{pmatrix}, \begin{pmatrix} w_i^{(1)} \\ w_i^{(2)} \end{pmatrix}\right) \text{ or } \bar{f}^{(p)}\begin{pmatrix} w_i^{(1)} \\ w_i^{(2)} \end{pmatrix}}$$

$$+ \frac{1}{N}\left(\sum_{i=1}^N \overbrace{\frac{1}{2} \parallel \begin{pmatrix} v_i^{(1)} \\ v_i^{(2)} \end{pmatrix} - \begin{pmatrix} w_i^{(1)} \\ w_i^{(2)} \end{pmatrix} \parallel_V^2}^{} + \overbrace{\lambda \parallel q_i \parallel_1}^{:=f_i^{(s)}(q_i)} \right) + \overbrace{\frac{\gamma_\alpha}{2} \parallel q \parallel_2^2}^{:f^\alpha(q)},$$

$$\text{s.t.} \begin{cases} v^{(1)} = L^{(1)}u^{(1)} \\ v^{(2)} = L^{(2)}u^{(2)} \\ v_i^{(1)} = R_i u^{(1)} \\ v_i^{(2)} = R_i u^{(2)} \end{cases} \text{and} \begin{cases} w^{(1)} = D^{(1)}\alpha \\ w^{(2)} = D^{(2)}\alpha \\ q_i = W_i \alpha_i \\ q = W\alpha \end{cases}, \tag{8}$$

where we introduced separate copies of the transformed image reconstructions $u^{(1)}$ and $u^{(2)}$ as well as of the patch coefficients and α denotes the stacked up coefficients of all patches (which allows imposing spatial coherence onto the α_i through W if desired). Following [11] we can use SDMM to solve (8).

For the dictionary-based sparse coding we have three sets of transformed variables, $u^{(1)}$, $u^{(2)}$ and the α copies. The images may even be of different dimensionalities (for example when dealing with a color and a gray-scale image). In our implementation of SDMM, we use $L^{(1)} = L^{(2)} = I$ and $W_i = W = I$.

Dictionary Learning. We use a dictionary based approach and hence need to be able to learn a suitable dictionary from the data. We use alternating optimization. Assuming that the coefficients α_i and the measured patches $\{p_i^{(1)}, p_i^{(2)}\}$ are given, we compute the current best least-squares solution for the dictionary as

$$D = (\sum_{i=1}^N p_i \alpha_i^T)(\sum_{i=1}^N \alpha_i \alpha_i^T)^{-1}. \tag{9}$$

The optimization with respect to the α_i terms follows (for each patch independently) the SDMM algorithm. Since the local dictionary learning approach assumes that patches to learn the dictionary from are given, the only terms remaining from Eq. (8) are, $\bar{f}_i^{(p)}$ and $f_i^{(s)}$. Hence the problem completely decouples with respect to the coefficients α_i and we obtain

$$E = \frac{1}{N}\left(\sum_{i=1}^N \bar{f}_i^{(p)}\begin{pmatrix} w_i^{(1)} \\ w_i^{(2)} \end{pmatrix} + f_i^{(s)}(q_i) \right), \tag{10}$$
$$\text{s.t. } w_i^{(1)} = D^{(1)}\alpha_i, \ w_i^{(2)} = D^{(2)}\alpha_i, \ q_i = \alpha_i.$$

Sparse Coding. Sparse coding follows the same numerical solution approaches for dictionary learning. However, since the dictionaries are known at the sparse coding stage, no alternating optimization is necessary and we can simply solve for $u^{(1)}$ and $u^{(2)}$ using SDMM. The difference is that for sparse coding for image analogies the measurement of the second image $f^{(2)}$ is unknown. Hence, $f_D^{(2)}(v^{(2)})$ is absent from the optimization and the reconstructed $u^{(2)}$ is the prediction.

3   Results

We (i) reconstruct the "missing" analogous image and (ii) consistently denoise the image to be registered with. We consider affine registration in our experiments, but the method is applicable to other transformation models. The key is that training image pairs represent expected appearance variations well.

3.1   Data

We use four pairs of 2D correlative SEM/confocal images containing 100 nm gold fiducials. The confocal image is the same in the four datasets and the SEM images are from the same area as the confocal image but for different views and magnifications. We also have six pairs of TEM/confocal images of mouse brains with resolutions 582.24 pixels per μm and 7.588 pixels per μm respectively.

3.2   Registration of SEM/Confocal Images (with Fiducials)

Pre-processing. The confocal image is denoised by the sparse representation-based denoising method [7]. We use a landmark based registration on the fiducials to get the gold standard alignment result.

Image Analogies (IA) Results. We applied the standard image analogies method and our method. We trained the dictionaries using a leave-one-out method. In both image analogy methods we use 10×10 patches, and in our proposed method we randomly sample 20000 patches and learn 800 dictionary elements in the dictionary learning phase. We choose $\gamma = 0.2$ and $\lambda = 1$ in (6). In Fig. 3, both IA methods can reconstruct the confocal image very well but our proposed method preserves more structure than the standard IA method.

Image Registration Results. We resampled the estimated confocal images with up to ± 600 $nm(15$ $pixels)$ in translation in the x and y directions (at steps of 1 pixel) and $\pm 15°$ in rotation (at steps of 1 degree) with respect to the gold standard alignment. Then we registered the resampled estimated confocal images to the corresponding original confocal images. Tab. 1 summarizes the registration results over all these experiments. Our method outperforms the standard image analogy method as well as a direct use of mutual information on the original images in terms of registration accuracy. Both image analogy methods achieve subpixel accuracy.

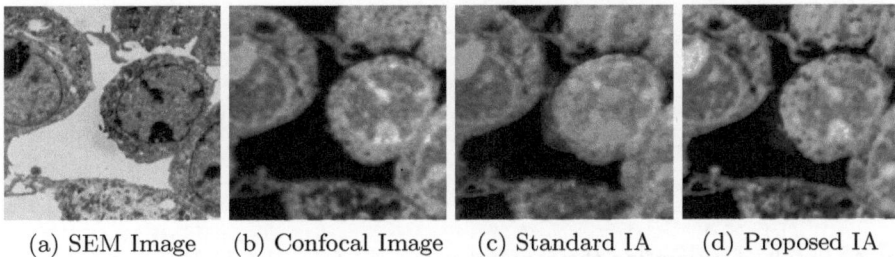

(a) SEM Image   (b) Confocal Image   (c) Standard IA   (d) Proposed IA

Fig. 3. Results of estimating a confocal (b) from an SEM image (a) using the standard image analogy (c) and our proposed sparse image analogy method (d)

Table 1. Registration errors on translation and rotation(translation t_x and t_y are in nm, pixel size is $40nm$; rotation r is in degree; $RMS = \sqrt{t_x^2 + t_y^2}$)

case		r	std_r	t_x	t_y	RMS	std_{RMS}
	Our method	0.171	0.191	14.687	28.451	33.5482	6.4561
1	Standard IA	**0.134**	0.252	15.26	27.677	**32.6751**	8.4876
	Original SEM/confocal	0.401	0.157	30.584	85.708	94.2085	8.0601
	Our method	**0.165**	0.258	15.537	26.462	**30.6862**	6.5831
2	Standard IA	0.268	0.212	14.756	28.238	32.0217	6.8241
	Original SEM/confocal	0.557	0.530	56.392	70.312	90.5242	6.2284
	Our method	**0.246**	0.537	19.924	80.512	**83.7206**	7.1757
3	Standard IA	0.368	0.511	20.548	79.821	84.7861	6.8433
	Original SEM/confocal	0.368	0.372	33.452	109.054	114.469378	9.3514
	Our method	**0.226**	0.583	17.069	19.024	**26.3190**	6.3156
4	Standard IA	0.232	0.640	13.954	25.35	29.9319	6.2327
	Original SEM/confocal	1.27	0.776	46.278	58.724	75.3439	5.4435

3.3 Registration of TEM/Confocal Images (without Fiducials)

Pre-Processing. We extracted the corresponding region of the confocal image and resample both confocal and TEM images to an intermediate resolution. The final resolution is 14.52 pixels per μm, and the image size is about 200×200 pixels. The datasets are already roughly registered based on manually labeled landmarks with a similarity transformation model.

Image Analogies Results. We tested the standard image analogy method and our proposed sparse method. For both image analogy methods we use 15×15 patches, and for our method we randomly sample 20000 patches and learn 900 dictionary elements in the dictionary learning phase. We choose $\gamma = 0.01$ and $\lambda = 1$ in (6). The image analogies results in Fig. 4 show that our proposed method preserves more local structure than the standard image analogy method.

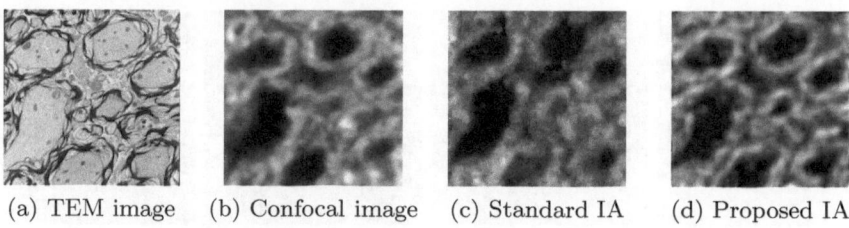

(a) TEM image   (b) Confocal image   (c) Standard IA   (d) Proposed IA

Fig. 4. Result of estimating the confocal image (b) from the TEM image (a) for the standard image analogy method (c) and the proposed sparse image analogy method (d) which shows better preservation of structure

Table 2. Image Registration Results (in μm, pixel size is 0.069 μm)

case		Our method MAE	STD	Standard IA MAE	STD	Original TEM/Confocal MAE	STD	Landmark MAE	STD
1	SSD	0.3174	0.2698	**0.3119**	0.2622	0.3353	0.2519	0.2705	0.1835
	MI	0.3146	0.2657	**0.3036**	0.2601	0.5161	0.2270		
2	SSD	0.3912	0.1642	**0.3767**	0.2160	2.5420	1.6877	0.3091	0.1594
	MI	0.4473	0.1869	0.4747	0.3567	**0.4140**	0.1780		
3	SSD	0.4381	0.2291	1.8940	1.0447	**0.4063**	0.2318	0.3636	0.1746
	MI	**0.3864**	0.2649	0.4761	0.2008	0.4078	0.2608		
4	SSD	0.4451	0.2194	**0.4416**	0.2215	0.4671	0.2484	0.3823	0.2049
	MI	0.4554	0.2298	**0.4250**	0.2408	0.4740	0.2374		
5	SSD	**0.3271**	0.2505	1.2724	0.6734	0.7204	0.3899	0.2898	0.2008
	MI	**0.3843**	0.2346	0.4175	0.2429	0.4030	0.2519		
6	SSD	0.7832	0.5575	**0.7169**	0.4975	2.2080	1.4228	0.3643	0.1435
	MI	0.7259	0.4809	1.2772	0.4285	**0.7183**	0.4430		

Image Registration Results. We manually determined $10 \sim 15$ corresponding landmark pairs on each dataset to establish a gold standard for registration. The same type and magnitude of shifts and rotations as for the SEM experiment are applied. The image registration results based on both image analogies methods are compared to the landmark based image registration results using mean absolute errors (MAE) and standard deviations (STD) of the absolute errors on all the corresponding landmarks. We use both SSD and mutual information (MI) as similarity measure. The registration results are displayed in Tab. 2. The landmark based image registration result is the best result achievable given the affine transformation model. We show the results for both image analogy methods as well as using the original TEM/confocal image pairs[2]. Tab. 2 shows that the MI based image registration results are similar among the three methods and also close to the landmark based registration results (best registration results).

---

[2] We inverted the grayscale values of original TEM image for SSD based image registration of original TEM/confocal images.

For SSD based image registration, our proposed method is more robust than the other two methods for the current datasets, for example, using the standard image analogies method results in large MAE values in case 3 and case 4 while using the original TEM/confocal images for registration results in large MAE values in case 2 and case 6. While our method does not currently give the best results for all the cases available to us, it appears to be the most consistent with results close to the best among all the methods investigated for all cases.

4   Conclusion

We developed a multi-modal registration method for correlative microscopy. The method is based on image analogies with a sparse representation model. It estimates the transformation from one modality to another based on training datasets of two different modalities. Our image registration results suggest that the sparse image analogy method can improve registration accuracy.

Our future work includes additional validation on a larger number of datasets from different modalities. Our goal is also to estimate the local quality of the image analogy result. This quality estimate could then be used to weight the registration similarity metrics to focus on regions of high confidence. We will also apply our sparse image analogy method to 3D images, which is straightforward.

Acknowledgments. This research is supported by NSF EECS-1148870, NSF EECS-0925875, NIH NIHM 5R01MH091645-02 and NIH NIBIB 5P41EB002025-28.

References

1. Caplan, J., Niethammer, M., Taylor II, R.M., Czymmek, K.J.: The power of correlative microscopy: multi-modal, multi-scale, multi-dimensional. Current Opinion in Structural Biology (2011)
2. Fronczek, D., Quammen, C., Wang, H., Kisker, C., Superfine, R., Taylor, R., Erie, D.A., Tessmer, I.: High accuracy FIONA-AFM hybrid imaging. Ultramicroscopy (2011)
3. Yang, S., Kohler, D., Teller, K., Cremer, T., Le Baccon, P., Heard, E., Eils, R., Rohr, K.: Nonrigid registration of 3-D multichannel microscopy images of cell nuclei. IEEE Transactions on Image Processing 17(4), 493–499 (2008)
4. Hertzmann, A., Jacobs, C.E., Oliver, N., Curless, B., Salesin, D.H.: Image analogies. In: The 28th Annual Conference on Computer Graphics and Interactive Techniques, pp. 327–340. ACM (2001)
5. Wells III, W.M., Viola, P., Atsumi, H., Nakajima, S., Kikinis, R.: Multi-modal volume registration by maximization of mutual information. Medical Image Analysis 1(1), 35–51 (1996)
6. Bruckstein, A.M., Donoho, D.L., Elad, M.: From sparse solutions of systems of equations to sparse modeling of signals and images. SIAM Review 51(1), 34–81 (2009)
7. Elad, M.: Sparse and redundant representations: from theory to applications in signal and image processing. Springer (2010)

8. Boyd, S., Parikh, N., Chu, E., Peleato, B., Eckstein, J.: Distributed optimization and statistical learning via the alternating direction method of multipliers. Machine Learning 3(1), 1–123 (2010)
9. Boulanger, J., Kervrann, C., Bouthemy, P., Elbau, P., Sibarita, J.B., Salamero, J.: Patch-based nonlocal functional for denoising fluorescence microscopy image sequences. IEEE Transactions on Medical Imaging 29(2), 442–454 (2010)
10. Roy, S., Carass, A., Prince, J.: A Compressed Sensing Approach for MR Tissue Contrast Synthesis. In: Székely, G., Hahn, H.K. (eds.) IPMI 2011. LNCS, vol. 6801, pp. 371–383. Springer, Heidelberg (2011)
11. Combettes, P.L., Pesquet, J.C.: Proximal splitting methods in signal processing. In: Fixed-Point Algorithms for Inverse Problems in Science and Engineering, pp. 185–212. Springer (2011)

Author Index